# Ensuring Medical Care
## for the Aged

# Pension Research Council

# PENSION RESEARCH COUNCIL PUBLICATIONS

*Monograph Series*

The Social Aspects of Retirement—*Otto Pollak*
Positive Experiences in Retirement—*Otto Pollak*

*Other Volumes*

Fundamentals of Private Pensions—*Dan M. McGill*
Concepts of Actuarial Soundness in Pension Plans—*Dorrance C. Bronson*
Ensuring Medical Care for the Aged—*Mortimer Spiegelman*

# Ensuring Medical
## Care for the Aged

by
MORTIMER SPIEGELMAN, F.S.A.

Published for the
PENSION RESEARCH COUNCIL
Wharton School of Finance and Commerce
University of Pennsylvania

by

RICHARD D. IRWIN, INC.
Homewood, Illinois

vi

# PURPOSE OF THE COUNCIL

The Pension Research Council of the Wharton School was created in 1952 for the purpose of sponsoring nonpartisan research in the area of private pensions. It was formed in response to the urgent need for a better understanding of the private pension movement. Private pensions have experienced a phenomenal growth during the last two decades, but their economic, political, and social implications are yet to be explored. They seem destined to play a major role in the quest for old-age economic security, but the nature of that role can be ascertained only on the basis of a more enlightened evaluation of the capabilities and limitations of the private pension mechanism. It was to conduct an impartial study into the facts and basic issues surrounding private pensions, under the auspices of an academic and professional group representing leadership in every phase of the field, that the Council was organized.

Projects undertaken by the Council are broad in scope and predominantly interpretive rather than technical in nature. In general, attention is concentrated on areas which are not the object of special investigation by other research groups. Its research studies are conducted by mature scholars drawn from both the academic and business spheres. Research results are published from time to time in a series of books and monographs.

# FOREWORD

ONE of the most complex and controversial problems facing the United States today is the determination of the best structure for providing and financing medical care for the expanding population. There are many facets to this problem, some going to the very heart of traditional medical practices. At the moment, public attention is focused on that phase of the over-all problem concerned with the financing of medical care for the aged segment of the population. For the current aged, the problem is complicated by the combination of a relatively high rate of utilization of medical care and a lessened income. The Pension Research Council saw in this situation a possible threat to the adequacy of retirement benefits and, as a step toward gauging the magnitude of the problem and the development of possible solutions, authorized this study. It did so in full knowledge of the fact that the issues go far beyond the confines of a pension plan or, for that matter, of the medical care needs of the aged population.

In this volume, Mr. Spiegelman, an eminent and highly respected student of population and medical statistics, brings together all of the meaningful data on medical care for the aged and, through a series of penetrating interpretations, adds a new dimension of meaning to these data. He presents a wealth of information on the economic status of the aged, including current income and asset resources; their health status; the utilization of hospital and medical services by the aged; and the extent of their medical care expenditures. He portrays the scope of coverage of medical care expenditures of the aged under existing voluntary and governmental mechanisms. Finally, he explores the broad approaches to providing medical care for the aged, including voluntary health insurance, extension of the federal OASDI program

ix

to cover medical care expenditures of aged beneficiaries, and a national health service. He makes no proposals of his own, preferring to let the facts speak for themselves.

Mr. Spiegelman is a Fellow of the Society of Actuaries, of the American Statistical Association, and of the American Public Health Association. He is a member of the International Congress of Actuaries, of the International Union for the Scientific Study of Population, and of the Social Science Research Council. He is the author of *Introduction to Demography* and *Significant Mortality and Morbidity Trends in the United States Since 1900;* co-author of *Length of Life* and *Money Value of a Man;* and author of numerous articles on population and health topics in scientific and professional journals. He has served on many institutional and scientific committees and is currently Chairman of the Statistics Section of the American Public Health Association and of its Committee on Vital and Health Statistics Monographs. He has been affiliated with the Metropolitan Life Insurance Company throughout his professional life, presently holding the title of Associate Statistician.

The Council is proud to present the results of Mr. Spiegelman's latest research. It is hoped that this volume will contribute toward a fuller understanding of the problems involved in ensuring medical care for the aged and, more important, will point the way to the most beneficial solution to these problems.

The views expressed in this volume are those of the author and do not necessarily represent the views of all members of the Council.

DAN M. McGILL

PHILADELPHIA, PA.
   March, 1960

# PREFACE

Issues concerning the provision of medical care for the aged in the United States have been shaped by various scientific, social, and economic developments. The rapidity and growing complexity of these changes has led to an urgent search for facts and figures to define the issues adequately and to provide bases for a solution. Many isolated facets of the problem have been studied, reported in scientific and professional journals, and discussed in meetings and conferences. The present volume is designed to give an integrated and comprehensive picture of the essential findings from these various sources.

To this end, many tables of pertinent data have been prepared and, where needed, figures have been incorporated in the text. Since statistics are used frequently and extensively in discussions of medical care for the aged, it was felt that an account should be included of the pitfalls and qualifications in their interpretation; too frequently figures are taken at face value. It was also felt necessary to pay some attention to definitions, since commonly used terms may be given different meanings by different people. Background material has been introduced at some points, the principal examples being a brief account of the present status of medical services for the aged and the development of voluntary health insurance. Other sources are quoted directly where the original was eminently authoritative, where the point was exceptionally well stated, or where it was desired to avoid misinterpretation.

It is hoped that this volume will be useful in the consideration of proposals for providing medical care for the aged. The author has not made any proposal of his own, since his purpose was merely to bring together the many specialized studies bearing upon the issues. In judging a proposed solution to a social problem, it is important to consider its social consequences. What appears to be an obvious solution is not necessarily the best, nor is the best solution often obvious.

Valuable comments and suggestions were received from many to whom the author submitted parts or the whole of his manuscript. Special thanks are due Mr. J. F. Follmann, Jr., Director of Information and Research at the Health Insurance Association of America, for a critical review of the draft, particularly the sections relating to insurance mechanisms. To Dr. Dan M. McGill, Frederick H. Ecker Professor of Life Insurance at the University of Pennsylvania and Research Director of the Pension Research Council, the author is indebted for sustained interest in watching the development of the volume and for advice regarding its organization. The author is also indebted to other members of the Pension Research Council who made valuable suggestions. The specialists who commented on the sections relating to their fields include: Dr. Odin W. Anderson, Research Director of the Health Information Foundation, and Messrs. Paul Sheatsley and J. J. Feldman of the National Opinion Research Center at the University of Chicago on the sections relating to attitudes based upon their surveys; Miss Pearl Bierman, Medical Care Consultant with the American Public Welfare Association, on the section relating to medical care programs for the indigent; Dr. Herbert E. Klarman, Director of the Hospital Council of Greater New York, on the sections describing medical services for the aged; Mr. Robert J. Myers, F.S.A., Chief Actuary of the Social Security Administration, on the sections relating to social security in Chapter 7. Among the many consulted on frequent occasions were Mrs. Agnes W. Brewster, Medical Economist with the Social Security Administration, and Dr. Walter Polner, formerly of the American Medical Association. The author owes many thanks to those associates in the Metropolitan Life Insurance Company who aided in several phases of this undertaking. Miss Catherine M. Natelli rendered valuable assistance at all stages by taking care of many details. The manuscript gained appreciably by the editing of Mr. Jacob Baar.

The author alone, however, bears the final responsibility for the opinions expressed and the shortcomings which remain.

MORTIMER SPIEGELMAN

NEW YORK
March, 1960

# CONTENTS

# LIST OF TABLES

# Introduction

1

A SURVEY of cultures in various stages of civilization—from the primitive to our own—has led to the observation that,[1]

Five wishes seem to be shared by aging people everywhere: to live as long as possible, to hoard their waning energies, to share in the continuing affairs of life, to safeguard their seniority rights, and to have as easy and honorable relief from life as possible.

In these wishes, health is dominant. The record of increasing longevity in countries of the Western world is ready evidence that large numbers now have promise of long life. This is the achievement of an economic progress which has raised the standard of living, provided the resources for advances in the medical sciences, and improved health status generally. Currently, most persons enter old age in sufficiently good health so that they can take part in some purposeful activity. Even among those who incurred significant impairments during midlife or earlier, medical advance has enabled large proportions to survive to old age.

Although morbidity data to describe the trend in the health status of the aged are lacking, an insight is provided by the declining mortality at the higher ages since the beginning of the century. Improvement in the health status of the aged may also be inferred from the general rise in the standard of living, one feature of which is an advance in nutrition. Whether or not the mental health of the aged has changed in any degree over the years it is impossible to say.

---

[1] L. W. Simmons, "An Anthropologist Views Old Age," *Public Health Reports,* Vol. 72, p. 290 (April, 1957).

The rate of admission to mental institutions fails as an index, since it is affected by such extraneous influences as the availability of facilities and trends in diagnosis and treatment.

Notwithstanding the apparent improvement in the general health of the aged, their medical care problems have grown rapidly. These flow, in the first place, from recent medical progress, with its rapid gains in the fields of prevention, diagnosis, therapy, and rehabilitation. Secondly, progress in medicine and the growing demands for costly facilities, services, and drugs have brought with them substantial increases in the medical care bill. Although economies are being sought, the prospect is for a continuing upward trend in such costs. These issues, while not unique to the aged, affect them more than the others in the population because of their greater medical care needs.

The medical care problems of the aged have also been affected by social and economic trends, most of which stem from the growing urbanization of the population.[2] Thus, the shift from rural to urban life has changed the pattern of family living, including the ability if not the attitude of families to meet their responsibilities to the aged.[3] In the typical small urban home, there may not be room for the dependent aged; on the other hand, the aged person may not want to leave an accustomed environment. Among the economic trends affecting the well-being of the aged, and particularly their medical care, is the rapid inflation since World War II. This has depreciated the purchasing power of the dollar, so that the lifelong savings of the aged and their fixed income can hardly accomplish their intended

---

[2] W. E. Moore, "The Aged in Industrial Societies," *The Aged and Society,* Industrial Relations Research Association, December, 1950, p. 24.

[3] H. D. Sheldon, *The Older Population* (New York: John Wiley & Sons, 1958), pp. 5–8 and 94–102; W. J. Cohen, "Social Aspects of Aging," *International Social Science Review,* No. 3, p. 34 (October, 1957), United Nations, Department of Social and Economic Affairs; R. J. Havighurst, "A World View of Gerontology," *Journal of Gerontology,* Vol. 13, supplement to April, 1958 issue, p. 2.

purposes. Thus placed at a disadvantage compared with the population at the productive ages, whose income is responsive to inflation, the aged of the present and the future have a great stake in a stabilized currency. On a community scale, these social and economic changes affecting the medical care problems of the aged are being accentuated by their increasing numbers. The problems are, in fact, among the leading social issues of the day.

Evidently, there are many interrelated facets to the medical care problems of the aged. An insight into these problems requires an understanding of the demography of the aged, their social characteristics, their economic status, their health status, their attitudes toward their health problems, and their record for utilization of medical care services. Lastly, there is the important matter of financing the medical care costs of the aged. Each of these facets will be surveyed not only with respect to the current situation, but also with regard to trends.

# Demographic, Social, and Economic Characteristics of the Aged

# 2

SINCE AGING is a continuing process, variable from one individual to another, no single chronological age can be selected to define the threshold of "old age."[1] However, for purposes of description and discussion, convention will be followed, and the aged will be considered here as those at ages 65 years and over.[2] Only characteristics bearing on the medical care problems of the aged are described in this chapter. It will become evident that the aged are a very heterogeneous group in many respects. Large numbers are still active in employment or housework as they enter "old age" and enjoy a full family life. For many, this favorable state continues well into the later years. As these later years advance, they bring with them, increasingly, restriction in activity, the break-up of the immediate family, and needs for medical care.

## DEMOGRAPHIC CHARACTERISTICS

*Number, Age, and Sex.* The growth in the numbers of the aged provides one indication, among others, of the increasing

---

[1] R. S. Cavan, E. W. Burgess, R. J. Havighurst, and H. Goldhammer, *Personal Adjustment in Old Age* (Chicago: Science Research Associates, Inc., 1949), chap. i.

[2] World Health Organization, Regional Office for Europe, *Advisory Group on the Public Health Aspects of the Aging of the Population, Oslo, 28 July–2 August, 1958,* Report dated 30 December, 1958, p. 5.

4

magnitude of their medical care problems. Thus, in 1959 the number at ages 65 and over totaled more than 15 million, a rise of 6½ million since 1940. A rise equally great is expected by 1975, when almost 22 million will be at ages 65 and over. Also, the numbers of the aged have increased more rapidly than for the rest of the population, and the present outlook is that this trend will continue. Table 2.1 shows that those at

TABLE 2.1

SHIFTS IN THE AGE AND SEX DISTRIBUTION OF THE POPULATION
OF THE UNITED STATES SINCE 1920 WITH PROJECTION TO 1980

| Year | Population, Thousands | | Per Cent of Total at Ages | | Ratio: Females per 100 Males | | | |
|---|---|---|---|---|---|---|---|---|
| | All Ages | Ages 65 and Over | 65 and Over | 75 and Over | All Ages | Under Age 65 | Ages 65–74 | Ages 75 and Over |
| Census Data | | | | | | | | |
| 1920 | 105,711 | 4,933 | 4.7 | 1.4 | 96.1 | 96.0 | 93.9 | 110.9 |
| 1930 | 122,775 | 6,634 | 5.4 | 1.6 | 97.6 | 97.5 | 95.9 | 108.8 |
| 1940 | 131,820 | 8,969 | 6.8 | 2.0 | 99.1 | 98.7 | 101.3 | 113.2 |
| 1950 | 151,132 | 12,194 | 8.1 | 2.6 | 100.8 | 99.9 | 107.3 | 121.1 |
| 1959 | 177,103 | 15,380 | 8.7 | 3.0 | 102.1 | 100.4 | 114.9 | 132.8 |
| Projected Data | | | | | | | | |
| 1965 | 193,643 | 17,638 | 9.1 | 3.3 | 102.6 | 100.4 | 121.7 | 139.5 |
| 1970 | 208,199 | 19,549 | 9.4 | 3.5 | 102.9 | 100.3 | 125.3 | 146.5 |
| 1975 | 225,552 | 21,872 | 9.7 | 3.7 | 103.0 | 100.0 | 127.1 | 153.0 |
| 1980 | 245,409 | 24,526 | 10.0 | 3.8 | 102.9 | 99.5 | 128.9 | 157.4 |

Note: Data for 1940–1980 include armed forces overseas; projections are based upon assumption of relatively high birth rates.

Source: 1920 and 1930: *U.S. Census of Population: 1950*, Vol. II, *Characteristics of the Population*, Part 1, U.S. Summary, Chapter B, Washington, D.C., 1952, p. 93 (not adjusted for ages unknown); 1940–1980: *Current Population Reports*, P-25, No. 98, p. 15; No. 187, pp. 16, 17–21 (Series III); No. 193, p. 9.

ages 65 and over constituted 6.8 per cent of the total population in 1940 and 8.7 per cent in 1959; this may rise to 9.7 per cent by 1975.

Among the aged, the proportion at the extreme ages is also

rising. Of the total at 65 and over, 30 per cent were at ages 75 and over in 1940 and 35 per cent in 1959; the trend may continue to 38 per cent by 1975. In the rising numbers and proportions of aged, females are gaining more rapidly than males. At ages 65–74 years, females have outnumbered males since 1940; the excess amounted to 15 per cent in 1959, with the outlook of a 27 per cent margin by 1975. The differences are even greater at ages 75 and over, with females exceeding males by more than 30 per cent in 1959, and the prospect is that by 1975 the excess may amount to more than 50 per cent.

*Marital Status.*   Mortality data tell us that the married have lower death rates than the unmarried, particularly among men. This is usually attributed not only to the selection of the healthier lives for marriage, but also to the stability and better care associated with married life. Hence, disruption of family life by death, a frequent occurrence in old age, presents many social and economic problems that may affect the health status of the surviving spouse.

According to the data in Table 2.2, which relate to the 1950 census of population, over one fourth of the males at ages 65–69 are not married and most of these are widowers. The proportion of males unmarried increases to almost one third at ages 70–74 years, and mounts to almost one half at ages 75 and over. For females, the corresponding proportions unmarried—predominantly widows—are appreciably greater, namely more than half at ages 65–69, almost two thirds at ages 70–74, and over four fifths at and above ages 75.

## SOCIAL CHARACTERISTICS

The attitude toward hospital and medical care utilization by the aged may be strongly influenced by many social characteristics, such as place of residence, educational attainment, and living arrangements.

*Living Arrangements.*   Persons living alone or without relatives in a household are more likely to be sent to a hos-

TABLE 2.2

CHARACTERISTICS AND LIVING ARRANGEMENTS OF THE POPULATION BEFORE AND AFTER AGE 65, BY SEX, UNITED STATES, CENSUS OF APRIL 1950

| Characteristics | Males at Specified Ages | | | | Females at Specified Ages | | | |
|---|---|---|---|---|---|---|---|---|
| | 20–64 | 65–69 | 70–74 | 75 and Over | 20–64 | 65–69 | 70–74 | 75 and Over |
| **Marital Status** | | | | | | | | |
| Total, per cent | 100.0 | 100.0 | 100.0 | 100.0 | 100.0 | 100.0 | 100.0 | 100.0 |
| Married | 77.5 | 74.0 | 67.5 | 52.4 | 77.7 | 48.9 | 36.6 | 18.7 |
| Widowed | 2.1 | 15.0 | 22.3 | 38.5 | 7.2 | 41.1 | 53.3 | 71.2 |
| Divorced | 2.3 | 2.3 | 1.9 | 1.3 | 2.9 | 1.6 | 1.1 | 0.6 |
| Single | 18.1 | 8.7 | 8.3 | 7.8 | 12.2 | 8.4 | 9.0 | 9.5 |
| **Living Arrangements** | | | | | | | | |
| Total, per cent | 100.0 | 100.0 | | 100.0 | 100.0 | 100.0 | | 100.0 |
| Living in families | 88.9 | 81.6 | | 76.2 | 91.6 | 75.5 | | 68.9 |
| Head | 72.4 | 71.6 | | 54.2 | 6.0 | 13.6 | | 14.5 |
| Wife | — | — | | — | 70.5 | 39.3 | | 15.0 |
| Other relative | 16.5 | 10.0 | | 22.0 | 15.1 | 22.6 | | 39.4 |
| Living alone or with no relative in household | 9.6 | 16.2 | | 19.0 | 7.7 | 22.6 | | 25.3 |
| Inmates of institutions | 1.5 | 2.2 | | 4.8 | 0.7 | 1.9 | | 5.8 |
| In mental hospitals | 0.6 | 1.1 | | 1.3 | 0.5 | 1.0 | | 1.5 |
| In homes for aged and dependents | 0.1 | 0.9 | | 3.2 | 0.1 | 0.8 | | 4.2 |
| Others | 0.8 | 0.2 | | 0.3 | 0.1 | 0.1 | | 0.1 |
| **Residence** | | | | | | | | |
| Total, per cent | 100.0 | 100.0 | 100.0 | 100.0 | 100.0 | 100.0 | 100.0 | 100.0 |
| Urban | 66.4 | 61.8 | 59.8 | 57.7 | 68.9 | 67.4 | 67.3 | 66.8 |
| Rural nonfarm | 19.7 | 20.9 | 23.2 | 25.9 | 18.6 | 20.1 | 21.2 | 21.9 |
| Rural farm | 13.9 | 17.3 | 17.0 | 16.4 | 12.5 | 12.5 | 11.5 | 11.3 |
| **Migration** | | | | | | | | |
| Total, per cent | 100.0 | 100.0 | | 100.0 | 100.0 | 100.0 | | 100.0 |
| Nonmovers | 78.4 | 89.6 | | 89.4 | 81.2 | 89.6 | | 89.2 |
| Movers within county | 12.3 | 5.9 | | 5.9 | 11.5 | 6.0 | | 5.8 |
| Others | 9.3 | 4.5 | | 4.7 | 7.3 | 4.4 | | 5.0 |

TABLE 2.2—*Continued*

| Characteristics | Males at Specified Ages | | | | Females at Specified Ages | | | |
|---|---|---|---|---|---|---|---|---|
| | 20–64 | 65–69 | 70–74 | 75 and Over | 20–64 | 65–69 | 70–74 | 75 and Over |
| Education (School Years Completed) | | | | | | | | |
| Total, per cent....... | 100.0 | 100.0 | | 100.0 | 100.0 | 100.0 | | 100.0 |
| Under 5.......... | 9.2 | 24.0 | | 26.3 | 7.5 | 19.5 | | 20.1 |
| 5–11.............. | 52.0 | 56.5 | | 54.7 | 50.1 | 58.4 | | 57.9 |
| 12 or more........ | 35.9 | 15.7 | | 13.8 | 40.3 | 19.1 | | 17.1 |
| Not reported...... | 2.9 | 3.8 | | 5.2 | 2.1 | 3.0 | | 4.9 |
| Nativity (White) | | | | | | | | |
| Total, per cent....... | 100.0 | 100.0 | 100.0 | 100.0 | 100.0 | 100.0 | 100.0 | 100.0 |
| Native-born....... | 90.6 | 73.5 | 74.8 | 75.1 | 91.1 | 77.8 | 78.0 | 78.1 |
| Foreign-born...... | 9.4 | 26.5 | 25.2 | 24.9 | 8.9 | 22.2 | 22.0 | 21.9 |

Source: U.S. Bureau of the Census, *U.S. Census of Population: 1950*, Vol. IV, *Special Reports*, Washington, D.C., 1953 and later.

pital when ill, or to receive more attention from the physician, than those who have the benefits of family life. According to the 1950 census data in Table 2.2, the proportions living in families are over four fifths for males at ages 65–74, and over three fourths at ages 75 and over. Although the corresponding proportions are lower for females, they are still appreciable, namely three fourths at ages 65–74, and over two thirds at ages 75 and over. In 1959, according to a survey by the Bureau of the Census, 81 per cent of aged males and 69 per cent of aged females were family members; 16 per cent and 29 per cent respectively were living alone or with nonrelatives, and the rest were in institutions.

However, these census data are hardly adequate for an insight into the role that family and neighborly relationships have in the care of the aged. A number of local surveys have indicated a tendency for the aged to live near their married children or other relatives, to be visited frequently by them, and to receive close attention at times of illness.[3] Such aid may reduce the need for care in facilities outside the home and, equally important, it may provide a spiritual comfort lacking in an institution. The same surveys have shown a tendency for friends and neighbors to give some attention in the absence of relatives. In summarizing, a committee of the World Health Organization reports that, "Wherever careful studies have been carried out in the industrialized countries, the lasting devotion of children for their parents has been amply demonstrated. The great majority of old people are in regular contact with their children, relatives or friends."[4]

The importance of adequate and suited housing for the health and well-being of the aged has been made abundantly clear.[5] Among the many findings from experience is the advantage of allowing the aged to live in an accustomed environment rather than locating them in a separate community. However, it has been found desirable to design their living accommodations to allow for their infirmities.[6]

*Residence and Migration.* The accessibility of hospital and medical care facilities to the aged is not much different than for younger people. About three fifths of the males at ages 65 and over live in urban centers, somewhat less than one fourth in rural nonfarm places, and about one sixth in rural farm areas. In the case of females at ages 65 and over,

---

[3] *The Aging of Three Parishes,* National Conference of Catholic Charities, Washington, D.C. (see the detailed report of each parish); R. G. Brown, "Family Structure and Social Isolation," presented at the Annual Meeting of the American Sociological Society, Chicago, September 5, 1959; P. Townsend, *The Family Life of Old People* (Glencoe, Ill.: The Free Press, 1957); *Old Age in Rhode Island,* Report of the Governor's Commission to Study Problems of the Aged, Providence, July, 1953, p. 7.

[4] Sixth Report of the Expert Committee on Mental Health, *Mental Health Problems of Aging and the Aged,* World Health Organization, Geneva, 1959, p. 7.

[5] *Housing the Elderly: A Review of Significant Developments,* Housing and Home Finance Agency, Office of the Administration, Washington, D.C., April, 1959.

[6] Sixth Report of the Expert Committee on Mental Health, *op. cit.,* p. 23.

about two thirds live in urban centers and less than one eighth are on the farm.

As might be expected, the aged do not change residence as readily as younger people. According to the census of 1950, only one tenth of those 65 and over moved during the previous year, compared with one fifth for adults under 65. This situation suggests that the elderly have a good opportunity to become aware of the hospital and medical care facilities available in their community in time of need. The recently retired who have moved to another community must generally establish new medical contacts.

*Education.*    The aged in our country today had less schooling than did younger adults. At the time of the 1950 census, only one seventh of the males at ages 65 and over had completed 12 or more years at school; for males under 65 more than one third had gone that far. The same pattern will be observed for females in Table 2.2; however, the extent of their schooling is somewhat greater than among males. It is fair to assume from these data that our aged, in the years ahead, will show a continuing rise in educational attainment. Thus, according to projections by the Bureau of the Census, the proportion of population aged 65 and over with at least four years of high school will rise from 18 per cent in 1950 to 26 per cent in 1970 and further to 35 per cent in 1980.[7]

Since we are a health-conscious nation, subject to a constant stream of health literature, our growing corps of aged will undoubtedly have an increasing sense of personal hygiene. Also, with their advantage in education, compared with the aged of today, they will not only have a better knowledge of the medical care benefits and facilities at their disposal, but will also have become accustomed to making use of them. For the same reason, the aged in coming years should respond more readily to medical guidance and instruction. The effect of the increasing proportion of native born

[7] Bureau of the Census, *Current Population Reports, Population Characteristics,* Series P-20, No. 91, January 12, 1959.

among our aged upon their health status and medical care problems will correspond very closely to that of their rising educational level.

*The Veteran Population.*  The aging population of war veterans will introduce an increasingly important element in the medical care problems of the aged in the years ahead because of their rights to services from the federal government under prescribed circumstances.[8] Of the participants of all wars of the United States living in 1957, totaling over 22½ million, only 4.6 per cent were at ages 65 and over. Although these veterans will decrease to little more than 20 million by 1971, almost 10 per cent of this total will be at ages 65 and over (Table 2.3). These aged veterans[9] will then

TABLE 2.3
ESTIMATED AGE DISTRIBUTION OF VETERAN POPULATION, EXCLUDING
PEACETIME VETERANS, 1957–86

| Age | 1957 | Projected Data | |
|---|---|---|---|
| | | 1971 | 1986 |
| All ages, number (thousands)... | 22,560 | 20,257 | 15,107 |
| per cent............... | 100.0 | 100.0 | 100.0 |
| Under age 65............... | 95.4 | 90.1 | 63.0 |
| 65–74................... | 4.2 | 4.6 | 30.7 |
| 75 and over............. | .4 | 5.3 | 6.3 |

Source: Veterans Administration, Department of Medicine and Surgery, and Bureau of the Budget, Hospital Programs, Labor and Welfare Division, *Current and Projected Veteran Patient Load Through 1986*, June 4, 1958, Table 2, p. I-11.

constitute about one fourth of all males over age 65 and about one tenth of the aged of both sexes. By 1986, over one third of the surviving veterans will be at least 65 years of age.

## ECONOMIC CHARACTERISTICS

A picture of the resources available to the aged to meet their costs of medical care may be pieced together from

---

[8] See p. 228.

[9] A small number of females is included.

several studies of their economic status. Chapters 6 and 7 describe present mechanisms for meeting the costs of medical care in old age.

*Sources of Income.* In December, 1958, out of a total population of 15.38 million at ages 65 and over, about one fourth received current income as earners or wives of earners. About 70 per cent of the aged were in receipt of a life income from such federal programs as Old-Age and Survivors Insurance, the Railroad Retirement program, Veterans' compensation and pensions, and government employees' retirement programs. Table 2.4 shows that 2.510 million aged, or one sixth of the total, then received income from public assistance. A miscellaneous class of about one tenth of the total were either without income or had income from sources other than those already specified. These data may be supplemented by findings from a survey of persons 65 and over, made in the spring of 1957 by the National Opinion Research Center (NORC), on their resources in 1956.[10] During that year, 6 per cent of the aged received pensions from an employer (11 per cent for males and 2 per cent for females), 23 per cent had some income from interest, dividends, annuities, and insurance, 20 per cent received rent from house or property, and 8 per cent had a regular cash income from someone outside their household.

The decade from 1948 to 1958 witnessed some marked changes in the sources of money income of the aged. Very largely as a result of extensions in the scope of Old-Age and Survivors Insurance, the proportion in receipt of money income from social insurance and related programs rose from 20 per cent to 68 per cent during these ten years (Table 2.4). At the same time, those on public assistance decreased from

---

[10] E. Shanas, *Financial Resources of the Aging,* Research Series 10, Health Information Foundation, New York, 1959. The proportions with income from employment, social insurance and related programs, and from public assistance in this survey were similar to those in Table 2.4. In the NORC survey, the *main* sources of income for the aged were: employment, 31 per cent; social insurance and related programs, 34 per cent; public assistance, 14 per cent; pensions from employer, 2 per cent; interest, etc., 6 per cent; rent, 7 per cent; someone outside household, 4 per cent; no money income, 2 per cent.

TABLE 2.4

DISTRIBUTION OF POPULATION AT AGES 65 AND OVER RECEIVING MONEY
INCOME FROM SPECIFIED SOURCES, UNITED STATES, 1948 AND 1958[a]

| Source of Money Income[b] | Number (Thousands) December 1958 | | | Per Cent Distribution Both Sexes | |
|---|---|---|---|---|---|
| | Both Sexes | Males | Females | June 1958 | June 1948 |
| 1. Population ages 65 and over. . . | 15,380 | 6,990 | 8,390 | 100.0 | 100.0 |
| 2. Employment. . . . . . . . . . . . . . . | 3,680 | 2,110 | 1,570 | 26.0 | 33.2 |
| Earners. . . . . . . . . . . . . . . . | 2,810 | 2,110 | 700 | 20.2 | 25.4 |
| Nonworking wives of earners | 870 | — | 870 | 5.8 | 7.8 |
| 3. Social insurance and related programs[c]. . . . . . . . . . . . . . . . . | 10,830 | 5,420 | 5,410 | 68.2 | 20.2 |
| Old-Age, Survivors, and Disability Insurance. . . . . . . . | 9,230 | 4,590 | 4,640 | 58.2 | 12.7 |
| Railroad retirement program | 590 | 300 | 290 | 3.8 | 2.6 |
| Government employees' retirement programs. . . . . . . | 790 | 420 | 370 | 4.9 | 2.6 |
| Veterans' compensation and pensions. . . . . . . . . . . . . . . | 1,240 | 710 | 530 | 7.6 | 3.0 |
| 4. Public assistance[d]. . . . . . . . . . . | 2,510 | 940 | 1,570 | 16.6 | 20.8 |
| 5. No money income or income solely from other sources. . . . . | 1,610 | 240 | 1,370 | 9.9 | 29.4 |
| 6. Income from more than one source specified on lines 2–4. . . | 3,250 | 1,720 | 1,530 | 20.7 | 3.6 |
| OASDI and employment[e]. . . | — | — | — | 12.5 ⎫ | |
| Other programs and employment[e]. . . . . . . . . . . . . . . . | — | — | — | 4.0 ⎭ | 2.3 |
| Old-age assistance and OASDI. . . . . . . . . . . . . . . | — | — | — | 4.0 ⎫ | |
| Other assistance and OASDI or related programs. . . . . . | — | — | — | .2 ⎭ | 1.3 |

[a] 1958 data relate to the continental United States, Alaska, Hawaii, Puerto Rico, and the Virgin Islands; 1948 data for continental United States. Persons with income from sources specified may also have received money income from others, such as interest, dividends, private pensions or annuities, or cash contributions from relatives.

[b] Because persons frequently have income from more than one of the sources specified, the sum of persons shown on lines numbered 2–5 exceeds the total number in the population (line 1). The estimates of persons with income from more than one source are developed from survey data. They are therefore subject to sampling and reporting errors, as well as the error inherent in projection of survey findings to additional population groups and different dates, errors which are relatively more significant in the case of small estimates.

[c] Persons with income from more than one of the programs listed are counted only once. Estimates of women beneficiaries under programs for government employees and veterans include the estimated number of beneficiaries' wives not in direct receipt of benefits.

[d] Old-age assistance recipients and persons aged 65 and over receiving aid to the blind or to the permanently and totally disabled, including a small number receiving vendor payments for medical care but no direct cash payment.

[e] Excludes a small number with income from employment and OASDI and another insurance or related program, because the figures on line 3 have already been adjusted for overlap among the insurance and related programs.

Source: L. A. Epstein, "Money Income of Aged Persons: A 10-Year Review, 1948 to 1958," *Social Security Bulletin*, June, 1959, p. 3.

21 per cent to 17 per cent of the aged, and those without money income or income from other sources fell from 29 per cent to only 10 per cent. Extensions of OASI coverage were also a factor in the decline of the proportion receiving income as earners or as wives of earners from 33 per cent in 1948 to 26 per cent in 1958.

*Employment Status.* Although a relatively large number of men past 65 are still at work, the proportion decreases rapidly with advance in age. Table 2.5 shows that in March, 1957, one half of the men at ages 65–69 were still employed, but this fell to less than two fifths at ages 70–74, and to only one sixth at ages 75 and over; the corresponding proportions are much lower for women. Self-employment is a significant influence in continuing an active career into the higher ages, almost two fifths of the employed being so engaged at ages 65–69 and nearly one half at ages 70 and over. Well over half of the aged self-employed males were in agriculture. However, among all employed males past 65, over one fourth were working part time. In the case of employed women at the older ages, substantially more than one fourth have jobs in private households. About two fifths of all employed women worked part time.

It is usual to point to a decline in labor-force participation by the aged since the beginning of the century. Some of this change may be due to the shift from an agricultural to an industrialized economy. Sheldon also suggests that:

In terms of health, an interpretation of this historic decline in labor force participation is tenable only on the assumption that the progress in medical science and the reduction in mortality during the past half-century have permitted larger and larger numbers of the physically inadequate to survive to a ripe old age.[11]

*Retirement.* Retirement is influenced by many factors, of which one of the most significant is health status.[12] Evi-

---

[11] H. D. Sheldon, *The Older Population* (New York: John Wiley & Sons, 1958), p. 53.

[12] G. F. Streib and W. E. Thompson in *The New Frontiers of Aging* (eds. W. Donahue and C. Tibbitts) (Ann Arbor: University of Michigan Press,

## TABLE 2.5

EMPLOYMENT STATUS AND WORK EXPERIENCE BEFORE AND AFTER AGE 65, BY SEX, UNITED STATES, 1957

| Status | Males at Specified Ages | | | | Females at Specified Ages | | | |
|---|---|---|---|---|---|---|---|---|
| | 14–64 | 65–69 | 70–74 | 75 and Over | 14–64 | 65–69 | 70–74 | 75 and Over |
| **Employment Status*** | | | | | | | | |
| Total population, per cent | 100.0 | 100.0 | 100.0 | 100.0 | 100.0 | 100.0 | 100.0 | 100.0 |
| Civilian labor force | 86.9 | 53.0 | 39.0 | 16.7 | 38.5 | 18.6 | 11.8 | 3.9 |
| Employed | 83.1 | 50.5 | 37.8 | 16.2 | 36.8 | 18.0 | 11.2 | 3.9 |
| In agriculture | 8.2 | 11.0 | 11.9 | 3.7 | 1.4 | 1.3 | 0.6 | 0.6 |
| In nonagricultural industries | 74.9 | 39.5 | 25.9 | 12.5 | 35.4 | 16.7 | 10.6 | 3.3 |
| Unemployed | 3.8 | 2.5 | 1.2 | 0.5 | 1.7 | 0.6 | 0.6 | † |
| Not in labor force | 13.1 | 47.0 | 61.0 | 83.3 | 61.5 | 81.4 | 88.2 | 96.1 |
| Unable to work | 1.1 | 5.3 | 8.7 | 13.3 | 0.5 | 2.2 | 3.5 | 15.2 |
| Others | 12.0 | 41.7 | 52.3 | 70.0 | 61.0 | 79.2 | 84.7 | 80.9 |

**Class of Worker‡**

| Status | Males at Specified Ages | | | Females at Specified Ages | | |
|---|---|---|---|---|---|---|
| | 14–64 | 65–69 | 70–74 and 75 and Over | 14–64 | 65–69 | 70–74 and 75 and Over |
| Total employed, per cent | 100.0 | 100.0 | 100.0 | 100.0 | 100.0 | 100.0 |
| In agriculture | 10.2 | 23.8 | 31.2 | 4.0 | 8.6 | 12.7 |
| Wage and salary | 2.7 | 2.7 | 3.9 | 0.7 | 0.6 | † |
| Self-employed | 6.4 | 21.1 | 27.3 | 0.6 | 4.4 | 8.3 |
| Unpaid family worker | 1.1 | † | † | 2.7 | 3.6 | 4.4 |
| In nonagricultural industries | 89.8 | 76.2 | 68.8 | 96.0 | 91.4 | 87.3 |
| Wage and salary | 78.8 | 58.8 | 49.6 | 88.3 | 77.8 | 69.7 |
| In private households | 0.7 | 1.8 | 2.0 | 9.6 | 24.8 | 33.2 |
| Government workers | 10.0 | 9.6 | 8.8 | 13.9 | 13.8 | 6.5 |
| Others | 68.1 | 47.4 | 38.8 | 64.8 | 39.2 | 30.0 |
| Self-employed | 10.8 | 17.4 | 19.2 | 5.2 | 11.5 | 14.7 |
| Unpaid family worker | 0.2 | † | † | 2.5 | 2.1 | 2.9 |

**Full-time or Part-time Work Status§**

| Status | Males 14–64 | Males 65 and Over | Females 14–64 | Females 65 and Over |
|---|---|---|---|---|
| Total employed, per cent | 100.0 | 100.0 | 100.0 | 100.0 |
| Total at work | 97.0 | 93.8 | 97.0 | 95.1 |
| Worked full-time survey week | 85.4 | 66.6 | 69.7 | 51.5 |
| Worked part-time survey week | 11.6 | 27.2 | 27.3 | 43.6 |
| Usually work full time | 5.3 | 5.5 | 5.0 | 3.7 |
| Usually work part time | 6.3 | 21.7 | 22.3 | 39.9 |
| Economic reasons | 1.1 | 2.4 | 2.5 | 2.9 |
| Other reasons | 5.2 | 19.3 | 19.8 | 37.0 |
| With a job but not at work | 3.0 | 6.2 | 3.0 | 4.9 |

**Per Cent of Specified Marital Category in Labor Force***

| Status | 14–64 | 65–69 | 70–74 | 75 and Over | 14–64 | 65–69 | 70–74 | 75 and Over |
|---|---|---|---|---|---|---|---|---|
| Single | 59.0 | 32.8 | 35.5 | 10.1 | 48.1 | 38.7 | 27.8 | 10.8 |
| Married, spouse present | 96.8 | 55.5 | 41.0 | 20.1 | 31.4 | 8.3 | 5.6 | 2.6 |
| Other marital status | 79.6 | 44.6 | 30.6 | 12.1 | 58.8 | 25.7 | 12.7 | 3.2 |

* Data relate to survey week during March. The figures for employment status at ages 70–74 and 75 and over were estimated by the author from the marginal totals in the source.

† Less than 0.05 per cent.

‡ Data relate to survey week during April.

§ Data relate to survey week during May.

Note: These estimates are derived from sample surveys and are subject to sampling variation which may be relatively large, particularly where the percentages are based on a small number of cases. Data relate to civilian population.

Source of basic data: Bureau of the Census, *Current Population Reports, Labor Force*, Series P-57, No. 177, April, 1957, and Series P-50, No. 76, November, 1957; and unpublished data supplied by the Bureau of the Census.

dence of the role of health as a factor influencing retirement is found in a survey of the general population conducted by the Bureau of the Census in April, 1952. At that time, 60 per cent of the men at ages 65 and over no longer in the labor force stated that they retired voluntarily for reasons of health.[13] That reason was given by only one fifth of the retired who had professional and technical careers, by almost two fifths of those who had been clerical workers, and by about two thirds of the men who spent most of their lives in agriculture and as operatives. For most other occupational groups, more than half retired for reasons of health. However, these proportions may be influenced by the frequency with which formal retirement plans may be present in the occupation. Thus, only negligible proportions of the aged in 1952 formerly in agriculture retired through a formal plan; on the other hand, well over one fourth of those formerly clerical workers had the benefit of a retirement plan. Among aged retired women who had worked since they were age 50, almost half gave health as the reason for their retirement.[14] Commenting on the high proportions at the older ages who claim to be unable to work, Sheldon states that:

. . . there can be no easy statement as to the exact degree by which disability contributes to retirement. Among older men, in their own terms, it looms relatively large; if, on the other hand, the questions are focused on specific disabilities to which names can be given, or the existence of which stands up under cross examination, the proportion retired by disability is considerably lower.[15]

With the growth of formal retirement plans and the expansion of the Old-Age and Survivors Insurance system

---

1957), chap. xiv. The authors comment on their findings from the Cornell Study of Occupational Retirement; see also W. E. Thompson and G. F. Streib, "Situational Determinants: Health and Economic Deprivation in Retirement," *Journal of Socal Issues,* Vol. 14, No. 2, p. 18 (1958).

[13] P. O. Steiner and R. Dorfman, *The Economic Status of the Aged* (Berkeley and Los Angeles: University of California Press, 1957), p. 48.

[14] P. O. Steiner and R. Dorfman, *op. cit.,* pp. 50 and 63.

[15] H. D. Sheldon, *op. cit.,* p. 45.

since the time of the April, 1952 survey, the proportions retiring for reasons of health have undoubtedly changed, perhaps to lower figures. Strictly, retirement should be considered as complete withdrawal from the labor force, with no intent to return. However, many who, for any reason, leave the labor force for the first time re-enter it later. For example, in 1955 and 1956, 4 per cent of all old-age beneficiaries under the Old-Age and Survivors Insurance system had their benefits suspended because they engaged in some covered employment that provided an income over that permitted by the retirement test.[16] Also, the average age at retirement under the Old-Age and Survivors Insurance system, namely 68 years for men during 1953 to 1955, is actually only the age at which initial claim is made for entitlement to old-age benefit. Somewhat less than two fifths of the men making their initial claim during this period were 65 years of age.

Questions have also been raised regarding the effect of retirement upon health. As for indications provided by mortality data, Myers attributes the relatively high death rates in the early years after retirement, as observed in a number of pension plans, to a tendency for workers in poor health to retire as soon as possible, and for those in good health to continue at work if retirement is not compulsory.[17] Thompson and Streib also noted that ". . . people in poor health tend to retire, and not that retirement affects health. It should be noted, of course, that our data does *not* necessarily refute the notion that a radical withdrawal from sustaining activities results in a decline of health."[18] Also pertinent in this connection is the theory of Hinkle and Wolff that stresses produced by difficulties in adapting to a new

---

[16] R. J. Myers, "Some Implications of a Retirement Test in Social Insurance Systems," *Proceedings of the Conference of Actuaries in Public Practice,* Vol. 7, p. 337 (October, 1957).

[17] R. J. Myers, "Factors in Interpreting Mortality After Retirement," *Journal of the American Statistical Association,* Vol. 49, p. 499 (September, 1954).

[18] *Op. cit.,* p. 33.

environment may become manifest in outbreaks of illness among persons highly susceptible to illness.[19] The applicability of this theory to the recently retired, in view of their newly changed daily environment, is worth considering.[20]

The accumulation of further physical ailments since retirement is made apparent in the survey of April, 1952. Whereas 60 per cent of the aged men not then in the labor force retired for reasons of health, 78 per cent of them stated they were not well enough to work, as may be noted in Table 2.6. The proportion of males stating they were not well

TABLE 2.6

PROPORTION OF MEN AGED 65 AND OVER NOT WELL
ENOUGH TO WORK ACCORDING TO LONGEST OCCUPATION,
LABOR FORCE STATUS, AND ANNUAL INCOME,
UNITED STATES, APRIL, 1952

| Longest Occupation, Labor Force Status, Annual Income | Per Cent Not Well Enough to Work |
|---|---|
| All men 65 and over | 45 |
| With longest occupation as | |
| Professional and technical | 15 |
| Farmers and farm managers | 46 |
| Nonfarm managers and proprietors | 29 |
| All others | 52 |
| Men 65 and over not in the labor force | 78 |
| With a 1951* income of | |
| Nothing | 80 |
| Less than $1,000 | 80 |
| $1,000–$2,499 | 74 |
| $2,500–$4,999 | 62 |
| $5,000 and over | 44 |

* The income is that of the individual in case of unrelated males and that of couples in case of married males.

Source: Derived from Tables 4.1, 4.2, and 4.3 of P. O. Steiner and R. Dorfman, *The Economic Status of the Aged* (Berkeley and Los Angeles: University of California Press, 1957).

enough to work was 80 per cent where there was no income in 1951 or where the income was less than $1,000; at the other extreme, the proportion was 44 per cent where the

[19] L. E. Hinkle and H. G. Wolff, "The Nature of Man's Adaptation to His Total Environment and the Relation of This to Illness," *Archives of Internal Medicine,* Vol. 99, p. 442 (March, 1957).

[20] This was suggested in a communication from Dr. R. T. Monroe.

income was $5,000 or more. Although the proportions may differ in a more recent situation, the general pattern is not likely to change substantially. Since these incomes relate to 1951, while the health status relates to April, 1952, the low proportions of those not well enough to work among the higher-income groups may be due to relatively larger contingents of the more recently retired among them. On the other hand, those in the lower-income groups may be more heavily weighted with the older persons farther removed from their working days.

*Annual Income—General Population.* Whatever the source, most aged persons are in receipt of some money income to meet their current needs, including medical care, in whole or in part.[21] Most income data are derived from census reports and field surveys and are to be used with some caution since such sources "generally produce underestimates of the amounts of income and of the number of income recipients."[22] Table 2.7, derived from sample surveys of the general population, shows that in 1957, the proportion of individual aged males with any money income was not much less than for all males at ages 20 and over, 95.2 per cent compared with 97.5 per cent.[23] Moreover, the proportion for the aged has risen considerably; in 1947 it was only 84.5 per cent. However, among aged males with income in 1957, the median received was only $1,421, compared with $3,684 for all males. An improving economic status for the aged is evident not only in the rising proportion with money income, but also in their higher income level. Thus, the median money income for aged males with income in 1957 was almost 50 per cent greater than for 1947. Also significant is

---

[21] In a sample of persons 65 and over surveyed in the spring of 1957 by the National Opinion Research Center, 45 per cent regarded their financial status the same as at age 60; 15 per cent considered it better and 37 per cent worse (E. Shanas, *op. cit.*).

[22] H. P. Miller, *Income of the American People* (New York: John Wiley & Sons, 1955), p. 145.

[23] For a definition of money income as used in the reports of the Bureau of the Census, see H. P. Miller, *op. cit.*, p. 133.

TABLE 2.7

TOTAL MONEY INCOME AT THE OLDER AGES, UNITED STATES

| Status | Total United States | Urban | Rural Nonfarm | Rural Farm |
|---|---|---|---|---|
| | Per Cent of Persons with Income | | | |
| Males | | | | |
| Ages 20 and over, 1957 | 97.5 | 97.6 | 97.9 | 96.0 |
| Ages 65 and over, 1957 | 95.2 | 95.5 | 95.6 | 93.5 |
| 1950 | 89.9 | 90.3 | 88.4 | 90.2 |
| 1947 | 84.5 | 83.5 | 82.2 | 89.4 |
| Females | | | | |
| Ages 20 and over, 1957 | 53.9 | 57.2 | 49.9 | 42.0 |
| Ages 65 and over, 1957 | 71.8 | 72.2 | 74.0 | 64.7 |
| | Median Income for Persons with Income | | | |
| Males | | | | |
| Ages 14 and over, 1957 | $3,684 | $4,082 | $3,712 | $1,570 |
| Ages 65 and over, 1957 | 1,421 | 1,615 | 1,207 | 1,018 |
| 1950 | 986 | 1,272 | 851 | 586 |
| 1947 | 956 | 1,225 | 818 | 725 |
| Females | | | | |
| Ages 14 and over, 1957 | 1,199 | 1,429 | 932 | 467 |
| Ages 65 and over, 1957 | 741 | 804 | 665 | 445 |
| | Median Income, 1957 | | | |
| Families headed by persons | | | | |
| Of all ages | $4,971 | $5,359 | $4,894 | $2,490 |
| At ages 65 and over | 2,490 | 3,000 | 2,217 | 1,606 |
| Individuals not living with any relative | | | | |
| Individuals of all ages | 1,496 | 1,716 | 1,037 | 945 |
| Individuals aged 65 and over | 918 | 992 | 786 | 711 |

Note: These estimates are derived from sample surveys and are subject to sampling variation which may be relatively large, particularly where the figures are based on a small number of cases.

Source: Bureau of the Census, *Current Population Reports, Consumer Income*, Series P-60.

the fact that nearly three fourths of the aged women in 1957 had some money income, but the median was rather low.[24] Since the family acts as a unit in time of need on the part

---

[24] See also L. A. Epstein, "Money Income Distribution of the Aged," *Research and Statistics Note No. 14,* Division of Program Research, Social Security Administration, Washington, D.C., May 13, 1959.

of any of its members, data regarding the median income of all families including persons at ages 65 and over would be pertinent in considering resources available for the medical care costs of the aged.[25] For such families, where younger persons may be at the head, the median incomes would generally be higher than for families headed by the aged. For example, the median income of all families in the United States during 1951 was $3,709.[26] Of these families, 13 per cent were headed by a person aged 65 or over, and for them the median income was $1,956. However, over 17 per cent of all families had at least one member at ages 65 or over, and among the latter nearly two thirds had only one aged member. For those families with only one such aged member, whether or not the family head, the median income was $3,177, or only about one sixth less than that for all families. On the other hand, for those families with two or more such members the median was less than half that for all families, namely $1,712.[27] It may be surmised that a large proportion of the latter families are made up solely of two aged members.

Since data for the study of trends in income for *all* families containing aged persons are not available, it is usual to study the situation of families headed by the aged. The contributors to these family incomes are not only the family heads who may be working, but also other family members with employment. In 1957, the median income of families headed by persons at ages 65 and over was $2,490, just half that for family heads of all ages.[28] The lower income after age 65 is

---

[25] D. S. Brady, "Individual Incomes and the Structure of Consumer Units," *American Economic Review,* Vol. 48, p. 269 (May, 1958).

[26] Bureau of the Census, *Current Population Reports, Consumer Income,* Series P-60, No. 12, June, 1953.

[27] Unpublished data supplied by the Bureau of the Census from the April, 1952 Current Population Survey on the income of families in 1951.

[28] The Federal Reserve Board reports, from the Survey of Consumer Finances, that spending units whose head is 65 years or older had, among them, 25 per cent with a money income of less than $1,000 before taxes in 1957 and 17 per cent with $4,000 or more. The respective comparable proportions in 1951 were 36 per cent and 13 per cent. A spending unit includes "all persons living in the same dwelling unit and related by blood, marriage

due to a number of factors, the principal one being full or partial withdrawal from the labor force in old age. However, it is important to note that in the later years of life, family needs are less, particularly because dependent children have left the home and the size of families is smaller. Moreover, the aged are permitted income tax deductions in addition to those allowed younger people.

Among families headed by the aged, the median income in 1957 in urban centers, where the majority live, was $3,000. This fell to $2,217 in rural nonfarm places, and to $1,606 in rural farm areas, where less than one sixth of the aged have their homes. Income in kind may be a significant item for the support of the family in rural farm areas, and to some extent in rural nonfarm places. For the aged not living with any relative, the median incomes are quite low; their principal sources of funds are, very likely, Old-Age and Survivors Insurance benefits and/or Old-Age Assistance.

*Annual Income—Aged Beneficiaries of Old-Age and Survivors Insurance.* With a large fraction of the aged in receipt of benefits under the Old-Age and Survivors Insurance program of the Social Security system, the results of a 1957 survey provide an insight into the current resources of most retired people and their dependents. The findings therefore exclude data relating to the aged in receipt of public assistance only, those with annual earnings of more than $1,200 in covered employment, and all other aged not in receipt of OASI benefits. During September through November, 1957, a sample of the old-age beneficiaries was questioned with regard to their income within the year prior to interview. The results, summarized in Table 2.8, are subject to the usual qualification regarding understatement for income data gathered by field surveys.[29] The married couples in receipt of

or adoption, who pool their incomes to meet major expenses; also persons living alone."

[29] For a critique of this survey, see K. T. Schlotterbeck, U.S. House, Committee on Ways and Means, *Hospital, Nursing Home, and Surgical Benefits for OASI Beneficiaries* (Hearings . . . 86th Cong., 1st sess., July, 1959), p. 132.

TABLE 2.8

AMOUNT AND SOURCES OF INCOME OF AGED BENEFICIARIES OF OLD-AGE AND
SURVIVORS INSURANCE WITHIN SURVEY YEAR PRIOR TO DATE OF INTERVIEW
DURING SEPTEMBER–NOVEMBER, 1957

| Source of Income | Married Couples | Single Retired Workers | | Aged Widows |
| | | Males | Females | |
| --- | --- | --- | --- | --- |
| Total money income[a]......... | 100.0% | 100.0% | 100.0% | 100.0% |
| Under $1,500.............. | 24.2 | 66.6 | 68.3 | 79.1 |
| $1,500–$2,999.............. | 45.1 | 25.5 | 26.1 | 16.3 |
| $3,000 and over........... | 30.7 | 8.0 | 5.6 | 4.4 |
| Median.................. | $2,249 | $1,170 | $1,106 | $882 |
| Per cent with other money income than OASI benefits[a]... | 91.1% | 78.6% | 85.8% | 75.4% |
| Income of those with other money income........... | 100.0% | 100.0% | 100.0% | 100.0% |
| Under $600.............. | 24.8 | 47.6 | 48.5 | 54.6 |
| $600–$1,499.............. | 34.4 | 36.8 | 37.2 | 32.9 |
| $1,500 and over........... | 40.6 | 15.7 | 14.1 | 12.5 |
| Median.................. | $1,237 | $652 | $629 | $525 |
| Per cent with independent money retirement income other than OASI benefits[b]... | 68.5% | 52.3% | 59.2% | 56.8% |
| Income of those with independent retirement income..... | 100.0% | 100.0% | 100.0% | 100.0% |
| Under $150.............. | 26.5 | 31.6 | 45.4 | 40.6 |
| $150–$899.............. | 35.1 | 36.2 | 36.8 | 36.6 |
| $900 and over.............. | 38.3 | 32.3 | 17.9 | 22.8 |
| Median.................. | $595 | $463 | $223 | $303 |
| Per cent with asset income[c].... | 58.9% | 37.9% | 52.7% | 52.1% |
| Income of those with asset income.................. | 100.0% | 100.0% | 100.0% | 100.0% |
| Under $75................. | 35.6 | 45.5 | 43.0 | 39.0 |
| $75–$299................. | 25.3 | 27.6 | 27.9 | 22.0 |
| $300 and over.............. | 39.1 | 26.9 | 29.2 | 38.8 |
| Median.................. | $180 | $96 | $106 | $149 |
| Per cent with income from earnings[d]...................... | 39.1% | 29.0% | 36.8% | 14.6% |
| Income of those with earnings.. | 100.0% | 100.0% | 100.0% | * |
| Under $600.............. | 32.0 | 50.7 | 50.3 | * |
| $600–$1,499.............. | 37.2 | 26.4 | 36.8 | * |
| $1,500 and over........... | 30.6 | 23.0 | 12.6 | * |
| Median.................. | $989 | $588 | $596 | * |

TABLE 2.8—*Continued*

| Source of Income | Married Couples | Single Retired Workers | | Aged Widows |
| --- | --- | --- | --- | --- |
| | | Males | Females | |
| Per cent with income from employer and union pensions[e].. | 25.3% | 18.8% | 11.2% | 2.4% |
| Income of those with employer and union pensions....... | 100.0% | 100.0% | * | * |
| Under $600............... | 33.9 | 41.9 | * | * |
| $600–$1,499.............. | 44.1 | 49.0 | * | * |
| $1,500 and over........... | 22.0 | 8.9 | * | * |
| Median................... | $835 | $696 | * | * |
| Per cent with income from veterans' compensation and pensions[f]..................... | 6.0% | 7.3% | 3.8% | 5.9% |
| Median income from veterans' compensation and pensions.. | $1,074 | * | * | * |
| Per cent with income from public assistance[g].............. | 7.3% | 14.2% | 13.2% | 11.8% |
| Income of those with public assistance................ | 100.0% | 100.0% | 100.0% | * |
| Under $300............... | 14.9 | 33.3 | 20.2 | * |
| $300–$599................ | 28.1 | 39.3 | 33.7 | * |
| $600 and over............. | 56.9 | 27.4 | 46.2 | * |
| Median................... | $670 | $427 | $566 | * |
| Per cent with contributions from persons outside the household[h].................... | 4.8% | 4.6% | 12.2% | 11.4% |

\* Fewer than 100 persons in sample.

[a] Represents cash receipts from all sources except sale of property, tax refunds, large cash gifts, lump-sum inheritances and insurance payments, and cash contributions by relatives within the household. Includes, if known, the value of bills, except medical, paid by relatives outside the household.

[b] Represents money income from employer, union, and veterans' pensions; rents, interest, dividends, and annuities; and income from trust funds and other reasonably permanent sources.

[c] Represents interest, dividends, and rental income.

[d] Represents wages and salaries, net income from farm and nonfarm self-employment, and income from boarders or lodgers.

[e] Represents money income received as retirement pay from public or private employee-benefit plans, railroad retirement benefits, and union pensions financed entirely by members.

[f] Represents money income received from the Veterans Administration.

[g] Represents money income from old-age assistance, aid to the blind, aid to the permanently and totally disabled, and general assistance.

[h] Represents cash contributions by persons outside the household and, if known, the value of bills, except medical, paid by persons outside the household.

Source: "Income of Old-Age and Survivors Insurance Beneficiaries: Highlights from Preliminary Data, 1957 Survey," *Social Security Bulletin*, August, 1958, p. 17.

benefit reported a median total annual income of $2,249 from all sources, while the single retired workers had only half that amount; aged widows had a median income of $882.

Over 90 per cent of the aged couples had some money income from sources other than their Old-Age and Survivors Insurance benefits; for the single retired and the aged widows, the proportion was over 75 per cent. For those with other money income, the median amount received from such sources by couples was $1,237, just about double that of single retired workers. Over two thirds of the couples and over one half of the single retired and the aged widows had some current retirement money income from their own independent sources other than OASI benefits, the median amounts so received being practically $600 for couples, about $460 for retired males, $220 for retired females, and $300 for aged widows. About half of the aged beneficiaries had income from assets in the form of interest, dividends, and rents, but the median amounts involved were rather small. Although drawing OASI benefits, about one third of these aged had some income from earnings; however, only one seventh of the aged widows had additional income from this source.

One fourth of the aged couples had an income from employer or union pensions, with a median of $835. Income from these sources went to nearly one fifth of the retired single males. For some of the aged OASI beneficiaries, the amounts received had to be supplemented by public assistance. Such supplements were given to 7 per cent of the couples, 14 per cent of retired single males, 13 per cent of retired single females, and 12 per cent of the aged widows. Barely 5 per cent of the aged couples and retired single male beneficiaries received contributions from outside their household, but among retired single female and aged widow beneficiaries about 12 per cent had such aid.

*Assets—General Population.* Current income is not the sole resource of the aged for their costs of medical care. In fact, at the higher ages, when income is reduced, an important resource is the savings that have accumulated over a working lifetime.[30] Considering only financial assets, as defined in the Survey of Consumer Finances for the Federal Reserve Board, Table 2.9 shows that 31 per cent of the spending units headed by aged persons had no such holdings in early 1957.[31] However, this does not portray adequately the asset position of the aged since many are living in spending units of which they are not the head. Among all spending units, 24 per cent were without financial assets. Furthermore, this picture of the resources of the aged is far from complete because it excludes, among others, such commonly held assets as homes, farms, and equities in life insurance policies. Notwithstanding these shortcomings, Table 2.9 is informative by showing that 35 per cent of the spending units headed by aged persons had financial assets of $2,000 or more, compared with 24 per cent for all spending units.

The first resource used for medical expenditures is undoubtedly current income and whatever insurance benefits may be available. Then, as further funds are needed, recourse may be made to liquid assets, loans and other assistance, and finally to nonliquid assets. The Survey of Consumer Finances showed that, according to their definition of liquid assets, 73 per cent of the spending units headed by aged persons had access to some ready funds early in 1958, and 40 per cent had ready access to $2,000 or more. The liquid financial position of these spending units headed by the aged is improving rapidly, for only four years earlier, in 1954, the respective proportions were 68 per cent and 31 per cent. A ready resource for the costs of medical care, not included among financial assets by the Survey of Consumer Finances, is the loan provision in life insurance. According to a sample survey conducted in 1957, life insurance was owned by 56

---

[30] A. Kemp, L. W. Martin, and C. Harkness, "Some Observations on Financial Assets of the Aged and Forand-Type Legislation," *Journal of the American Medical Association,* Vol. 171, p. 1228 (October 31, 1959).

[31] The financial assets are defined in the footnote to Table 2.9. See the footnote on page 21 for the definition of a spending unit.

TABLE 2.9

DISTRIBUTION, ACCORDING TO AMOUNT OF FINANCIAL ASSETS, OF ALL
SPENDING UNITS AND OF THOSE HEADED BY PERSONS AGED 65 AND OVER,
UNITED STATES, EARLY IN VARIOUS YEARS

| Amount of Assets | All Financial Assets* | | Liquid Assets† | | | |
|---|---|---|---|---|---|---|
| | All Spending Units | Spending Units Headed by Aged | All Spending Units | | Spending Units Headed by Aged | |
| | 1957 | 1957 | 1954 | 1958 | 1954 | 1958 |
| Total, per cent.......... | 100 | 100 | 100 | 100 | 100 | 100 |
| No assets............. | 24 | 31 | 26 | 26 | 32 | 27 |
| $1–$500.............. | 30 | 14 | 28 | 31 | 18 | 17 |
| $500–$2,000.......... | 21 | 18 | 24 | 22 | 19 | 17 |
| $2,000–$5,000........ | 12 | 17 | 13 | 12 | 18 | 20 |
| Over $5,000.......... | 12 | 18 | 9 | 9 | 13 | 20 |
| Not ascertained....... | 1 | 2 | — | — | — | — |

* All financial assets include stocks, marketable U.S. government bonds, and corporate, state, and local government bonds, plus liquid assets. This definition excludes such other assets as direct investments in businesses, farms, real estate, stocks in privately owned corporations, currency, and equities in life insurance policies and retirement funds.

† Liquid assets include U.S. government savings bonds, checking and savings accounts, and shares in savings and loan associations and in credit unions.

Source: Survey of Consumer Finances, Federal Reserve Board.

per cent of the spending units at ages 65 and over.[32] Such life insurance protection can be a very significant factor in meeting the costs of terminal illness.

Spending units headed by the aged are relatively free of short or intermediate term debt, according to the Survey of Consumer Finances, as shown in Table 2.10. Thus, early in 1958, 73 per cent of these spending units had no such debt, compared with 41 per cent for all spending units. Also, the aged spending units were much less heavily in debt in this way, only 6 per cent owing $500 or more, compared with 28 per cent for all units.

[32] J. L. Miner, *Life Insurance Ownership Among American Families, 1957,* Survey Research Center, Institute for Social Research, University of Michigan, Ann Arbor; *The Life Insurance Public,* Institute of Life Insurance, New York, February, 1957.

TABLE 2.10

DISTRIBUTION, ACCORDING TO SHORT AND INTERMEDIATE TERM CON-
SUMER DEBT,* OF ALL SPENDING UNITS AND OF THOSE HEADED BY
PERSONS AGED 65 AND OVER, UNITED STATES IN EARLY 1951 AND 1958

| Amount of Debt | All Spending Units | | Spending Units Headed by Aged | |
|---|---|---|---|---|
| | 1951 | 1958 | 1951 | 1958 |
| Total, per cent............100 | 100 | 100 | 100 |
| No debt.................. 51 | 41 | 80 | 73 |
| $1–$200................. 25 | 17 | 13 | 17 |
| $200–$500............... 11 | 13 | 3 | 4 |
| $500–$1,000............. 7 | 13 | 2 | 5 |
| Over $1,000.............. 5 | 15 | 1 | 1 |
| Not ascertained........... 1 | — | 1 | — |

* Excluding charge accounts and mortgage and business debt.
Source: Survey of Consumer Finances, Federal Reserve Board.

An insight into the relation between asset holdings and
current income among the aged is provided by a sample survey of the population relating to 1951. The pertinent data
are summarized in Table 2.11. In this survey, income and
assets are defined differently from the Survey of Consumer
Finances.[33] It is particularly interesting to find that, among
all those reporting no receipts in 1951 or receipts under $500,
the proportions with assets of $3,000 or more were appreci-
able. For example, the proportion was over one third for
unmarried aged persons without receipts; where the receipts
were under $500, the proportion was about one fourth. At
the other extreme, well over one third of the unmarried aged
without receipts were also without assets. Over one half of
the unmarried aged males with receipts of less than $500 had
no assets; for unmarried aged females, the proportion was
almost one third, and for aged couples, over one fourth.
With the generally high level of employment and income
prevailing since 1951, a more recent picture would very
likely show smaller proportions of aged without assets and
larger proportions with assets of $3,000 or more.

---

[33] The definitions used in the 1951 survey are set forth in the footnote
to Table 2.11.

TABLE 2.11

LIVING ARRANGEMENT AND NET VALUE OF TOTAL ASSETS OF PERSONS AGED
65 AND OVER ACCORDING TO TOTAL RECEIPTS, UNITED STATES, 1951

| Total Receipts* | Per Cent Distribution of Couples or Individuals According to Total Receipts | Per Cent Living with Relatives | Per Cent Distribution According to Net Value of Total Assets* | | | | |
|---|---|---|---|---|---|---|---|
| | | | None | Less than $500 | $500 to $999 | $1,000 to $2,999 | $3,000 or more |
| | | | Couples† | | | | |
| Total.............. | 100.0 | 31.1 | 13.3 | 5.7 | 3.6 | 7.5 | 69.9 |
| None............ | 4.8 | § | § | § | § | § | § |
| Under $500...... | 10.1 | 46.1 | 27.7 | 18.1 | 6.0 | 6.0 | 42.2 |
| $500–$999....... | 19.3 | 29.7 | 20.1 | 11.7 | 5.8 | 5.8 | 56.6 |
| $1,000–$1,499.... | 16.1 | 27.6 | 20.4 | 5.0 | 4.5 | 6.3 | 63.8 |
| $1,500–$2,499.... | 20.8 | 31.4 | 8.1 | 1.4 | 3.3 | 9.5 | 77.6 |
| $2,500–$4,999.... | 21.0‖ | 26.8 | 3.3 | 1.4 | .9 | 12.2 | 82.2 |
| | | | Males Not Married‡ | | | | |
| Total.............. | 100.0 | 49.8 | 34.2 | 6.1 | 9.9 | 9.1 | 40.8 |
| None............ | 13.7 | 74.6 | 37.5 | 1.6 | 9.6 | 12.8 | 38.4 |
| Under $500...... | 23.0 | 50.9 | 51.8 | 12.5 | 4.5 | 8.0 | 23.2 |
| $500–$999....... | 28.7 | 40.0 | 42.3 | 4.6 | 15.9 | 7.6 | 29.6 |
| $1,000–$1,499.... | 13.1‖ | 53.1 | 22.2 | 7.9 | 11.1 | 7.9 | 50.8 |
| | | | Females Not Married‡ | | | | |
| Total.............. | 100.0 | 61.5 | 27.2 | 15.4 | 9.3 | 8.2 | 39.8 |
| None............ | 25.6 | 83.7 | 35.4 | 12.5 | 11.7 | 6.4 | 34.0 |
| Under $500...... | 30.4 | 66.4 | 32.4 | 21.0 | 9.2 | 8.6 | 28.9 |
| $500–$999....... | 27.1 | 45.5 | 26.3 | 15.8 | 9.9 | 8.3 | 39.8 |
| $1,000–$1,499.... | 6.3‖ | 40.0 | 13.2 | 14.8 | 4.9 | 4.9 | 62.2 |

* Total receipts is the sum of total income, occasional cash gifts, lump-sum receipts, such as insurance payments or inheritance, and use of savings or assets to meet living expenses. Assets include money in the bank or cash savings, the face amount of life insurance, stocks and bonds, and a home or other property in which $3,000 or more is invested.

† Married couples include those in which the male member is 65 and over, irrespective of the age of the wife; this excludes couples with wives 65 and over but with husbands below that age.

‡ Those not married include the single, widowed, divorced, and persons separated from their spouse.

§ Percentages not computed because sample includes less than 50 cases.

‖ Couples over $5,000 = 7.9%; males not married over $1,500 = 21.5%; females not married over $1,500 = 10.6%.

Source: Tables 302 and 304 of P. O. Steiner and R. Dorfman, *The Economic Status of the Aged* (Berkeley and Los Angeles: University of California Press, 1957).

For the aged with little or no money receipts and without assets, a medical episode of even small order is catastrophic unless assistance is available from relatives, friends, or some private or public agency. However, the tendency is for those with low receipts to live with relatives. In 1951, this was found to be the case for 84 per cent of the unmarried women and 75 per cent of the unmarried men without receipts; where the receipts were under $500, the respective figures were 66 per cent and 51 per cent.[34] It is possible that many of those not living with relatives had none.

After reviewing the economic position of the aged in 1951, Steiner and Dorfman conclude that:

Although the total amount of assets held by the aged seem large relative to *annual* medical payments, the large group without assets, the probable recurrence of medical expenses, and the use of assets for many purposes, including current living expenses, caution against too optimistic an evaluation of the adequacy of assets to meet medical expenses.[35]

This conclusion with regard to the aged may be applicable to many who live alone and are without relatives, but it does not take full account of the resources available for medical care from relatives not in the household.

The significance of noncash help to the aged from others was evidenced in the survey of the National Opinion Research Center made in the spring of 1957.[36] Reporting on the situation among the aged during 1956, they found that 24 per cent of the men and 39 per cent of the women had some noncash assistance. This aid was for medical or dental care only among 6 per cent of the men and 5 per cent of the women; another 3 per cent of the men and 8 per cent of the women received aid for medical or dental care in conjunction with aid for food and/or clothing.

The NORC survey made special inquiries into the resources available to the aged in case they had a large medical

---

[34] P. O. Steiner and R. Dorfman, *op. cit.*, Table 302, p. 283.

[35] P. O. Steiner and R. Dorfman, *op. cit.*, p. 145.

[36] E. Shanas, *op. cit.*, p. 9.

expense, using $500 as an example.[37] According to this survey, 79 per cent of the aged had access to one or more types of assets to meet medical expenses of that size beyond those covered by hospital or health insurance (Table 2.12). Although this does not necessarily imply that both of an aged couple would have access to the same resource in the

TABLE 2.12

Assets and Sources of Funds Available to Pay a $500 Medical Bill by Persons Aged 65 and Over, United States, Spring of 1957

| Type of Asset; Source of Funds | Per Cent Reporting Such Asset or Source of Funds | | |
|---|---|---|---|
| | Both Sexes | Males | Females |
| Type of asset* | | | |
| With assets of one or more types | 79 | 81 | 78 |
|   Own home or real estate | 55 | 58 | 53 |
|   Life insurance | 35 | 39 | 32 |
|   Savings | 54 | 58 | 51 |
|   Stocks and bonds | 19 | 21 | 18 |
|   Help of children or relatives | 3 | 2 | 4 |
| With assets of only one type | | | |
|   Own home or real estate | 12 | 12 | 12 |
|   Life insurance | 4 | 3 | 5 |
|   Savings | 9 | 9 | 9 |
|   Stocks and bonds | — | — | — |
|   Help of children or relatives | 1 | — | 2 |
| Without assets | 21 | 20 | 22 |
| Source of funds† | | | |
|   Savings | 40.2 | 44.4 | 36.6 |
|   Current income | 17.0 | 19.1 | 15.2 |
|   Life insurance | 1.0 | 1.0 | 1.1 |
|   Mortgage on house or property | 7.2 | 8.4 | 6.1 |
|   Hospital or health insurance | 7.6 | 8.7 | 6.6 |
|   Children or relatives | 14.6 | 9.2 | 19.3 |
|   Public assistance or charitable aid | 8.2 | 8.2 | 8.3 |
|   Other | 0.7 | 0.6 | 0.8 |
|   Could not pay such a bill | 9.6 | 7.2 | 11.6 |

\* This refers to assets that would be used for large medical expenses beyond those covered by hospital or health insurance.

† More than one source might be reported by a person.

Source: E. Shanas, *Financial Resources of the Aging*, Research Series 10 (New York: Health Information Foundation, 1959).

---

[37] E. Shanas, *op. cit.*, p. 9.

unusual case where they would need it at the same time, it is reasonable to infer that it would be available to either at any one time. In the total, 55 per cent had their own home or real estate as available assets and almost a like proportion (54 per cent) could count on savings, 35 per cent owned life insurance, 19 per cent had stocks and bonds, and 3 per cent could rely on help from children or relatives. However, the home or real estate represented the sole asset that could be used for a $500 medical expense outgo by 12 per cent of the aged. Savings were the only asset for 9 per cent of the aged, life insurance for 4 per cent, and 1 per cent could count only on children or relatives. Among the aged, 21 per cent had no assets they could use to pay medical expenses amounting to $500 for an episode of illness or injury.

Somewhat different from the resources *available* for a large medical care bill are the sources of funds that *would* be used. Savings represent the most common source of funds the aged would use to pay a medical bill of $500, this being cited by 40 per cent of the respondents in the NORC survey (Table 2.12). Current income would be used as a source by 17 per cent of the aged, almost 8 per cent would count on hospital or health insurance, 7 per cent would mortgage a home or property, and 1 per cent would use their life insurance equity. Nearly 15 per cent of the aged would go to their children or relatives for funds to pay a $500 medical bill, 8 per cent would ask for public assistance or charitable aid, and almost 10 per cent stated that they would have no way of paying a bill of that size.

If a picture of the resources available to the aged for a large medical bill were on hand for 1937, or for 1947, it would undoubtedly differ greatly from that drawn by the NORC survey in the spring of 1957. It may easily be conjectured that the more recent situation would show a greater availability of assets, more savings, and a sharp rise in hospital and health insurance; on the other hand it would show a smaller reliance on children or relatives, or on public assistance or charitable aid. Very likely, a survey for 1967 would show, compared with 1957, much greater reliance by the aged on their own resources for a large medical bill and appreciably less on children, relatives, and public or charitable assistance.

*Assets—Aged Beneficiaries of Old-Age and Survivors Insurance.* A more penetrating picture of the asset position of the retired aged is provided by the 1957 survey of the aged beneficiaries of the Old-Age and Survivors Insurance program, already referred to. The findings in this regard are summarized in Table 2.13. Generally, the asset holdings of the retired—in terms of net worth, liquid assets, and home ownership—are greatest for married couples, smaller for aged

TABLE 2.13

ASSETS AND NET WORTH OF AGED BENEFICIARIES OF OLD-AGE AND SURVIVORS INSURANCE ON DATE OF INTERVIEW DURING SEPTEMBER–NOVEMBER, 1957

| Asset Item | Married Couples | Single Retired Workers | | Aged Widows |
| --- | --- | --- | --- | --- |
| | | Males | Females | |
| Net worth* | 100.0% | 100.0% | 100.0% | 100.0% |
| Negative | 3.5 | 4.7 | 4.6 | 3.8 |
| Zero | 8.3 | 32.5 | 24.5 | 23.4 |
| Positive | 88.2 | 62.7 | 71.0 | 72.8 |
| Under $3,000 | 15.0 | 24.1 | 24.9 | 17.4 |
| $3,000–$4,999 | 8.8 | 8.2 | 8.4 | 6.6 |
| $5,000–$9,999 | 18.6 | 12.3 | 15.3 | 16.5 |
| $10,000 and over | 45.1 | 18.0 | 21.2 | 32.0 |
| Not ascertained | .5 | .1 | 1.1 | .5 |
| Median | $8,786 | $803 | $2,077 | $4,385 |
| Liquid assets† | 100.0% | 100.0% | 100.0% | 100.0% |
| None | 27.6 | 48.9 | 38.7 | 39.7 |
| Some | 72.4 | 51.1 | 61.3 | 60.3 |
| Under $500 | 11.6 | 11.7 | 14.6 | 11.0 |
| $500–$2,999 | 25.5 | 17.3 | 22.5 | 21.5 |
| $3,000–$4,999 | 8.4 | 8.2 | 9.1 | 8.5 |
| $5,000 and over | 25.7 | 13.6 | 14.1 | 18.9 |
| Not ascertained | 1.0 | .5 | 1.1 | .5 |
| Median | $1,271 | $37 | $371 | $457 |
| Per cent owning homes | | | | |
| Farm and nonfarm | 70 | 32 | 33 | 46 |
| Nonfarm only | 65.2 | 30.7 | 32.7 | 44.8 |

TABLE 2.13—*Continued*

| Asset Item | Married Couples | Single Retired Workers | | Aged Widows |
| --- | --- | --- | --- | --- |
| | | Males | Females | |
| Amount of equity in nonfarm home owned‡ | | | | |
| All owners...................... | 100.0% | 100.0% | 100.0% | 100.0% |
| Under $3,000................. | 10.8 | 27.3 | 17.8 | 8.5 |
| $3,000–$4,999............... | 14.3 | 19.8 | 19.4 | 14.5 |
| $5,000–$9,999............... | 40.3 | 32.4 | 37.6 | 43.6 |
| $10,000 and over............ | 34.7 | 20.6 | 24.5 | 33.4 |
| Not ascertained............. | — | — | .8 | — |
| Median.....................$8,100 | | $5,458 | $6,650 | $8,090 |
| Per cent owning life insurance..... | 70.7 | 47.6 | 52.2 | 49.8 |
| Face value of life insurance | | | | |
| All owners...................... | 100.0% | 100.0% | 100.0% | 100.0% |
| Under $1,000................. | 21.1 | 41.8 | 66.8 | 70.9 |
| $1,000–$1,999............... | 33.9 | 31.6 | 27.7 | 24.0 |
| $2,000–$2,999............... | 18.8 | 11.0 | 4.1 | 3.5 |
| $3,000 and over............. | 25.8 | 15.3 | 1.3 | 1.6 |
| Not ascertained............. | .3 | .3 | — | — |
| Median.....................$1,848 | | $1,254 | $792 | $744 |
| Per cent with borrowings on life insurance................. | 2.3 | 1.8 | .7 | 1.3 |

* Represents the difference between the value of selected assets and total reported debt. Assets represent money at home (except amounts held for current operation expenses), bank deposits, all types of stocks and bonds, loans to others, equity in an owner-occupied home and other real estate, full or part interest in a nonfarm unincorporated business or privately held corporation, and the market value of a professional practice, patents, and copyrights. Liabilities represent balances owed on installment purchases; bills past due on open accounts and for rent, taxes, interest on mortgages, and medical care; and borrowings on securities and unsecured borrowings.

† Represents money at home (except amounts held for current operation expenses), checking accounts, savings accounts in banks, postal savings, shares in savings and loan associations and credit unions, all types of stocks and bonds, mortgages on real estate, and loans to others.

‡ Owner's estimate of current value of home, less any mortgage or other debt on home.

Source: "Assets and Net Worth of Old-Age and Survivors Insurance Beneficiaries: Highlights from Preliminary Data, 1957 Survey," *Social Security Bulletin*, January, 1959, p. 3.

widows, still smaller for single females retired from work, and least for single males retired from work. It should be noted that the definitions of assets in this survey differ from those of the 1951 survey of the general population and of the Survey of Consumer Finances.[38]

[38] The definition of assets in this survey is set forth in the footnote to Table 2.13.

Only about 4 per cent of the aged beneficiaries had liabilities in excess of their assets. However, the proportion reporting no assets varied from somewhat over 8 per cent for married couples to about 24 per cent for aged widows and single females retired from work, and to nearly 33 per cent for retired single males. Among those with assets, the net worth was about $8,800 or more for half of the married couples, $4,400 for aged widows, $2,100 for retired single females, but only $800 for retired single males (median amounts).

Liquid assets were held by almost three fourths of the married couples, three fifths of the aged widows and retired single females, and over one half of the retired single males. For one half of the married couples with liquid assets, the amount available was over $1,300 or more (median amount). The median liquid assets were substantially smaller for other aged beneficiaries: about $460 for aged widows, over $370 for retired single females, but only $37 for retired single males. Thus, there are sizable proportions among the current aged beneficiaries with some liquid asset, but among those with such assets the amounts are rather small.

Over two thirds of the married couples among the aged beneficiaries and about one half of the unmarried owned some life insurance. Only about 1 or 2 per cent had borrowed on it. However, the amounts of insurance held were generally small. Home ownership was relatively common among the married couples, about two thirds being so situated. On the other hand, homes were owned by less than half of the widows and under one third of the retired single workers.

***Income and Saving.***    Since the concern is with trends as well as the recent situation, it is worth examining the course of disposable personal income and personal saving in the United States. This may provide a clue regarding the capacity for those now at the productive ages to save for their costs of medical care in old age. For this purpose, reference will be made to estimates of personal saving originated in the

Department of Commerce.[39] The definition of saving from this source differs from those used in the surveys previously cited. In fact, the question of what constitutes savings is answered so differently by various compilers that a wide range of estimates has been produced. The data from the Department of Commerce in Table 2.14, which extend from 1929

TABLE 2.14

DISPOSABLE INCOME* AND PERSONAL SAVINGS† OF THE PEOPLE OF THE UNITED STATES, 1929–58

| Year | Billions of Dollars | | Per Capita Personal Saving, Dollars | Year | Billions of Dollars | | Per Capita Personal Saving, Dollars |
| | Disposable income | Personal saving | | | Disposable income | Personal saving | |
|---|---|---|---|---|---|---|---|
| 1929 | 83.1 | 4.2 | 34 | 1944 | 146.8 | 36.9 | 267 |
| 1930 | 74.4 | 3.4 | 28 | 1945 | 150.4 | 28.7 | 205 |
| 1931 | 63.8 | 2.5 | 20 | 1946 | 160.6 | 13.5 | 95 |
| 1932 | 48.7 | −.6 | −5 | 1947 | 170.1 | 4.7 | 33 |
| 1933 | 45.7 | −.6 | −5 | 1948 | 189.3 | 11.0 | 75 |
| 1934 | 52.0 | .1 | 1 | 1949 | 189.7 | 8.5 | 57 |
| 1935 | 58.3 | 2.0 | 16 | 1950 | 207.7 | 12.6 | 83 |
| 1936 | 66.2 | 3.6 | 28 | 1951 | 227.5 | 17.7 | 115 |
| 1937 | 71.0 | 3.7 | 29 | 1952 | 238.7 | 18.9 | 120 |
| 1938 | 65.7 | 1.1 | 8 | 1953 | 252.5 | 19.8 | 124 |
| 1939 | 70.4 | 2.9 | 22 | 1954 | 256.9 | 18.9 | 116 |
| 1940 | 76.1 | 4.2 | 32 | 1955 | 274.4 | 17.5 | 106 |
| 1941 | 93.0 | 11.1 | 83 | 1956 | 290.5 | 21.1 | 125 |
| 1942 | 117.5 | 27.8 | 206 | 1957 | 305.1 | 20.7 | 121 |
| 1943 | 133.5 | 33.0 | 241 | 1958 | 311.6 | 21.0 | 121 |

* Personal income net of so-called direct personal taxes.
† Estimated by residual method; that is, disposable income less expenditures on consumer goods and services.

Source: Disposable income and personal saving from U.S. Department of Commerce; per capita personal saving computed by author.

to 1958, have not been adjusted to allow for changes in the purchasing power of the dollar. Since the depth of the depression in the early 1930's, there has been a rather steady upward trend in disposable income.[40] The rise has been partic-

---

[39] The saving figures are residual after expenditure on consumer goods and services and after so-called direct personal taxes have been deducted from personal income. As a residual estimate the saving figures are only indicative, rather than precise.

[40] This relates to consumer income less so-called direct personal taxes.

ularly rapid since 1950, from $207.7 billion that year to $311.6 billion in 1958.

Except for the war years, personal savings since 1951 have been substantially larger than ever before, averaging not far from 20 billion or about 7 per cent of disposable income. In order to take account of the increasing size of population, Table 2.14 also shows the per capita personal saving for each year since 1929. Most of the present aged (1959) were in their prime productive period during the decade from 1930 to 1939; in each of these years the per capita personal saving was less than $30. On the other hand, for each year but one since 1951, per capita saving ranged between $110 and $125. Evidently, people now in their productive years have a greater capacity to save for their costs of medical care in old age than those in the 1930's. Specific influences pointing to an improving financial status of our aged are the growth of pension funds, the expansion of life insurance, and also the extension of the Social Security program.[41] The recent trend toward home ownership is also a factor in the same direction. The intrinsic urge to save for old age, which manifests itself in many ways, is generally for means to take care of the usual expenses of daily life. Also to be considered in this connection are the medical exigencies in old age which may involve unusually high costs. This consideration is particularly important with regard to the remaining years of the surviving spouse, since many will then be living alone or without relatives in the household.

*The Family Cycle.* Compared with their elders, the generation presently in its most productive years has not only the benefit of much larger savings each year, but also the advantage of a longer period during which savings are possible. For most families, the potentials for saving are

---

[41] M. Civic, *Income and Resources of Older People* (New York: National Industrial Conference Board, 1956), p. 28. For a discussion of the effect of the extension of the Social Security system, see *Hospitalization Insurance for OASDI Beneficiaries,* Report submitted to the Committee on Ways and Means by the Secretary of Health, Education, and Welfare, Washington, D.C., April 3, 1959, p. 11.

greatest after the responsibility to children ceases. A measure of the trend in this regard is the median age of the husband at the marriage of the last child; this decreased from 52.8 years in 1940 to 50.3 years in 1950.[42] In other words, that part of the working lifetime during which the capacity for saving is at its height has increased by 2.5 years. During this terminal period in the labor force, earnings tend to remain high, although below the peak.[43]

## CONCLUSION

Facile conclusions are frequently drawn from readily available data, whereas further search would provide a more complete picture. Thus, the census sources that describe the decrease, with advance in age, in the proportion of aged living in families have nothing to say on the extended family, which includes relatives of the aged who live nearby and with whom they have frequent contact. Although the picture with regard to the extended family is far from complete, surveys show the persistence of strong ties between the generations after children have left the parental home and also with other relatives. These surveys have made evident, furthermore, that in case of illness or at other times of need, friends and neighbors are often ready with assistance. Without such aid from relatives, friends, and neighbors—even though it may entail some sacrifices on their part—the community would have thrown upon it a task of extraordinary magnitude.

In the same vein, the usual economic data relating to the aged are hardly sufficient for an adequate picture of the resources available to them in time of need. The role of both the immediate and the extended family is lost in accounts which describe the relatively low average current income of aged individuals. Closer examination shows that many aged

---

[42] P. C. Glick, *American Families* (New York: John Wiley & Sons, 1957), Table 33, p. 54.

[43] H. P. Miller, *op. cit.*, p. 64.

with small or no incomes may indeed have assets of their own and live in families headed by younger persons. Similarly, lessened family needs are seldom brought into evidence in conjunction with data portraying the lower average income of families headed by the aged.[44] Most such families no longer have the responsibility of dependent children, generally require little in the way of expenditure for household goods, and are in a period of dissaving rather than of saving.

Treating the current aged as an undifferentiated aggregate glosses over the marked variation in economic status between those just past the threshold of old age and those who survive into the 80's. At the more advanced ages today are individuals who spent most of their working lifetime during a period of relatively low earnings, including the severe depression of the 1930's. Their opportunities for savings were limited, inflation depreciated the intrinsic value of any fixed income they may have, relatively small proportions are beneficiaries of our Old-Age and Survivors Insurance program, and their benefits are quite low when compared with those at the less advanced ages.[45] Thus, the economic situation of those at the extreme ages currently clouds the picture of those aged 65 and over as a whole.

In contrast to the economic situation of the very old is that of individuals who have recently entered the ranks of the aged. Their later productive years were spent in a period of prosperity; there was opportunity to save; and the period of maximum saving was greater than it had been for their predecessors because the last child left home earlier in the family cycle. Also, much larger proportions of them than of persons at the extreme ages are beneficiaries of OASI and their benefits are greater. In addition, the rapid postwar

---

[44] Z. Campbell, "Spending Patterns of Older Persons," *Management Record,* Vol. 21, p. 85 (March, 1959); S. Goldstein, "Consumer Patterns of Aged Spending Units," *Journal of Gerontology,* Vol. 14, p. 328 (July, 1959); and R. D. Millican, "Two Factor Analyses of Expenditures of the Aged," *Journal of Gerontology,* Vol. 14, p. 465 (October, 1959).

[45] *Social Security Bulletin, Annual Statistical Supplement, 1957,* p. 33, Social Security Administration, Washington, D.C.

growth of private pension programs is bringing into the ranks of the aged increasing numbers of pension recipients.[46] There are, further, the many aged who continue full-time or part-time work well past their 65th birthday. Taking census data at their face value, the decade from 1947 to 1957 witnessed not only a drop in the proportion of aged males without income from 15 per cent to less than 5 per cent, but also a 50 per cent rise in the median income of those with income. On the whole, the economic situation of people aged 65 and over has improved greatly during the postwar period. An even more marked improvement is in sight for many years ahead as those currently at the extreme ages leave the scene and the increasing numbers benefiting from postwar prosperity enter old age.

The conclusions from this survey of the demographic, social, and economic characteristics of the aged may be aptly summarized by quoting from a report of the World Health Organization: ". . . although the aging of populations creates certain serious problems, there has been a tendency to magnify the dangers that are likely to arise."[47]

---

[46] A. M. Skolnik and J. Zisman, "Growth in Employee-Benefit Plans, 1954–1957," *Social Security Bulletin,* March, 1959, and W. M. Van Eenam, "Private Pension and Deferred Profit-Sharing Plans, 1957–1958," *Research and Statistics Note No. 25,* Division of Program Research, Social Security Administration, September 9, 1959.

[47] Sixth Report of the Expert Committee on Mental Health, *op. cit.,* p. 5.

# The Health Status and            3
# Health Attitudes
# of the Aged

THE DESIGN and distribution of health services in a community must necessarily conform to its health needs and also give consideration to its health attitudes. In both respects, the aged have many characteristics markedly different from the rest of the population; these are discussed in this chapter on the basis of recent data. An understanding of these data requires, of course, consideration of the circumstances under which they were gathered. The element of sampling variability enters into most data presented, since these are derived largely from surveys made on samples of population. Unless otherwise stated, these surveys usually exclude the institutional population of the area under consideration.

It is also important to recognize that data are descriptive only of the situation in which they were compiled. Applicability to another situation (that is, another community or the same community at another time, or in the presence of a changed mechanism for financing or providing medical care) requires careful study. The use of averages also calls for a note of caution, since an average can easily mask a wide range of individual variations.

## CHANCES OF SURVIVAL

During the century there has been a very marked increase in the chances of survival through the productive years and,

to a lesser extent, in the years after retirement. Table 3.1
shows that on the basis of mortality conditions in 1900–1902,
only one half of the white males at age 20 could expect to
reach age 65; with mortality conditions of 1957, the chances

TABLE 3.1

CHANCES OF SURVIVING THROUGH A WORKING LIFETIME TO AGE
65 AND TEN YEARS THEREAFTER; WHITE POPULATION BY SEX,
UNITED STATES, 1957 AND 1900–1902

| Age | White Males | | White Females | |
|---|---|---|---|---|
| | 1957 | 1900–1902 | 1957 | 1900–1902 |
| | Chances per 1,000 of Surviving from Specified Age to Age 65 | | | |
| 20.............. | 680 | 514 | 824 | 555 |
| 30.............. | 692 | 551 | 830 | 593 |
| 40.............. | 707 | 604 | 841 | 645 |
| 50.............. | 748 | 685 | 867 | 718 |
| | Chances per 1,000 of Surviving from Age 65 to Age 75 | | | |
| 65.............. | 589 | 545 | 728 | 579 |
| | Expectation of Life, Years | | | |
| 20.............. | 49.9 | 42.2 | 55.7 | 43.8 |
| 40.............. | 31.4 | 27.7 | 36.6 | 29.2 |
| 65.............. | 12.7 | 11.5 | 15.4 | 12.2 |
| 75.............. | 7.9 | 6.8 | 9.1 | 7.3 |

are more than two in three. For those men who reach age 65,
the chances of surviving ten years further went up from a
little more than 1 in 2 to 3 in 5. Also, at age 65, the expectation of life for white males in the United States rose from
11.5 years to 12.7 years, and at age 75 from 6.8 to 7.9 years.
For white females, the corresponding figures are not only
greater than for white males, but their improvements have
also been the more rapid. Such relatively small gains in expectation of life at the higher ages, as compared with the
younger ages, are readily explained. With a human life span

limited to about 110 years, the margin for improvement in expectation of life diminishes as that limit is approached.

The part that preventive measures for the control of disease have had in increasing the chances of survival is well known. Not so clearly recognized is the role of medical and surgical advances in increasing the average lifetime of the population. For example, these advances have prolonged the lives of untold numbers of diabetics, cancer patients, and persons with various heart conditions. There is every indication that the future will see further increases in the chances of survival. Preventive measures are still a major factor in health promotion, and medical and surgical knowledge will continue to advance, with benefit to impaired lives. However, the growing medical needs of the aged arise, in part, out of the medical advances that prolong impaired lives, as pointed out by Page with regard to one condition: "Enough patients with severe hypertensive disease are now being kept alive so that clinical manifestations of the associated vascular disease are looming larger and larger."[1]

It has been observed that at the younger ages mortality in the United States is lower than in most other countries of the Western world but that this advantage is lost with advance in age. This unique situation of the United States may be due not only to preventive health measures of special benefit to the younger ages, but also to advances in medical care which prolong the lifetime of those with physical impairments, such as diabetes. By carrying forward large numbers of impaired lives, the proportion of them at the older ages in the United States may be greater than in other countries, with a corresponding adverse effect upon its mortality record for that period of life.[2] Thus, conclusions from inter-

---

[1] I. H. Page, "A Clinical Evaluation of Antihypertensive Drugs," *Bulletin of the New York Academy of Medicine,* Vol. 33, p. 261 (April, 1957).

[2] M. Spiegelman, "An International Comparison of Mortality Rates At the Older Ages," *Proceedings of the World Population Conference, Rome, 1954,* Vol. 1, p. 289 (New York: United Nations Department of Economic and Social Affairs, 1955).

national comparisons of mortality and longevity in old age must be tempered by considering the stage to which the countries have developed their medical resources as well as the mode of life of their populations.

## HEALTH STATUS

A report of the World Health Organization states that, "Heredity, as well as economic circumstances and social environment, influence physiological and pathological changes in aging and are important factors in determining the health status of the aged."[3] The influence of heredity on health status has not yet been probed deeply, although some important starts have been made.[4] Investigations of the biology of aging are being intensified and have been reported in many sources.[5] However, morbidity data describing the health status of the aged are available in relatively few sources. For the most part, they represent the findings of surveys in selected communities. These results are fragmentary, seldom comparable from one area to another, and generally treat those at ages 65 and over as a single group, so that a detailed account of morbidity in old age is rarely available. The usual survey technique is to have trained lay enumerators, using specially designed questionnaire forms, secure information regarding health status and medical care utilization by interviews with a sample of individuals or households selected to represent the community. In the course of time, the United

---

[3] World Health Organization, Regional Office for Europe, *Advisory Group on the Public Health Aspects of the Aging of the Population, Oslo, 28 July–2 August, 1958,* Report dated 30 December, 1958, p. 7.

[4] A. Scheinfeld, *The New You and Heredity* (Philadelphia: J. B. Lippincott Co., 1950). For a general review, see V. A. McKusick *et al.,* "Medical Genetics—1958," *Journal of Chronic Diseases,* Vol. 10, p. 256 (October, 1959).

[5] N. W. Shock, *Trends in Gerontology* (2d. ed., Stanford University: Stanford University Press, 1957), chaps. ix and x; see also L. Szilard, "On the Nature of the Aging Process," *Proceedings of the National Academy of Sciences,* Vol. 45, p. 30 (January, 1959).

States National Health Survey program, which started interviewing in 1957, will accumulate a sizable body of detail on these matters for the general population of the country.[6]

*The Limitations of Sickness Surveys.* A fundamental consideration in interpreting the data from any sickness survey is the concept of morbidity that was used. Persons claiming an illness, whether or not accompanied by physical signs, are usually included among the sick. A survey may also include, according to specifications, persons with known defects, either congenital or acquired, and also those with diseases and impairments that do not interfere with daily activity, such as defects of vision, minor orthopedic defects, and quiescent chronic diseases. In some surveys, the statement regarding a morbid condition is checked by referring to the attending physician or to a hospital record. However, unless screening examinations and clinical examinations by a physician are also a feature of the survey, it will miss cases with latent or incipient disease of which the person affected is unaware, examples being diabetes and early tuberculosis.[7] The range of morbid conditions reflected in a sickness survey may therefore be very wide, covering on the one hand definitely recognized cases of serious illness, and on the other hand not only those cases of minor indisposition that do not

---

[6] The principal sources prior to 1957 are: A. W. Brewster and D. McCamman, *Health Costs of the Aged,* Division of Research and Statistics, Social Security Administration, Washington, D.C., May, 1956; S. D. Collins, *Long-Time Trends in Illness and Medical Care,* Public Health Monograph No. 48, Public Health Service, Washington, D.C., 1957; S. D. Collins, J. L. Lehmann, and K. S. Trantham, *Surgical Experience in Selected Areas of the United States,* Public Health Monograph No. 38, Public Health Service, Washington, D.C., 1956; idem, *Major Causes of Illness and of Death in Six Age Periods* and *Sickness Experience in Selected Areas of the United States,* Public Health Monograph Nos. 30 and 25, Public Health Service, Washington, D.C., 1955; G. St. J. Perrott *et al., Illness and Health Services in An Aging Population,* Public Health Service Publication No. 170, Washington, D.C., 1952.

[7] R. E. Trussell, J. Elinson, and M. L. Levin, "Comparison of Various Methods of Estimating the Prevalence of Chronic Disease in a Community—The Hunterdon County Study," *American Journal of Public Health,* Vol. 46, p. 173 (February, 1956).

interfere with usual activity, but also cases of persons unaware of their disease.[8]

Subjective elements are also present in the reporting of
sickness. An elderly worker may tend to minimize an illness,
particularly when jobs are scarce, in fear that its recognition
may cost him his job. Another elderly worker may imagine
an illness or magnify a minor case if it will bring him an early
retirement without substantial financial loss. Among the retired, there are undoubtedly some high-spirited individuals
who refuse to recognize an illness even though aware of
symptoms, and there are also those who claim illness for
the attention it brings. The study of morbidity among the
retired is further complicated by the fact that the economic
incentive to minimize a disability is not as great as at the
productive ages.

The quality of the sickness survey is affected if the respondent to the enumerator is answering for some one else
in the household, as may happen for the aged, for then the
information is secondhand or not known at all. An insight
into this matter was obtained from a survey conducted by the
National Opinion Research Center (NORC), with the support of the Health Information Foundation, in which a
sample of the aged population in the United States was interviewed for themselves.[9] For this survey, which relates to
illnesses during April and May, 1957, those interviewed were
asked to report any condition that "bothered" him or her
during a four-week period. The prevalence of illness in this
survey is compared, in Table 3.2, with that in two other surveys where the respondent could have been either the aged
person himself or some one else in the household reporting

---

[8] For a description of the concept of morbidity used in the U.S. National
Health Survey, see *Concepts and Definitions in the Health Household-Interview Survey,* Public Health Service, Washington, D.C., September, 1958,
p. 11.

[9] E. Shanas, "Self-Reports of Illness in a Study of Older People," presented before the Population Association of America, May 3, 1958.

for him. "Illness" was defined in substantially the same terms in the three surveys. The comparison shows that the illness prevalence rate at ages 65 and over in the NORC survey of 1957 was appreciably higher than that in the California Health Survey of 1954–55 and the New York City survey of 1952. This differential is attributed, in large measure, to

TABLE 3.2

ILLNESS PREVALENCE ACCORDING TO THREE SURVEYS AMONG PERSONS AT AGES 65 AND OVER, BY SEX

| Survey | Illness Period Preceding Interview, Weeks | Illnesses per 100 Persons | | |
|---|---|---|---|---|
| | | Both Sexes | Males | Females |
| United States, May–June, 1957* | 4 | 86.5 | 85.3 | 87.5 |
| California Health Survey, May 1954–April, 1955† | 4 | 70.5 | 66.9 | 73.6 |
| New York City, March–June, 1952‡ | 8 | 61.7 | 55.0 | 67.3 |

* From a survey conducted by the National Opinion Research Center sponsored by the Health Information Foundation and reported by E. Shanas.

† *Health in California*, Department of Public Health, State of California, Berkeley, 1957, Table 7, p. 86.

‡ *Health and Medical Care in New York City* (Cambridge: Harvard University Press, 1957), p. 74.

Source: Adapted from E. Shanas, "Self-Reports of Illness in a Study of Older People," presented before the Population Association of America, May 3, 1958.

the fact that the aged were reporting for themselves in the NORC survey, but not necessarily so in the others. In her account of this survey, Shanas states that, "Where other household members may neglect to report chronic conditions of long standing for aged family members, such family members themselves are eager to report such conditions."

The training of the survey enumerator also has a bearing on the results of a household survey of morbidity, since his understanding and recording of the facts may differ from those supplied him. When the physician has a part in the survey, much depends upon the intensity of his examination, his training, and his understanding of diagnostic standards, where such exist. It has been shown that diagnostic tests may be interpreted differently by experts.[10] The qualifications noted in this and the preceding paragraphs give special meaning to the statement of the Commission on Chronic Illness that, "A measure of the true prevalence of disease in the population would include all conditions detectable by the best available techniques appropriate to the purpose."[11]

The principal advantage of a health survey conducted by trained lay interviewers on a representative sample of a population, without recourse to medical or hospital records and also without any supplemental medical tests or examinations, is threefold.[12] First, it presents a picture of the morbidity a population recognizes in itself. Second, the population states the disability incurred. Third, it provides information regarding the extent and kinds of medical care sought.

*Definitions—Chronic Condition, Acute Condition, Disability.*    No concensus has been reached on the definition of any of these terms. The chronic conditions have been variously defined according to the purposes to be served. Thus, on one occasion the Commission on Chronic Illness, without defining "normal," used the definition:[13]

Chronic disease comprises all impairments or deviations from normal which have one or more of the following characteristics: are permanent; leave residual disability; are caused by nonreversible pathological alteration; require special training of the patient for rehabilitation; may be expected to require a long period of supervision, observation, or care.

---

[10] C. L. Chiang, J. L. Hodges, Jr., and J. Yerushalmy, "Statistical Problems in Medical Diagnoses," *Proceedings of the Third Berkeley Symposium on Mathematical Statistics and Probability* (ed. J. Neyman), Vol. IV, *Biology and Problems of Health* (Berkeley and Los Angeles: University of California Press, 1956).

[11] Commission on Chronic Illness, *Chronic Illness in a Large City, The Baltimore Study,* Vol. IV (Cambridge: Harvard University Press, 1957), p. 20.

[12] For a discussion of the collection of morbidity statistics by survey methods, see M. Spiegelman, *Introduction to Demography* (Chicago: Society of Actuaries, 1955), p. 117.

[13] Commission on Chronic Illness, *Prevention of Chronic Illness,* Vol. I (Cambridge: Harvard University Press, 1957), p. 4, and *Chronic Illness in a Rural Area,* Vol. III, pp. 149–51 and 185–87.

This definition implies that the chronic condition would be ascertained by a clinical evaluation. However, for purposes of a household interview, the Commission adopted the definition[14] that:

A chronic condition was one which met one or more of the following criteria:
1. Started 3 months or more prior to the interview.
2. Was stated by the respondent to cause "repeated trouble."
3. Was one of 33 conditions on a list read to the respondent and defined as chronic, or was reported in response to general questions about any chronic condition or ailment, impairment or handicapping condition.

Very similar, but not identical, are the criteria for inclusions in the category of chronic conditions used in the California Health Survey of 1954–55 and the continuing National Health Survey program in that each included conditions lasting more than three months and also used a check list of conditions.[15] It is important to recognize that these various definitions of chronic conditions include many of minor significance, such as hay fever.

The acute conditions are those conditions not classed as chronic. The California Health Survey included among the acute conditions any illness or injury that "bothered" a person during a four-week period, while the National Health Survey excluded from its records any that did not involve either medical attendance or restriction of activity.

Disability may result from either, or both, an acute or chronic condition. On the other hand, there are a great many cases of acute and chronic conditions that are not disabling; this will be referred to again later in the chapter. Disability is generally defined in terms of the impact of a morbid con-

[14] Commission on Chronic Illness, *Chronic Illness in a Large City, The Baltimore Study, op. cit.,* p. 493.

[15] *Health in California,* Department of Public Health, State of California, Berkeley, 1957, pp. 17 and 75; U.S. National Health Survey, *Concepts and Definitions in the Household-Interview Survey,* pp. 16 and 19, and *Chronic Respiratory Conditions Reported in Interviews, July 1957–June 1958,* p. 1, Public Health Service, Washington, D.C., September, 1958, and December, 1959.

dition upon usual activity. Thus, a condition may be regarded as disabling if it merely "bothers," as in the California Health Survey, or, taking a somewhat more restricted viewpoint, as in the National Health Survey, if it produced "any temporary or long-term reduction of a person's activity." A shade more restricted than the latter is the definition of disability of the Commission on Chronic Illness for its household survey in Baltimore according to which a condition is regarded as disabling if it kept a person away from a usual daily activity. At the older ages, these concepts of disability may not be as definitively applied in a survey as at the younger ages since the usual activity may be obscure if it does not involve work for income.[16] However, this difficulty is not present in the same degree if a bed stay is involved at home, in the hospital, or in the nursing home. The prevalence and duration of disability among the aged give some idea, though indirect, of the drain of severe and prolonged illness upon resources available for their medical care.

*The Frequency of Acute and Chronic Conditions among the Aged.* According to the National Health Survey, the incidence of acute conditions among persons aged 65 and over of each sex during the year is only about three fifths of that for younger persons. The pertinent data for the general population of the United States during the period July, 1957–June, 1958 are shown in Table 3.3. Thus, for females the annual incidence of acute conditions was 282 per 100 persons at ages under 65, but at the higher ages the rate was only 169 per 100. However, the proportion of older persons

---

[16] The definition of disability for general population survey purposes differs from that frequently used in accident and sickness insurance, namely "inability of the insured to engage in any gainful occupation for which he is reasonably fitted"; see J. H. Miller *et al., Accident and Sickness Insurance Provided Through Individual Policies* (Chicago: Society of Actuaries, 1956), p. 15. Under Social Security, for entitlement to disability "freeze" or to periodic disability payments, disability is defined as "inability to engage in any substantial gainful activity by reason of any medically determinable physical or mental impairment which can be expected to result in death or to be of long-continued and indefinite duration." (U.S. Senate, 84th Cong., 2d sess., Doc. No. 156, *Compilation of the Social Security Laws,* 1957, p. 77).

with some chronic condition was at least double that recorded at the younger ages. For example, chronic conditions were reported, at ages 65 and over, by 75 per cent of the males and 81 per cent of the females, compared with 36 per cent and 40 per cent respectively for the lower ages. Moreover, the older ages bring an accumulation of chronic condi-

TABLE 3.3

ANNUAL INCIDENCE OF ACUTE CONDITIONS AND PROPORTION OF PERSONS
WITH CHRONIC CONDITIONS BY AGE AND SEX, UNITED STATES,
JULY, 1957–JUNE, 1958

| Condition | Males | | | Females | | |
|---|---|---|---|---|---|---|
| | All Ages | Ages under 65 | Ages 65 and Over | All Ages | Ages under 65 | Ages 65 and Over |
| Acute, rate per 100 persons..... | 247.5 | 255.6 | 155.1 | 272.0 | 282.3 | 168.9 |
| Chronic, total, per cent of persons | 39.1 | 36.0 | 75.2 | 43.5 | 39.8 | 80.6 |
| 1 only.................... | 23.1 | 22.9 | 26.2 | 22.8 | 22.4 | 26.9 |
| 2 only..:................. | 9.3 | 8.3 | 21.3 | 10.7 | 9.8 | 19.9 |
| 3 or more................ | 6.7 | 4.8 | 27.7 | 10.0 | 7.6 | 33.8 |

Source: U.S. National Health Survey, *Acute Conditions, Incidence and Associated Disability, United States, July 1957–June 1958*, and *Limitation of Activity and Mobility Due to Chronic Conditions, United States, July 1957–June 1958*, U.S. Public Health Service, Washington, D.C., 1958 and 1959.

tions. Among persons 65 and over, the proportion with three or more such conditions was 28 per cent for males and 34 per cent for females, each about five times the proportion at the younger ages. However, as already indicated, not all of these chronic conditions are of major significance; this is also discussed further in later pages.

*Specific Acute Conditions among the Aged.* The incidence and associated disability for specific acute conditions in the general population of the United States for the year beginning with July, 1957 is summarized in Table 3.4; the data are derived from a report of the National Health Survey. The respiratory conditions accounted for practically two thirds of all acute illnesses for all ages and also for ages 65 and over. Although the incidence of the acute conditions as a whole was lower among the aged, for a few specific condi-

tions the aged had no advantage over the rest of the population. For example, the annual incidence of acute conditions of the digestive system was the same at ages 65 and over as

TABLE 3.4

ANNUAL INCIDENCE OF ACUTE CONDITIONS, DAYS OF RESTRICTED ACTIVITY, AND BED-DISABILITY DAYS BY AGE AND SEX, UNITED STATES, JULY, 1957–JUNE, 1958

| Condition Group | All Ages | | | Ages 65 and Over | | |
|---|---|---|---|---|---|---|
| | Both Sexes | Males | Females | Both Sexes | Males | Females |
| | Annual Incidence per 100 Persons | | | | | |
| All conditions.............. | 260.1 | 247.5 | 272.0 | 162.6 | 155.1 | 168.9 |
| Infectious and parasitic... | 22.9 | 21.8 | 24.0 | 2.6 | 1.3 | 3.7 |
| Upper respiratory........ | 91.2 | 82.7 | 99.3 | 58.2 | 61.3 | 55.5 |
| Other respiratory......... | 77.8 | 75.3 | 80.1 | 47.3 | 52.8 | 42.6 |
| Digestive system......... | 14.3 | 13.2 | 15.3 | 13.5 | 12.5 | 14.4 |
| Fractures, dislocations, sprains and strains..... | 7.3 | 8.9 | 5.8 | 10.0 | 7.9 | 11.8 |
| Open wounds and lacerations................. | 7.7 | 10.5 | 5.0 | 2.2 | 2.5 | 2.0 |
| Contusions and superficial injuries.............. | 5.8 | 5.7 | 6.0 | 7.6 | 2.3 | 12.1 |
| Other current injuries..... | 7.5 | 8.9 | 6.1 | 3.8 | 1.7 | 5.6 |
| All other conditions....... | 25.6 | 20.5 | 30.4 | 17.3 | 12.7 | 21.1 |
| | Annual Number of Days of Restricted Activity per 100 Persons | | | | | |
| All conditions.............. | 1,142 | 1,018 | 1,260 | 1,302 | 1,208 | 1,382 |
| Infectious and parasitic... | 113 | 108 | 118 | 31 | 17 | 42 |
| Respiratory.............. | 696 | 626 | 762 | 719 | 759 | 685 |
| Digestive............... | 47 | 39 | 54 | 87 | 62 | 108 |
| Injuries................. | 147 | 157 | 137 | 290 | 177 | 384 |
| All other conditions....... | 139 | 88 | 188 | 180 | 201 | 162 |
| | Annual Number of Bed-Disability Days per 100 Persons | | | | | |
| All conditions.............. | 519 | 454 | 580 | 509 | 479 | 534 |
| Infectious and parasitic... | 53 | 48 | 58 | 10 | 4 | 14 |
| Respiratory.............. | 352 | 321 | 382 | 301 | 349 | 260 |
| Digestive............... | 20 | 14 | 25 | 31 | 13 | 46 |
| Injuries................. | 43 | 43 | 43 | 103 | 57 | 143 |
| All other conditions....... | 50 | 27 | 73 | 64 | 56 | 71 |

Source: U.S. National Health Survey, *Acute Conditions, Incidence and Associated Disability, United States, July 1957–June 1958*, U.S. Public Health Service, Washington, D.C., 1958,

for all ages, namely 14 per 100. Aged females are particularly susceptible to fractures, dislocations, sprains, and strains and frequently experience contusions and superficial injuries. These, plus open wounds and lacerations and other current injuries, make up a rate of 31.5 per 100 females at ages 65 and over.

The acute conditions resulted in an annual average of 13 days of "restricted" activity per aged person; of this total, the respiratory conditions account for seven days and injuries for three days. Persons of all ages had the same average as the aged for the respiratory conditions; however, it was only half that of the aged for injuries. Both the aged and persons of all ages spent an annual average of five days per person in bed because of their acute conditions. For the aged, three days of the bed stay were for respiratory conditions and one for injuries.

*Specific Chronic Conditions among the Aged.*   Since the National Health Survey had not produced data for the chronic conditions with regard to age at this writing, the picture will be filled from the California Health Survey of 1954–55. For those 65 and over, the chronic conditions, as defined in this survey, were recorded at an annual incidence rate of almost three per person for males and four per person for females, compared with rates of two and over three respectively for all ages (Table 3.5). However, among the chronic illnesses experienced by the aged, only one fourth were regarded as disabling by the respondent. The annual incidence of disabling chronic conditions among the aged was 70 per 100 for males and 102 per 100 for females. These chronic conditions were of cardiovascular origin for one fifth of the male cases and one fourth of the female cases. A like proportion was attributed to diseases of the muscle, bone, and joint among females, but for males the proportion was less than one tenth. The respiratory conditions accounted for one sixth of all chronic conditions among aged females; for males, it was appreciably less.

On the basis of its liberal concept of disability, the Cali-

## TABLE 3.5

ANNUAL INCIDENCE OF CHRONIC CONDITIONS (TOTAL AND DISABLING) AND
DAYS OF DISABLING ILLNESS BY AGE AND SEX, CALIFORNIA HEALTH SURVEY,
MAY, 1954–APRIL, 1955

| Chronic Condition | All Ages | | Ages 65 and Over | |
|---|---|---|---|---|
| | Males | Females | Males | Females |
| **Annual Incidence per 100 Persons*** | | | | |
| All chronic conditions........ | 200.2 | 322.6 | 287.4 | 392.5 |
| Cardiovascular............. | 8.3 | 16.3 | 38.4 | 63.5 |
| Respiratory............... | 41.9 | 45.0 | 28.0 | 42.8 |
| Chronic sinusitis......... | 14.2 | 17.2 | 19.7 | 15.2 |
| Diseases of muscle, bone and joint................. | 23.2 | 37.7 | 49.8 | 69.3 |
| Arthritis and rheumatism.. | 9.5 | 16.5 | 36.3 | 48.4 |
| Back conditions.......... | 9.0 | 15.8 | 12.4 | 9.5 |
| Other.................. | 4.7 | 5.4 | 1.1 | 11.4 |
| Gastro-intestinal.......... | 27.3 | 34.5 | 54.8 | 62.6 |
| Indigestion............. | 6.4 | 4.7 | 12.4 | 8.5 |
| Constipation............ | 4.8 | 13.4 | 19.7 | 24.7 |
| Other.................. | 16.1 | 16.4 | 22.7 | 29.4 |
| Genito-urinary............ | 2.9 | 31.8 | 9.9 | 10.5 |
| Neoplasms................ | .9 | 3.1 | 2.1 | 2.9 |
| Eye, including blindness..... | 2.7 | 2.4 | 3.1 | 4.7 |
| Ear, including deafness...... | 3.5 | 5.5 | 6.2 | 7.6 |
| Migraine and headache..... | 15.0 | 34.3 | 15.5 | 21.8 |
| Asthma and hay fever...... | 20.1 | 21.6 | 20.7 | 8.5 |
| Accidents, current......... | 3.3 | 2.7 | 2.1 | 4.7 |
| All other................. | 51.1 | 87.7 | 56.8 | 93.6 |
| **Annual Incidence of Disabling Illness per 100 Persons*** | | | | |
| All chronic conditions........ | 47.4 | 80.6 | 69.5 | 102.4 |
| Cardiovascular............. | 3.0 | 5.7 | 13.5 | 25.6 |
| Respiratory............... | 16.3 | 17.7 | 5.2 | 16.1 |
| Diseases of muscle, bone and joint................. | 4.0 | 8.3 | 6.2 | 25.6 |
| Arthritis and rheumatism.. | 1.5 | 4.2 | 3.1 | 16.1 |
| All other................. | 24.1 | 48.9 | 44.6 | 35.1 |
| **Days of Disability per Person per Year** | | | | |
| All chronic conditions........ | 15.2 | 17.7 | 59.2 | 57.3 |
| Cardiovascular............. | 2.8 | 3.1 | 15.6 | 18.7 |
| Respiratory............... | 1.3 | 1.5 | 2.5 | 1.5 |
| Diseases of muscle, bone and joint................. | 3.4 | 3.8 | 12.2 | 14.3 |
| Arthritis and rheumatism.. | 1.0 | 1.7 | 5.9 | 8.0 |
| All other................. | 7.8 | 9.3 | 28.9 | 22.8 |

* The incidence rate refers not only to new cases occurring within the period of observation, but also to recurrences and relapses. A disabling illness causes at least one or more days of interruption of activity.

Source: *Health in California*, Department of Public Health, State of California, Berkeley, 1957, Tables 5, 6, and 9, pp. 85–87.

fornia Health Survey found that the average aged person had almost 60 days of disability per year, compared with about 16½ days for persons of all ages. About one half of the days of disability among the aged were due to cardiovascular conditions and diseases of the muscle, bone, and joint.

*A Clinical Evaluation of Chronic Conditions.* Recognizing the limitations of the usual type of sickness survey, in which lay interviewers obtain information from the population, the Commission on Chronic Illness undertook two surveys of its own, one on a random sample of the noninstitutionalized population of Baltimore and the other in Hunterdon County, New Jersey, a rural area. In the Baltimore survey the information obtained by trained lay interviewers was supplemented, for a subsample, by a review of records with private physicians and hospitals and by a complete diagnostic examination; those outside the subsample were given a series of diagnostic screening tests.[17] The results for the aged in this searching survey present a "measure of the true prevalence" of chronic disease, both manifest and non-manifest, in a population.[18] Unfortunately, in most instances, the sampling data for specific morbid conditions are too few to use as a basis for reliable rates.

Although this Baltimore survey does not represent the situation in the general population of the United States, it has the advantage of reflecting recent medical advances in diagnosis. For the purposes of this survey, the Commission on Chronic Illness defined the category of chronic disease in terms of a list of selected diagnostic entities. According to this criterion, Table 3.6 shows that the aged had four chronic

---

[17] Some of the difficulties in a study of this type are discussed by E. Chen and S. Cobb, "Further Study of the Nonparticipation Problems in a Morbidity Survey Involving Clinical Examination," *Journal of Chronic Diseases,* Vol. 7, p. 321 (April, 1958).

[18] The prevalence rates for a number of major diagnostic conditions (the neoplasms excepted) for the Baltimore survey were substantially higher than comparable rates for an average of six earlier surveys made by the more conventional procedures. However, these two bodies of data are not strictly comparable for a number of reasons; *Chronic Illness in a Large City, The Baltimore Study, op. cit.,* p. 498.

## TABLE 3.6

### PREVALENCE OF SELECTED CHRONIC CONDITIONS,* PERSONS WITH CHRONIC CONDITIONS, AND ESTIMATED NEEDS FOR MEDICAL CARE, BALTIMORE, MARYLAND, SEPTEMBER, 1953–APRIL, 1955

| Diagnosis | Cases per 100 Persons | | | Circumstance of Count | Rate per 100 Persons | | | Medical Care Needed‡ | Rate per 100 Persons | | |
|---|---|---|---|---|---|---|---|---|---|---|---|
| | All Ages | Under Age 65 | Ages 65 and Over | | All Ages | Under Age 65 | Ages 65 and Over | | All Ages | Under Age 65 | Ages 65 and Over |
| All diagnoses.......... | 156.7 | 137.9 | 404.2 | Persons with one or more chronic conditions Found in clinical evaluation........ | 64.9 | 62.6 | 95.4 | Consultation by specialist | 10.8§ | 10.3 | 17.0 |
| Males............... | 139.3 | 122.5 | 427.2 | | | | | | | | |
| Females............. | 172.3 | 152.3 | 390.6 | Reported for 12 months past in household survey. | 32.5 | 29.8 | 65.5 | Treatment by specialist | | | |
| White.............. | 163.5 | 139.6 | 412.0 | | | | | Surgical............ | 7.3 | 7.8 | 0.9 |
| Nonwhite........... | 138.7 | 133.7 | 331.7 | | | | | Psychiatric......... | 9.0 | 8.0 | 10.0 |
| Heart disease....... | 9.6 | 6.0 | 57.5 | Persons with one or more substantial chronic conditions found in clinical evaluation†... | 44.4 | 41.3 | 85.2 | | | | |
| Coronary artery disease and angina pectoris.. | 2.3 | 0.9 | 20.4 | | | | | Diet therapy......... | 10.0 | 9.0 | 29.4 |
| Hypertensive heart disease............. | 5.0 | 3.4 | 26.5 | | | | | | | | |
| Diabetes mellitus........ | 2.7 | 2.5 | 4.5 | | | | | | | | |
| Hernia of abdominal cavity............ | 3.7 | 2.3 | 21.2 | Persons with one or more conditions (acute or chronic) on day preceding household survey | | | | General medical care and supervision.......... | 100.0 | 100.0 | 100.0 |
| | | | | Bothered but not disabled........... | 11.5 | 10.8 | 20.1 | Periodic check-up only | 68.8 | 72.0 | 26.0 |
| Cataract (not causing blindness)........... | 1.7 | 0.7 | 15.6 | Disabled........... | 2.9 | 2.5 | 7.8 | Every six months.... | 6.5 | 6.3 | 9.7 |
| | | | | | | | | Every three months.. | 7.2 | 6.0 | 22.9 |
| | | | | | | | | Every two months.... | 10.2 | 9.5 | 20.4 |
| Arthritis............ | 7.5 | 4.2 | 51.5 | | | | | Every month........ | 6.3 | 5.2 | 20.3 |
| Osteoarthritis....... | 6.6 | 3.5 | 48.7 | | | | | Every two weeks or more often...... | 1.0 | 1.0 | 0.8 |

* The selected chronic conditions are those for which at least 15 cases were recorded at ages 65 and over in the clinical evaluation conducted on a subsample; however, the rates are based upon estimates from the subsample to approximate the number of cases in the entire sample of the population.

† This includes conditions which interfere with or limit activities or require care presently or likely in the future.

‡ Needs estimated not only at time of clinical evaluation, but also those expected within following year.

§ The source shows a rate of 9.4 which is obviously in error and also not in agreement with the figure on p. 197 of the source.

Note: The figures for ages under 65 were computed by the author from the basic data in the source.

Source: Commission on Chronic Illness, *Chronic Illness in a Large City, The Baltimore Study* (Cambridge, Mass.: Harvard University Press, 1957), Vol. IV, pp. 50–55, 195–200, 271, 281, and 527.

conditions per person, compared with 1.6 per person of all ages. An indication of the effect of the intensive case finding in this survey is provided by a comparison with an earlier survey of the Eastern Health District of Baltimore during 1938–43, which yielded only 0.2 chronic illnesses per person, one eighth of the recent rate. Almost 60 per cent of the aged in the later study were found to have heart disease; about half of these were hypertensive and over one third had coronary artery disease and angina pectoris. An arthritic condition, mostly osteoarthritis, was observed in little over one half of the aged. About one fifth of the aged suffered from a hernia of the abdominal cavity and nearly one sixth had a cataract not causing blindness. Almost 5 per cent had a diabetic condition. The number of chronic conditions per person, among the aged, was higher for males than for females, and also higher for whites than for nonwhites.

Altogether, 95 per cent of the aged had one or more chronic conditions according to clinical evaluation, compared with 63 per cent at ages under 65, and 65 per cent at all ages. The same clinical evaluation showed that 85 per cent of the aged had, on the day of the evaluation, one or more substantial chronic conditions interfering with the individual's activity or requiring care presently or likely in the future. However, in the household survey by lay interviewers, only 66 per cent of the aged were reported to have one or more chronic conditions during the 12 months preceding the interview, but this lower figure may understate the actual recognition of such conditions because of a memory loss by the respondent.

Thus, the usual sickness surveys conducted by lay interviewers, though well trained, may understate the actual prevalence of chronic disease among the aged by a considerable margin. On the other hand, in a discussion of the severity of chronic conditions, the Commission on Chronic Illness points out that ". . . many mild conditions require little care or a different kind of care than the moderate or severe conditions. At the same time, of course, it cannot be assumed that all severe conditions require care."[19] Indeed, Fry claims that "In assessing the health of the elderly it is much more important to base this on 'effective function' rather than on the incidence of various pathological states, which may never interfere with their daily lives."[20] This concept is evidently quite general, for a European advisory group of the World Health Organization "agreed that health in the aged is best measured in terms of function, and that degree of fitness rather than extent of pathology may be used as a measure of the amount of services the aged will require from the community."[21] The Baltimore study made it apparent that most chronic conditions evident in an intensive survey including a clinical evaluation do not result in substantial disability. Among the aged, 20 per cent stated that they were bothered but not disabled by one or more conditions (both acute and chronic) on the day preceding the interview, and only 8 per cent stated that they were so disabled that they were in bed, remained indoors, or were kept from usual activities.

The intricacies faced in gauging the medical needs of the aged are clearly implied by Zeman: "Nowhere in the whole range of medical experience, except in old age, does one find so many complex problems, so many pathologic lesions in 1 person, such bizarre clinical pictures and such unpredictable responses to treatment."[22] This situation gives emphasis to the statement of the Commission on Chronic Illness that ". . . translation of morbidity data into needs for service . . . for prolonged illness are complex and difficult procedures. They must be based on medical judgment regarding

[19] *Chronic Illness in a Large City, The Baltimore Study, op. cit.,* pp. 55–56 and 271.

[20] J. Fry, "Care of the Elderly in General Practice," *British Medical Journal,* September 21, 1957, p. 667.

[21] World Health Organization, Regional Office for Europe, *Advisory Group on the Public Health Aspects of the Aging of the Population, Oslo, 28 July–2 August, 1958,* Report dated 30 December, 1958, p. 8.

[22] F. D. Zeman, "Recent Contributions to the Medical Problems of Old Age," *New England Journal of Medicine,* Vol. 257, p. 369 (August 22, 1957).

diagnosis and the type and potential value of treatment and on assumptions regarding the organization of personnel and facilities."[23] This effort was made in the Baltimore study.[24] According to the judgment of the physicians in the evaluation clinic and the study director, also a physician, it was estimated that 21.1 per cent of the aged needed a physician's visit at least once a month, 20.4 per cent needed such care every two months, and 22.9 per cent every three months. Thus, almost two thirds of the aged were in need of a physician's attention at least every three months; for persons of all ages, the proportion was only one fourth. The clinical evaluation team also estimated that 17 per cent of the aged would need consultation by at least one kind of specialist within the year after the evaluation, that 10 per cent would be in need of psychiatric treatment within that period and about one per cent would require surgery.[25]

In summary, the results of this Baltimore survey make evident the inherent tendency of the usual sickness survey not employing a clinical evaluation to understate the true prevalence of chronic disease. In particular, the actual medical care needs of a population cannot be measured by its current rates of utilization of medical care services. Among the aged, as for the rest of the population, the demand for such services will undoubtedly grow with the development of new diagnostic, therapeutic and rehabilitation procedures and as measures are introduced that encourage them to give more attention to their health status.

*Disability in Relation to Family Income and Residence.* The prevalence of chronic conditions, as reported to the lay interviewers in the Baltimore study, was highest among individuals where the family income was under $2,000, but the

---

[23] *Chronic Illness in a Large City, The Baltimore Study, op. cit.,* p. 21.

[24] See also *Chronic Illness in a Rural Area, op. cit.,* p. 201.

[25] For an intensive study of unmet medical care needs in relation to age and social-economic status, see L. S. Rosenfeld, J. Katz and A. Donabedian, *Medical Care Needs and Services in the Boston Metropolitan Area,* United Community Services of Metropolitan Boston, Massachusetts, 1957.

decline just after that level is followed by a rise with income (Table 3.7). The same pattern was found in the rate of disability (counting cases with one or more days) at ages under 65. On the other hand, at ages 65 and over the disability rates were definitely greater at income levels over $4,000 than for the lower levels. Considering the shift in the pattern from

TABLE 3.7

DISABILITY DUE TO CHRONIC CONDITIONS* DURING A 12-MONTH PERIOD, ACCORDING TO ANNUAL FAMILY INCOME AND AGE, BALTIMORE, MARYLAND, SEPTEMBER, 1953–APRIL, 1955

| Extent of Disability | Annual Family Income | | | | |
|---|---|---|---|---|---|
| | Under $2,000 | $2,000–$3,999 | $4,000–$5,999 | $6,000 and Over | Un-known |
| | Annual Rate per 100 Persons | | | | |
| With one or more chronic conditions† | 41.7 | 29.1 | 32.2 | 36.0 | 28.6 |
| Disabled one day or more | | | | | |
| All ages | 14.5 | 8.9 | 9.5 | 11.6 | 9.7 |
| Kept from usual activity | 3.4 | 2.5 | 2.5 | 2.6 | 2.4 |
| Kept in bed | 11.2 | 6.4 | 7.1 | 9.0 | 7.3 |
| Ages under 65 | 13.5 | 8.4 | 9.0 | 10.7 | 8.1 |
| Ages 65 and over | 19.5 | 18.3 | 21.6 | 24.5 | 25.6 |
| Disabled more than 3 months | | | | | |
| All ages | 4.0 | 1.4 | 1.3 | 0.9 | 2.2 |
| Ages under 65 | 3.1 | 1.1 | 0.9 | 0.4 | 1.2 |
| Ages 65 and over | 7.8 | 6.9 | 8.6 | 8.2 | 11.4 |
| | Average Days per Person per Year | | | | |
| Disability | | | | | |
| All ages | 13.0 | 4.6 | 4.3 | 4.1 | 6.8 |
| Ages under 65 | 10.1 | 3.7 | 3.4 | 2.6 | 4.1 |
| Ages 65 and over | 25.6 | 22.5 | 24.8 | 26.4 | 32.7 |
| Bed | | | | | |
| All ages | 5.5 | 1.9 | 1.7 | 2.4 | 2.5 |
| Ages under 65 | 5.0 | 1.6 | 1.3 | 1.5 | 1.6 |
| Ages 65 and over | 7.9 | 7.9 | 9.1 | 16.6 | 10.9 |

* Chronic conditions included those regarded as such by the respondent and all other conditions of at least three months' duration.
† Disabling as well as nondisabling.
Note: The figures for ages under 65 were computed by the author from the basic data in the source.
Source: Commission on Chronic Illness, *Chronic Illness in a Large City, The Baltimore Study* (Cambridge, Mass.: Harvard University Press, 1957), Vol. IV, pp. 280–91.

the younger to the older ages, the inference was made "that disabling illness is more often a cause than an effect of low income."[26] This inference is also supported by observing that the average duration of disability varied little with income at ages over 65, but at the younger ages it decreased with rise in income.

Where the family income was under $4,000, the average annual bed stay was eight days per aged person; this rose to 16.6 days for the class with $6,000 and over. The greater average bed stay of the aged at the higher income levels may reflect a more liberal attitude toward utilization of health services than is found at the lower income levels. On the other hand, limited means at the lower income levels may tend to restrict utilization of these services; the facts in the situation are not known. Thus, it is possible that the educational level of the family head may be a more significant factor than income in shaping attitudes toward utilization of services.

The National Health Survey produced a picture with regard to bed stay somewhat like that of the Baltimore study (Table 3.8). For persons under age 65, the bed stay during the survey period fell steadily from an annual average of 9.9 days for family incomes under $2,000 to 5.7 days for incomes of $7,000 and over. However, at ages 65 and over, the average bed stay dropped from a high of 19.5 days for the lowest income group, but rose from its minimum to a level of 13.7 days for the class with incomes of $7,000 and over.

The data for bed stay with regard to place of residence in Table 3.8 show, on the whole, little variation between urban and rural residents. The only point of interest is that the average bed stay of urban males at ages 65 and over is about four days less than that of rural males.

*Impairments.* Increasingly with advance in age, disease, injury, and congenital conditions leave impairments as aftereffects; they also are the product of active chronic disease. However, impairments are not necessarily disabling. Thus,

---

[26] *Chronic Illness in a Large City, The Baltimore Study, op. cit.,* p. 291.

the National Health Survey included as impairments "certain chronic or permanent defects, disabling or not, representing, for the most part, decrease or loss of ability to perform certain functions, particularly those of the musculo-

TABLE 3.8

AVERAGE DAYS OF BED DISABILITY PER PERSON PER YEAR, UNITED STATES, JULY, 1957–JUNE, 1958

| Family Income; Residence; Major Activity | Ages under 65 | | | Ages 65 and Over | | |
|---|---|---|---|---|---|---|
| | Both Sexes | Males | Females | Both Sexes | Males | Females |
| Family income | | | | | | |
| Total............. | 7.0 | 6.0 | 7.9 | 16.3 | 16.0 | 16.6 |
| Under $2,000....... | 9.9 | 9.2 | 10.5 | 19.5 | 21.2 | 18.2 |
| $2,000–$3,999....... | 7.1 | 6.3 | 7.8 | 14.7 | 16.2 | 13.2 |
| $4,000–$6,999....... | 6.7 | 5.6 | 7.7 | 13.0 | 9.2 | 16.1 |
| $7,000 and over..... | 5.7 | 4.8 | 6.6 | 13.7 | 9.7 | 17.1 |
| Unknown.......... | 6.9 | 6.3 | 7.6 | 15.1 | 12.1 | 17.2 |
| | Ages 17 to 64 | | | Ages 65 and Over | | |
| Urban, total......... | 7.0 | 5.7 | 8.2 | 15.7 | 14.5 | 16.6 |
| Usually working..... | — | 4.4 | 6.2 | — | 6.1 | 5.5 |
| Keeping house...... | — | — | 8.9 | — | — | 13.4 |
| Other............. | — | 14.6 | 13.6 | — | 18.1 | 34.7 |
| Rural nonfarm, total... | 6.6 | 5.6 | 7.6 | 17.5 | 18.4 | 16.7 |
| Usually working..... | — | 4.6 | 6.5 | — | 3.9 | 4.0 |
| Keeping house...... | — | — | 7.4 | — | — | 12.5 |
| Other............. | — | 13.3 | 15.4 | — | 23.6 | 34.8 |
| Rural farm........... | 7.0 | 5.3 | 8.9 | 17.4 | 18.5 | 16.2 |
| Usually working..... | — | 4.2 | 8.1 | — | 8.8 | 3.0 |
| Keeping house...... | — | — | 9.0 | — | — | 8.8 |
| Other............. | — | 12.7 | 9.6 | — | 27.2 | 44.8 |

Source: U.S. National Health Survey, *Disability Days, United States, July 1957–June 1958*, Public Health Service, Washington, D.C., 1959. The data for ages under 65 were computed from the source by the author.

skeletal system and special senses." The principal impairment noted among older people is a defect of hearing, according to a survey of the noninstitutionalized population summarized in Table 3.9. Whereas hearing defects—ranging from a mild impairment to total deafness—were reported at a rate of 35 per 1,000 persons of all ages, for ages 65–74 years the rate was 129 per 1,000 and for ages 75 and over it was 256 per 1,000. Visual defects become increasingly significant with advance in age. The prevalence of blindness was nearly 6 per 1,000 at all ages, but 83 per 1,000 at ages 75 and over. Other visual defects were about equally prevalent at these

TABLE 3.9

PREVALENCE OF IMPAIRMENTS, BY AGE, UNITED STATES,
JULY, 1957–JUNE, 1958

| Type of Impairment | Rate per 1,000 Persons | | | Per Cent Distribution | | |
|---|---|---|---|---|---|---|
| | All Ages | Ages 65–74 | Ages 75 and Over | All Ages | Ages 65–74 | Ages 75 and Over |
| All impairments............ | 141.4 | 376.6 | 615.0 | 100.0 | 100.0 | 100.0 |
| Blindness................ | 5.7 | 25.9 | 83.3 | 4.0 | 6.9 | 13.5 |
| Other visual............. | 12.3 | 48.8 | 74.3 | 8.7 | 13.0 | 12.1 |
| Hearing................. | 34.6 | 129.2 | 256.4 | 24.4 | 34.3 | 41.7 |
| Speech defects........... | 6.5 | 6.8 | 6.1 | 4.6 | 1.8 | 1.0 |
| Paralysis................ | 5.6 | 15.9 | 34.4 | 3.9 | 4.2 | 5.6 |
| Absence, fingers, toes, only. | 8.5 | 22.6 | 17.4 | 6.0 | 6.0 | 2.8 |
| Absence, major extremities | 1.7 | 4.4 | 7.0 | 1.2 | 1.2 | 1.1 |
| Lower extremities*....... | 18.7 | 37.1 | 39.7 | 13.2 | 9.8 | 6.5 |
| Upper extremities*....... | 10.0 | 24.6 | 26.6 | 7.1 | 6.5 | 4.3 |
| Limbs, back, trunk†...... | 29.9 | 49.7 | 61.6 | 21.1 | 13.2 | 10.0 |
| All others.............. | 8.1 | 11.6 | 8.2 | 5.7 | 3.1 | 1.3 |

* Except paralysis and absence.
† Except extremities only; also except paralysis and absence.

Source: U.S. National Health Survey, *Impairments by Type, Sex, and Age, United States, July 1957–June 1958*, Public Health Service, Washington, D.C., April, 1959.

older ages. Impairments of the extremities and paralysis also rank high as impairments in late life.

*Dental Needs.* Data regarding the dental needs of aged persons are practically nonexistent. An indication of these needs is provided from the sample of adults screened in the Baltimore study. Among persons at ages 65–74 years of age, there were 21.4 missing teeth per person and 24.2 decayed, filled, or missing teeth per person. The comparable ratios for all persons under age 75 were 10.5 and 16.8 respectively.

## HEALTH ATTITUDES

"Individual initiative is vital in the prevention of chronic disease." This is the first recommendation of the Commission on Chronic Illness.[27] Every competent person has the responsibility to guard his health, not only against the more obvious hazards of the near future, but also against those that creep up in the later years. Since preventive measures are not always effective against chronic illness, the individual owes himself, at least, the protection that periodic health examinations provide by way of early detection and treatment in order to minimize disability or to forestall premature death. However, attitudes toward health maintenance and medical care are shaped during a lifetime and are not easily changed. They are strongly influenced by family traits and habits, and by the social and work environment. Furthermore, there is some evidence that the older person perceives his health status in terms of its relation to his daily activity.[28] He tends to recognize a state of health as poor only when it interferes with this activity. The attitude of the individual to his health problems may also be affected by the characteristics of the medical care facilities in the community.[29]

It is pertinent to ask, then: What are the health expectations for the later years by those now at the productive ages? How do the aged assess their health status? What attitudes do the aged have toward health maintenance? What are the attitudes of the aged toward the use of health services? And what are their attitudes in the financing of such services? The last question is discussed in Chapter 5.

*Self-Appraisal of Health Status by Adults.* Self-appraisal is often highly tinged with optimism. Thus, in a very small sample of persons at ages 70 and over, Tuckman and Lorge found that one eighth classified themselves as young, almost

[27] Commission on Chronic Illness, *Prevention of Chronic Illness,* Vol. I, *op. cit.,* p. 6.

[28] L. DiCicco and D. Apple, "Health Needs and Opinions of Older Adults," *Public Health Reports,* Vol. 73, p. 479 (June, 1958).

[29] E. Cohen, "Some Social Considerations About Research and Prolonged Hospital Stay," *Journal of Chronic Diseases,* Vol. 7, p. 264 (March, 1958).

one half as middle-aged, and about two fifths as old.[30] However, in another study of the aged, they found that five sixths considered the ages under 30 as the most favorable for health and a like proportion regarded the ages over 60 as the least favorable.[31]

Increasing dissatisfaction with one's state of health with aging was shown in a number of ways in an attitude survey conducted on a sample of the population of the United States in 1955 by the National Opinion Research Center (NORC) with the support of the Health Information Foundation (Table 3.10).[32] In this survey, 39 per cent of those at ages 65 and over reported themselves not satisfied with their state of health, compared with 18 per cent at ages 21 to 64 years. The proportion regarding their state of health as fair or poor rose to 57 per cent at ages 65 and over from 28 per cent at ages 21 to 64; those thinking about their health a great deal to 26 per cent from 16 per cent; and those talking about their health a great deal to 12 per cent from 6 per cent.[33] Apparently, the frame of mind of the aged concerning their state of health also influenced their thinking with regard to the general chances of having good health today as compared with 30 years ago. Only 67 per cent of those 65 and over thought they were better, compared with 85 per cent at ages 21 to 64 years.

Reporting on his studies, Tyhurst states:

---

[30] J. Tuckman and I. Lorge, "Classification of the Self as Young, Middle-aged, or Old," *Geriatrics,* Vol. 9, p. 534 (November, 1954).

[31] J. Tuckman and I. Lorge, "Old People's Appraisal of Adjustment Over the Life Span," *Journal of Personality,* Vol. 22, p. 417 (March, 1954).

[32] Data from this survey are being analyzed by J. J. Feldman and P. B. Sheatsley and will be reported in a forthcoming National Opinion Research Center publication; the data were kindly made available to the author by Dr. Odin W. Anderson, Director of Research, Health Information Foundation.

[33] For comparison: "Whereas an overwhelming majority of respondents had been blessed with good health when they were young, about one in six had poor health at the time the studies were made," *The Aging of Three Parishes,* National Conference of Catholic Charities, Washington, D.C., p. 5.

We have been impressed by the fact that, in the absence of other significant roles, some older or retired individuals resort to an assumption of the "sick role.". . . While it is clear that many older persons are not well, we have found that statements of poor health are often rationalizations of other issues.[34]

## TABLE 3.10

SELF-APPRAISAL OF HEALTH STATUS BY ADULTS, UNITED STATES, 1955

| Assessment Item | Age | | |
| --- | --- | --- | --- |
| | 21 and Over | 21 to 64 | 65 and Over |
| Present state of own health............100% | 100% | 100% |
| Satisfied............................ 79 | 82 | 61 |
| Not satisfied........................ 21 | 18 | 39 |
| Consider own state of health to be........100% | 100% | 100% |
| Excellent........................... 30 | 33 | 14 |
| Good............................... 38 | 39 | 29 |
| Fair................................ 25 | 23 | 34 |
| Poor............................... 7 | 5 | 23 |
| Think about own state of health........100% | 100% | 100% |
| A great deal........................ 17 | 16 | 26 |
| Fairly often........................ 20 | 20 | 18 |
| Only occasionally.................... 62 | 64 | 55 |
| Don't know......................... 1 | * | 1 |
| Talk about own state of health...........100% | 100% | 100% |
| A great deal........................ 6 | 6 | 12 |
| Fairly often........................ 11 | 10 | 13 |
| Only occasionally.................... 82 | 83 | 74 |
| Don't know......................... 1 | 1 | 1 |
| Chances of having good health today compared with 30 years ago............100% | 100% | 100% |
| Better............................. 84 | 85 | 67 |
| Worse.............................. 8 | 8 | 17 |
| About the same..................... 6 | 5 | 12 |
| Don't know......................... 2 | 2 | 4 |

* Less than 0.5 per cent.

Source: Unpublished data from 1955 survey by National Opinion Research Center sponsored by the Health Information Foundation; the figures for ages 21 to 64 were computed from source data by the author.

[34] J. S. Tyhurst, "The Neurologic and Psychiatric Aspects of the Disorders of Aging," *Proceedings of the Association for Research in Nervous and Mental Disease*, Vol. 35, p. 241 (Baltimore: Williams and Wilkins, 1956); see also W. Caudill, *Effects of Social and Cultural Systems in Reactions to Stress* (New York: Social Science Research Council, June, 1958), p. 17.

Nevertheless, on the whole, the self-appraisal of the aged with regard to their health status tends to be correlated with their actual state of health. An insight into this is provided in a survey of 500 persons over age 60 living in the Kips Bay–Yorkville Health District of New York City; the data are summarized in Table 3.11.

For purposes of study, health status in the Kips Bay–Yorkville study was determined by means of an index based upon time spent in bed because of illness during a year, deprivations due to poor health, the number of illnesses, and the reported presence of certain critical illnesses.[35] The data show a fair correlation between health status and self-rating as to health; 48 per cent of those in excellent health rated themselves in that status, and 55 per cent of those in poor health recognized their status.[36] However, among those of low social economic status, the proportions rating their health as excellent or good were smaller than for those of high social economic status, irrespective of their actual state of health. This situation is also reflected in the larger proportions among those of low social economic status who reported that they worried about health all or most of the time. Also, as expected, among those who rate their health as fair or poor, a greater proportion have high neurotic symptoms than among those who rate their health as excellent or good.

*Attitudes of the Aged toward Health Maintenance.* Most respondents in the 1955 survey of the National Opinion Research Center agreed that older people have to expect a lot of aches and pains. The proportion of the aged (79 per cent) agreeing in this was appreciably greater than at the main productive ages (62 per cent), as shown in Table 3.12. However, the attitude of the aged toward their health mainte-

---

[35] This index is not an objective evaluation of health status since the reporting for some of its elements may be influenced by an assumption of a "sick role" on the part of a number of the aged.

[36] For further evidence, in which the respondents' self-rating was compared with the physicians' rating, see E. A. Suchman, B. S. Phillips, and G. F. Streib, "An Analysis of the Validity of Health Questionnaires," *Social Forces,* Vol. 36, p. 223 (March, 1958).

## TABLE 3.11

HEALTH ATTITUDES IN RELATION TO HEALTH STATUS IN A STRATIFIED SAMPLE OF 500 PERSONS OVER AGE 60; KIPS BAY–YORKVILLE HEALTH DISTRICT OF NEW YORK CITY, NOVEMBER, 1952

| Health Attitude | Health Status | | | |
|---|---|---|---|---|
| | Good, Total | | Poor, Total | |
| | Excellent | Good | Fair | Poor |
| **Health self-rating** | | | | |
| All cases | 100% | 100% | 100% | 100% |
| Excellent | 48 | 25 | 10 | 6 |
| Good | 37 | 46 | 26 | 12 |
| Fair | 15 | 24 | 35 | 27 |
| Poor | — | 5 | 29 | 55 |
| High social economic status | 100% | | 100% | |
| Excellent or good | 80 | | 41 | |
| Fair or poor | 20 | | 59 | |
| Low social economic status | 100% | | 100% | |
| Excellent or good | 70 | | 24 | |
| Fair or poor | 30 | | 76 | |
| **Worry about health** | | | | |
| All cases | 100% | 100% | 100% | 100% |
| All of the time | — | 3 | 7 | 18 |
| Most of the time | — | 1 | 14 | 14 |
| Sometimes | 18 | 25 | 33 | 31 |
| Never | 82 | 71 | 46 | 37 |
| High social economic status | 100% | | 100% | |
| All or most of the time | 2 | | 17 | |
| Sometimes, never | 98 | | 83 | |
| Low social economic status | 100% | | 100% | |
| All or most of the time | 4 | | 29 | |
| Sometimes, never | 96 | | 71 | |
| **Futility feeling** | 100% | | 100% | |
| Low | 47 | | 29 | |
| Moderate | 46 | | 55 | |
| High | 7 | | 16 | |
| **Neurotic symptoms** | | | | |
| All cases | 100% | | 100% | |
| Low | 48 | | 23 | |
| Medium | 31 | | 32 | |
| High | 21 | | 45 | |
| Health self-rating excellent or good | 100% | | 100% | |
| Low | 52 | | 24 | |
| Medium | 31 | | 47 | |
| High | 17 | | 29 | |
| Health self-rating fair or poor | 100% | | 100% | |
| Low | 36 | | 22 | |
| Medium | 32 | | 26 | |
| High | 32 | | 52 | |

Source: B. Kutner, D. Fanshel, A. M. Togo, and T. S. Langner, *Five Hundred Over Sixty* (New York: Russell Sage Foundation, 1956), Tables 50, 51, 53, 54, 57, 68, and 70.

TABLE 3.12

ATTITUDES TOWARD HEALTH MAINTENANCE, UNITED STATES, 1955

| Attitude Question | Age | | |
|---|---|---|---|
| | 21 and Over | 21 to 64 | 65 and Over |
| Older people have to expect a lot of aches and pains | 100% | 100% | 100% |
| Agree | 65 | 62 | 79 |
| Disagree | 32 | 34 | 19 |
| Don't know | 3 | 4 | 2 |
| If a person is feeling all right, should he | 100% | 100% | 100% |
| Get physical examination anyway? | 80 | 83 | 58 |
| Or is it not worth trouble? | 19 | 16 | 39 |
| Don't know | 1 | 1 | 3 |
| Have you ever had a general physical examination? | 100% | 100% | 100% |
| Yes, regularly | 29 | 31 | 19 |
| Yes, occasionally | 58 | 58 | 57 |
| No, never | 13 | 11 | 24 |
| When you're not feeling well, do you ever talk with anyone else about whether you should see a doctor? | 100% | 100% | 100% |
| Yes | 44 | 46 | 31 |
| No | 56 | 54 | 69 |
| Thinking ahead over the next year, how likely do you think it is that you will be sick in bed for 3 or 4 days? | 100% | 100% | 100% |
| Very likely | 17 | 17 | 20 |
| Only fairly likely | 26 | 27 | 26 |
| Not likely at all | 49 | 50 | 36 |
| Don't know | 8 | 6 | 18 |
| Do you think there's anything you could do to prevent that sickness? | 100% | 100% | 100% |
| Yes | 29 | 30 | 23 |
| No | 66 | 65 | 71 |
| Don't know | 5 | 5 | 6 |
| If you had a chance to talk to a doctor for half an hour, at no cost, are there things about your own health you would like to ask him? | 100% | 100% | 100% |
| Yes | 44 | 44 | 40 |
| No | 54 | 54 | 59 |
| Don't know | 2 | 2 | 1 |
| Do you read health columns in newspapers, and newspaper articles about health? | 100% | 100% | 100% |
| Frequently | 23 | 23 | 21 |
| Only occasionally | 35 | 35 | 29 |
| Skip health columns | 20 | 21 | 19 |
| Don't read papers | 21 | 20 | 29 |
| Don't know | 1 | 1 | 2 |

TABLE 3.12—*Continued*

| Attitude Question | Age | | |
|---|---|---|---|
| | 21 and Over | 21 to 64 | 65 and Over |
| Have you read any magazine columns or articles about health and medicine in the last month? | 100% | 100% | 100% |
| Read, last month | 33 | 35 | 22 |
| Usually, not last month | 4 | 4 | 4 |
| Skip health articles | 13 | 12 | 17 |
| Don't read magazines | 47 | 46 | 55 |
| Don't know | 3 | 3 | 2 |
| Do you listen to radio or television programs dealing with health or medicine? | 100% | 100% | 100% |
| Frequently | 19 | 19 | 18 |
| Only occasionally | 35 | 36 | 31 |
| Skip health programs | 23 | 24 | 19 |
| Don't listen much | 21 | 19 | 30 |
| Don't know | 2 | 2 | 2 |
| Regarding articles, radio and television programs about health, do you feel there are | 100% | 100% | 100% |
| Too many? | 8 | 7 | 11 |
| Not enough? | 35 | 38 | 20 |
| About right? | 32 | 32 | 27 |
| Don't know | 25 | 23 | 42 |
| Would you say you take | 100% | 100% | 100% |
| Best possible care of your own health? | 58 | 56 | 74 |
| Or could do more? | 41 | 43 | 25 |
| Don't know | 1 | 1 | 1 |

Source: Unpublished data from the 1955 survey by the National Opinion Research Center sponsored by the Health Information Foundation; the figures for ages 21 to 64 were computed from source data by the author.

nance was not as favorable as that of younger people. For example, there was nearly a general consensus among those at the main productive ages that a person should get a general physical examination even if feeling well, 83 per cent so agreeing, but among the aged only 58 per cent thought so. On the other hand, relatively few acted as they thought in this regard, particularly among the aged, for only 19 per cent of them stated that they had a general physical examination regularly, compared with 31 per cent at the main productive ages.

Whereas 46 per cent of the younger persons consulted someone else about whether they should see a doctor when they were not feeling well, for the aged the proportion was 31 per cent. However, this lower proportion for the aged is very likely influenced by the fact that many live alone or without relatives in the household. Also, the aged were somewhat more pessimistic than younger people with regard to their outlook for health and the chances of preventing bad health, but the findings on these questions may be uncertain because many did not venture an answer. Even with this health outlook, somewhat fewer of the aged (40 per cent) than of younger persons (44 per cent) would use an opportunity to talk to a doctor at no cost about their health problems.

The aged apparently do not have as much interest as younger people in learning about health matters. According to Table 3.12, smaller proportions of those 65 and over than of persons under that age read health items in newspapers or magazines or turned to health programs on the television or radio. However, larger proportions of the aged also stated that they did not turn to any of these media at all. The lack of interest by the aged in newspapers and magazines may reflect, partly, their lower educational attainment compared with younger people and, perhaps, a loss of motivation by those with severe illness. Notwithstanding the attitude of the aged toward health news and physical check-ups, 74 per cent of them thought they were taking the best possible care of their own health, compared with 56 per cent at the younger ages.

As might be expected, the proportion of aged who have a regular physician is larger among those of high social economic status than among those not so well situated, according to findings from the Kips Bay–Yorkville study shown in Table 3.13. It is possible that further investigation would have shown, within each social economic status category, that the proportion of aged with a regular physician was greater for those with a better education. Among persons of high social economic status, the proportion with a regular physician was greater for those in fair or poor health than for those in excellent or good health; there was no such difference among those of low social economic status. Although

TABLE 3.13

ATTITUDES TOWARD USE OF HEALTH SERVICES IN A STRATIFIED SAMPLE OF
500 PERSONS OVER AGE 60; KIPS BAY–YORKVILLE HEALTH DISTRICT OF
NEW YORK CITY, NOVEMBER, 1952

| Attitude Toward Health Services | All Cases | | High Social Economic Status | | Low Social Economic Status | |
|---|---|---|---|---|---|---|
| | Health Status | | | | | |
| | Excellent or Good | Fair or Poor | Excellent or Good | Fair or Poor | Excellent or Good | Fair or Poor |
| Regular physician....... | 100% | 100% | 100% | 100% | 100% | 100% |
| Have................. | 64 | 61 | 74 | 82 | 55 | 52 |
| Do not have.......... | 36 | 39 | 26 | 18 | 45 | 48 |
| Have regular checkup.... | 100% | 100% | — | — | — | — |
| Twice or more a year... | 15 | 26 | — | — | — | — |
| Once a year........... | 33 | 31 | — | — | — | — |
| Seldom or never....... | 52 | 43 | — | — | — | — |
| Use of health resources | | | | | | |
| Isolated.............. | 100% | 100% | 100% | 100% | 100% | 100% |
| High resource use.... | 42 | 44 | 40 | 44 | 43 | 44 |
| Low resource use.... | 58 | 56 | 60 | 56 | 57 | 56 |
| Not isolated.......... | 100% | 100% | 100% | 100% | 100% | 100% |
| High resource use.... | 40 | 72 | 37 | 76 | 44 | 69 |
| Low resource use.... | 60 | 28 | 63 | 24 | 56 | 31 |
| Worry about health | | | | | | |
| All or most of the time. | 100% | 100% | — | — | — | — |
| High resource use.... | 51 | 63 | — | — | — | — |
| Low resource use.... | 49 | 37 | — | — | — | — |
| Sometimes, never...... | 100% | 100% | — | — | — | — |
| High resource use.... | 37 | 43 | — | — | — | — |
| Low resource use.... | 63 | 57 | — | — | — | — |
| Neurotic symptoms | | | | | | |
| Low symptoms........ | 100% | 100% | — | — | — | — |
| High resource use.... | 65 | 46 | — | — | — | — |
| Low resource use.... | 35 | 54 | — | — | — | — |
| Medium symptoms.... | 100% | 100% | — | — | — | — |
| High resource use.... | 57 | 47 | — | — | — | — |
| Low resource use.... | 43 | 53 | — | — | — | — |
| High symptoms....... | 100% | 100% | — | — | — | — |
| High resource use.... | 50 | 44 | — | — | — | — |
| Low resource use.... | 50 | 56 | — | — | — | — |

Note: The data in Tables 47 and 48 of the source were rearranged for this table.

Source: B. Kutner, D. Fanshel, A. M. Togo, and T. S. Langner, *Five Hundred Over Sixty*
(New York: Russell Sage Foundation, 1956), Tables 47, 48, 61, 64, and 69.

the proportion seeking a regular check-up twice or more a year among all aged persons in this study was greater for those in fair or poor health than for those in excellent or good health, about half of them seldom or never submitted to such examinations.

The apathy to regular physical check-up evidenced in both the Kips Bay–Yorkville study and the 1955 survey of the NORC also appeared in the Baltimore study. In the sub-sample of the latter study selected for clinical evaluation at no cost to themselves, among those who stated to the lay interviewer that they had no disease or only minor complications, 44 per cent did not show up.[37] This lack of concern with checks on health status in both the productive and later years results in a delay of medical care until symptoms become manifest—a frequent occurrence in old age. Only an intensive educational program can promote "Individual initiative . . . in the prevention of chronic disease."

The comparisons of the younger and older persons in the 1955 survey of the NORC justify some optimism as to the effectiveness of such an educational program. The present corps of aged hardly had, in their earlier years, the favorable social and economic environment experienced now by those at the main productive ages. The background of the present aged is different not only in education but also in culture, since a large proportion are foreign-born. As those now in their prime years enter old age, many will show the conservatism of their longer years; however, they will undoubtedly carry with them the health habits built up over a lifetime. Although these health habits are very likely better than those of preceding generations, there is still much that can be learned through an effective health education program.[38]

---

[37] *Chronic Illness in a Large City, The Baltimore Study, op. cit.,* p. 412; the figure relates to persons of all ages in Evaluation Group III. In this connection, see P. N. Borsky and O. K. Sagen, "Motivations Toward Health Examinations," *American Journal of Public Health,* Vol. 49, p. 514 (April, 1959).

[38] B. Kutner, "Health Education in Senior Citizens' Programs," *American Journal of Public Health,* Vol. 48, p. 622 (May, 1958).

*Attitudes of the Aged toward the Use of Health Services.* In a random sample of aged persons surveyed by the National Opinion Research Center in the summer of 1957, 85 per cent reported an illness or health complaint during the four weeks preceding their interview, but only one third of those so affected saw a physician about it. Commenting on the findings, Bugbee stated, "Economic factors seem to be a relatively minor element in this reluctance to see a physician. It is true that most people 65 and over are retired, and that their incomes are low compared with those of the working population. Yet only three out of every 100 older people said they had delayed because of cost." No information was provided regarding the morbid conditions of those who delayed. Bugbee continues, "Perhaps another reason for failing to seek medical attention is a feeling on the part of many older people that visiting a doctor or a hospital is tantamount to acknowledging an inability to cope with the inevitable illnesses of old age."[39] In fact, delay in seeking medical treatment may be conditioned by a wide complex of cultural and emotional influences.[40] Pertinent, in this connection, is the observation by Foster: "We know that in any culture a medical institution is a response not only to physiological conditions but to emotionally based and culturally defined conditions as well, . . ."[41]

The opinions of the aged regarding the quality of the hospitals in their community are not much different from those of younger people, according to the findings of the 1955 survey of the National Opinion Research Center; about two thirds in each age category considered the hospital facilities,

[39] *Progress in Health Services,* Vol. 8, p. 6 (April, 1959), Health Information Foundation, New York.

[40] R. A. King and J. B. Leach, "Habits of Medical Care," *Cancer,* Vol. 4, p. 221 (March, 1951); J. L. Titchener *et al.,* "Problem of Delay in Seeking Surgical Care," *Journal of the American Medical Association,* Vol. 160, p. 1187 (April 7, 1956); B. Kutner, H. B. Makover, and A. Oppenheim, "Delay in the Diagnosis and Treatment of Cancer: A Critical Analysis of the Literature," *Journal of Chronic Diseases,* Vol. 7, p. 95 (February, 1958).

[41] G. M. Foster, *Problems in Intercultural Health Programs* (New York: Social Science Research Council, April, 1958), p. 20.

in general, either excellent or good. Nevertheless, a substantially larger proportion of the aged (66 per cent) than of persons at the main productive ages (40 per cent) thought that no one should go to a hospital unless there is no alternative (Table 3.14). From this, Sheatsley suggests that "the

TABLE 3.14

ATTITUDES TOWARD THE USE OF HEALTH SERVICES, UNITED STATES, 1955

| | Age | | |
|---|---|---|---|
| Attitude Question | 21 and Over | 21 to 64 | 65 and Over |
| In general, the hospital facilities in the community are | 100% | 100% | 100% |
| Excellent | 22 | 23 | 17 |
| Good | 44 | 44 | 46 |
| Fair | 17 | 18 | 14 |
| Poor | 11 | 10 | 14 |
| Don't know | 6 | 5 | 9 |
| Nobody should go to a hospital unless there is no other way to be cared for properly | 100% | 100% | 100% |
| Agree | 43 | 40 | 66 |
| Disagree | 55 | 59 | 32 |
| Don't know | 2 | 1 | 2 |
| In general, the doctor service in the community is | 100% | 100% | 100% |
| Excellent | 23 | 24 | 20 |
| Good | 46 | 46 | 50 |
| Fair | 17 | 17 | 16 |
| Poor | 10 | 9 | 10 |
| Don't know | 4 | 4 | 4 |
| To get a doctor for a home visit at night or Sunday is | 100% | 100% | 100% |
| A great deal of trouble | 24 | 25 | 23 |
| A little trouble | 20 | 20 | 17 |
| No trouble at all | 48 | 48 | 51 |
| Don't know | 8 | 7 | 9 |
| Reasons for not seeing doctor when perhaps should* | 100% | 100% | 100% |
| Didn't know good doctor | 11 | 12 | 11 |
| Didn't think he could help | 9 | 8 | 15 |
| His office was too far away | 8 | 7 | 12 |
| Regular doctor | 100% | 100% | 100% |
| Have one now | 81 | 81 | 80 |
| Used to, not now | 10 | 10 | 13 |
| Never had one | 9 | 9 | 7 |
| First started seeing present regular doctor† | 100% | 100% | 100% |
| Last year | 8 | 8 | 10 |
| 1 year ago | 8 | 8 | 8 |
| 2 years ago | 9 | 9 | 8 |

TABLE 3.14—*Continued*

| Attitude Question | Age | | |
|---|---|---|---|
| | 21 and Over | 21 to 64 | 65 and Over |
| 3–4 years ago | 13 | 13 | 11 |
| 5–9 years ago | 26 | 27 | 23 |
| 10 or more years ago | 30 | 29 | 34 |
| Never | 6 | 6 | 6 |
| Last time saw present regular doctor for own health† | 100% | 100% | 100% |
| Less than 3 months ago | 31 | 30 | 39 |
| 3–5 months ago | 13 | 13 | 12 |
| 6–11 months ago | 15 | 15 | 12 |
| 1 year ago | 15 | 16 | 14 |
| 2 or more years ago | 20 | 20 | 17 |
| Never | 6 | 6 | 6 |
| Number of different doctors seen for own health in last year | 100% | 100% | 100% |
| None | 28 | 28 | 32 |
| 1 | 47 | 47 | 47 |
| 2 | 17 | 17 | 13 |
| 3–4 | 7 | 6 | 7 |
| 5 or more | 1 | 2 | 1 |
| Gone to second doctor for opinion without telling first doctor | 100% | 100% | 100% |
| Several times | 3 | 3 | 3 |
| Once or twice | 14 | 15 | 11 |
| No, but thought of it | 8 | 8 | 6 |
| Never thought of it | 75 | 74 | 80 |
| For those seeing a doctor for a condition last year Should he have been seen sooner? | 100% | 100% | 100% |
| Yes | 23 | 23 | 19 |
| No | 76 | 76 | 78 |
| Don't know | 1 | 1 | 3 |
| Would it have made any difference if he were not seen at all? | 100% | 100% | 100% |
| Yes | 79 | 80 | 77 |
| No | 16 | 16 | 17 |
| Don't know | 5 | 4 | 6 |
| For those with a condition last year who had not seen a doctor, think now one should have been seen | 100% | 100% | 100% |
| Yes | 19 | 20 | 18 |
| No | 77 | 77 | 77 |
| Don't know | 4 | 3 | 5 |
| Reaction to doctors seen in last year | 100% | 100% | 100% |
| Entirely satisfied | 89 | 90 | 87 |
| Not too satisfied | 11 | 10 | 13 |
| Reaction to doctor's orders in last year | 100% | 100% | 100% |
| Carried out | 91 | 90 | 97 |
| Not carried out | 9 | 10 | 3 |

TABLE 3.14—*Continued*

| Attitude Question | Age | | |
|---|---|---|---|
| | 21 and Over | 21 to 64 | 65 and Over |
| Have received medical care during last year from others than regular doctors | 100% | 100% | 100% |
| Yes | 10 | 11 | 9 |
| No | 90 | 89 | 91 |
| Would see other than regular doctors for some conditions in the future | 100% | 100% | 100% |
| Yes | 22 | 22 | 19 |
| No | 73 | 73 | 74 |
| Don't know | 5 | 5 | 7 |
| Have some time seen a specialist of some kind | 100% | 100% | 100% |
| Yes | 37 | 38 | 35 |
| No | 63 | 62 | 65 |
| Should make a practice of seeing dentist regularly | 100% | 100% | 100% |
| Yes | 88 | 91 | 74 |
| Not worth trouble | 11 | 8 | 24 |
| Don't know | 1 | 1 | 2 |
| Makes a practice of seeing dentist at least once a year | 100% | 100% | 100% |
| Yes | 37 | 40 | 16 |
| No | 63 | 60 | 84 |

* Since each respondent may give more than one reason, the percentages shown are not additive. All respondents, whether or not stating a reason, are taken as 100%.

† Answered only by those who now have a regular doctor.

Source: Unpublished data from the 1955 survey by the National Opinion Research Center sponsored by the Health Information Foundation; the figures for ages 21 to 64 were computed from source data by the author.

younger generation has been educated to a more favorable attitude toward hospitals" than their elders.[42] This attitude will very likely stay with the present younger generation into their later years.

The aged also had the same high opinion as younger people of the doctors in their community, 70 per cent rating them as either excellent or good. In addition, over two thirds in each age category thought they would have little or no trouble in having a doctor visit their home at night or on a Sunday. Only one ninth of the population in each age cate-

[42] P. B. Sheatsley, "Public Attitudes Toward Hospitals," *Hospitals,* May 16, 1957, p. 48; see also E. Freidson and J. J. Feldman, *The Public Looks at Hospitals,* Research Series 4 (New York: Health Information Foundation, 1958).

gory stated that they did not know a good doctor to visit when they should perhaps have seen one. However, on such occasions, the aged were more pessimistic than younger people with regard to the good the doctor might do, for 15 per cent of the former did not go for that reason, compared with 8 per cent for the latter. Understandably, a larger proportion of the aged (12 per cent) than of younger people (7 per cent) did not go to the doctor because his office was too far away.

Four fifths of both the younger and older people in the survey reported that they had a regular doctor and most had used his services for three or more years (about 70 per cent). Almost two thirds of the aged with a regular doctor saw him within the year prior to interview;[43] on the other hand, one sixth last saw him two or more years ago. Most of the aged apparently have confidence in the physician taking care of them. Although almost one third did not see any doctor about a health problem within the year before the survey, nearly half used only one during the period. Moreover, four fifths of the aged never thought of going to a second doctor for an opinion.

It was indicated earlier that most of the aged thought they were taking the best possible care of their health. This confidence is also reflected in the finding that nearly four fifths of the aged who reported seeing a doctor for some condition in the year before interview did not believe there would have been any advantage in seeing him sooner. On the other hand, over three quarters of those experiencing an ailment during the year which was not treated by a doctor stated that they saw no advantage in such attention.[44] However, almost

---

[43] About the same proportion was found in the U.S. National Health Survey for July–September 1957; see also p. 122 of Chapter 4.

[44] According to the May–June, 1957, survey of the National Opinion Research Center, as reported in *Progress in Health Services,* Vol. 8, p. 2 (April, 1959) (published by the Health Information Foundation), among persons 65 and over mentioning a health complaint but not seeing a physician, 44 per cent regarded their complaint as minor, 27 per cent did not believe the physician could help them, 6 per cent stated they did not have the money to pay a doctor, and 22 per cent gave no reason. These findings

all who saw a doctor within the year were satisfied with his treatment and carried out his orders. Less than one tenth of the aged had medical attention from others than regular doctors within the year before interview and nearly three quarters had no intention of seeking such attention in the future.[45]

With about three fifths of the aged edentulous, according to the United States National Health Survey,[46] it is not surprising that the NORC reported that 84 per cent of the aged did not make it a practice to see a dentist at least once a year.[47] However, the proportion was also high at the main productive ages, namely 60 per cent.

The Kips Bay–Yorkville survey of the aged showed that those who worry about their health all or most of the time make greater use of health services than those not so worrisome, irrespective of their actual health status (Table 3.13). However, among both the worrisome and the nonworrisome, the cases with fair or poor health status made greater use of health resources than those in excellent or good health. It is also interesting to find, in this survey, that among persons in excellent or good health, the proportion making a high use of health resources is greatest among those with low neurotic symptoms and least with high symptoms. Also, for those in excellent or good health, greater use was made than by persons of like neurotic status who were in fair or poor health. Furthermore, the extent of neurotic symptoms had little bearing on the use of health resources by those in fair or poor health.

---

relate to health complaints during a four-week period preceding the interview. Those with a health complaint who did not go for treatment constituted four fifths of all who did not see a doctor during this period.

[45] Pertinent, in this connection, is the finding in a local survey that the proportion of illnesses treated by nonmedical personnel is the greatest in the least favored social class; see E. L. Koos, *The Health of Regionville* (New York: Columbia University Press, 1954), chap. vi.

[46] U.S. National Health Survey, *Preliminary Report on Volume of Dental Care, United States, July–September 1957,* Public Health Service, Washington, D.C., March, 1958, Table D; see also page 128 of Chapter 4.

[47] E. Freidson and J. J. Feldman, *The Public Looks at Dental Care,* Research Series 6 (New York: Health Information Foundation, 1958), p. 6.

There is a possibility that the unmarried may express their desire for social contacts by an undue use of health services. Thus, in a small sample of aged persons of low social economic status in Boston, it was observed that those not married made a greater use of health services than the married, irrespective of health status.[48]

*The Role of Religion.*  In many individuals, reactions to health problems may be influenced by their religious attitudes. Barron suggests that:

Religion's gerontological task is essentially four-fold: (*a*) to help face impending death; (*b*) to help find and maintain a sense of meaningfulness and significance in life; (*c*) to help accept the inevitable losses of old age; and (*d*) to help discover and utilize the compensatory values that are potential in old age.[49]

With this goal, there is posed the question whether attitudes toward religion change with age and with one's state of health.[50]

---

[48] L. DiCicco and D. Apple, *op. cit.*

[49] M. L. Barron, "The Role of Religion and Religious Institutions in Creating the Milieu of Older People," *Organized Religion and the Older Person* (ed. D. L. Scudder) (Gainesville: University of Florida Press, 1958), p. 14; see also *The Aging of Three Parishes,* National Conference of Catholic Charities, Washington, D.C., and the detailed report of each parish.

[50] N. K. Covalt, "The Meaning of Religion to Older People—The Medical Perspective," *Organized Religion and the Older Person, op. cit.,* p. 78.

# Medical Care Utilization by the Aged

4

THE UTILIZATION of medical services in a community depends not only upon the health status and health attitudes of its population but, obviously, also upon the quantity, quality, and distribution of local medical resources. The aged are particularly affected in this regard by the fluid state of organization of their medical care in the light of continuing experiment. Since these developments are necessarily patterned to suit local needs and resources, and the approaches taken are therefore varied, they will be described only by a few broad generalizations.[1]

## MEDICAL SERVICES FOR THE AGED

Prevention, diagnosis, treatment, and rehabilitation constitute the elements of medical care at all ages. However, special medical problems are introduced in each of these elements at the older ages because of the high prevalence of chronic illness and the frequent presence of physical impairments that produce complications on the occurrence of acute illness. Whereas preventive measures are generally regarded as steps to eliminate disease, in the middle and later years they also encompass efforts to delay or even forestall physical deterioration when a chronic condition is present.[2] Prob-

---

[1] For other countries, see R. J. van Zonneveld, "Public Health and the Aged in Europe: Research and Programs," *Journal of Gerontology*, Vol. 13 (supplement to the April, 1958 issue), p. 68.

[2] D. Seegal and A. R. Wertheim, "Progress in Control of Chronic Disease," *Public Health Reports*, Vol. 73, p. 971 (November, 1958).

lems of diagnosis and treatment become much more complex,[3] and the primary purpose of rehabilitation is to restore the aged person to a point where he can at least take care of his personal needs.[4]

Emphasis on home care for the aged is found generally in discussions of their medical care problems, and local demonstrations have illustrated "the potentialities of visiting nurse services, homemaker services, housekeeper services, and home medical care programs as means to continued normal community living for the handicapped and the aged; and as ways of reducing hospital, nursing home, and clinic loads."[5] However, where the medical care needs of the aged have reached an advanced stage, the same demonstrations showed "the importance of integrating home, nursing home, general hospital, chronic disease facility, and outpatient clinic services in order to achieve continuity of care for the individual as appropriate to his changing needs." This concept is also contained in the recommendations of the Conference on the Care of Patients with Long-Term Illness,[6] and in the American Hospital Association Program for Care of Chronically Ill and Aged.[7]

*The Hospital.* Medical care for the aged, according to their needs and availability of services, is provided in general hospitals, chronic-disease hospitals, mental institutions, and tuberculosis hospitals.[8] Traditionally, the general hos-

---

[3] F. D. Zeman, "Recent Contributions to the Medical Problems of Old Age," *New England Journal of Medicine,* Vol. 257, p. 369 (August 22, 1957).

[4] Reference to some studies of the rehabilitation potential of the disabled aged is made by E. M. Snyder, *Public Assistance Recipients in New York State, January–February, 1957,* Interdepartmental Committee on Low Incomes, State of New York, October, 1958, p. 63.

[5] J. E. Cannon and E. L. Richie, *Community Views of Chronic Illness and Aging Problems and Needs,* Colorado State Department of Public Health, Denver, December 1, 1956.

[6] Sponsored by the American Hospital Association and the Public Health Service, Chicago, May 7–9, 1958.

[7] Approved by the Board of Trustees of the American Hospital Association, February, 1959.

[8] Commission on Chronic Illness, *Care of the Long-Term Patient,* Vol. II (Cambridge, Mass.: Harvard University Press, 1956), pp. 186–98.

pital is designed to care for the patient with a short-term illness or requiring surgery. Most of the chronic-disease hospitals are located in large urban centers and have as their function the care of the long-term patient. However, since many such patients suffer acute episodes of illness or have a need for surgery, the chronic-disease hospital is either under pressure to develop some facilities of the general hospital or to ally itself with one. This trend and the rapidly growing numbers with chronic illness have led some general hospitals to allocate part of their services to long-term patients.[9] Expanding in this way, by either allocating separate wings or beds to chronic-disease patients, the general hospital is able to serve better the medical needs of its community. Impetus to provide facilities for the long-term patients was given by the 1954 amendment to the Hill-Burton program originally enacted in August, 1946.[10]

Increasing hospital costs have stimulated studies for possible savings, many of which relate directly to the management of the patient. In particular, study is being given to the feasibility of organizing hospital services so that they may be adapted to suit the individual medical and nursing needs of the patient.[11] To the aged patient in a chronic-disease facility attached to a general hospital, a program of graduated care ensures service adapted to his current needs and with

---

[9] The situation facing municipal hospitals in New York City is described by H. A. Rusk, J. E. Silson, J. Novey, and M. M. Dacso in *Hospital Patient Survey*, The New York Foundation, July, 1956: "In brief, a very large number of patients in the municipal hospital system are elderly individuals suffering from chronic diseases of long duration. . . . On completion of their treatment . . . their re-integration into the community becomes a major problem. Many of these patients therefore remain in the hospital after they are otherwise ready for discharge."

[10] L. M. Abbe and A. M. Baney, *The Nation's Health Facilities, Ten Years of the Hill-Burton Hospital and Medical Facilities Program, 1946–1956,* Public Health Service, Department of Health, Education, and Welfare, Washington, D.C., 1958.

[11] J. C. Haldeman and F. G. Abdellah, "Concepts of Progressive Patient Care," *Hospitals,* Vol. 33, pp. 38 and 41 (May 16 and June 1, 1959); T. P. Weil and B. R. Cohen, "The Experience of a Hospital-Convalescent Center Relationship," *American Journal of Public Health,* Vol. 49, p. 778 (June, 1959).

due consideration to costs. Closely integrated with a scheme of graduated care within the hospital, arrangement could be made for a home care program.

*Home Care Programs.* Although semblances of organized home care programs for medical services are found in early records of the country, intensive efforts to promote such programs date from World War II.[12] This new development was spurred by the high costs of hospital care, the crowding of hospitals with long-term patients, the deleterious effects of lengthy hospital stay upon the patient, and the advantages of care in an accustomed family environment for those whose medical condition is suited to it.[13]

For the most part, home care programs were organized by hospitals to meet the needs of their indigent and medically indigent patients who no longer require the full battery of hospital services. According to the Commission on Chronic Illness, ". . . an organized home care program must have these essential characteristics: centralized responsibility for administration; coordination of services and resources; and the development and use of the patient care team to deal with the health needs of the patient." The hospital thus continues its medical supervision of the patient in his home by arranging for visits by a medical care team and by furnishing medicine, certain sickroom supplies and hospital equipment, laboratory tests, nursing, and rehabilitation.[14] The medical care team may consist of medical specialists, visiting nurses, therapists, social workers, and housekeepers.[15] Whenever

---

[12] Commission on Chronic Illness, Vol. II, *op. cit.,* pp. 63–81.

[13] E. J. Munter and M. Berke, "The Care of the Long-Term Patient: A Review of the Administration of Present Programs," *Journal of Chronic Diseases,* Vol. 7, p. 144 (February, 1958); *Aged Home Care Patients in New York City: Housing and Related Facilities Needed,* Bureau of Research and Statistics, New York State Division of Housing, Albany, N.Y., July, 1958, p. 26.

[14] *Organized "Home Care" Programs in the United States,* Council on Medical Service, American Medical Association, Chicago, December, 1956.

[15] W. H. Stewart, M. Y. Pennell, and L. M. Smith, *Homemaker Services in the United States, 1958,* Public Health Service Publication No. 644, Washington, D.C., 1958; M. Y. Pennell and L. M. Smith, "Characteristics of Families Served by Homemakers," *American Journal of Public Health,* Vol. 49, p. 1467 (November, 1959).

necessary, the patient is returned to the hospital. Experimentation is continuing with the home care program, one approach being to admit the patient directly to its service from the clinic without the requirement of a hospital stay.[16] Most of the patients on home care are aged persons.

Because of their success, the Commission on Chronic Illness states that:

Home care programs organized to provide auxiliary services to the private physician offer the most effective method yet devised for bringing to long-term patients at home and to their families the coordinated services required. Up to now they have usually been limited to only a few physicians in a community and for their needy patients. The experience of these programs should be utilized to devise ways to bring integrated auxiliary services to any physician for persons in all economic groups.

A home care program for all categories of patients, from the indigent to the private paying his own way, has been operating at the Reddy Memorial Hospital in Montreal, Canada, since 1950.[17] This arrangement, of course, does not preclude the development of special home care programs tailored to the needs of private patients.[18]

A simplified variant of the home care program has been experimented with; it provides visiting nurse service at home after early discharge of patients whose only further hospital need is for nursing attention.[19] The patient has the advantage of appraisal of his nursing needs before discharge, his home environment, and a reduction in his medical care

---

[16] M. Fraenkel, "Hospital-Home Care for the Aging," *Services for the Aging* (ed. I. L. Webber) (Gainesville: University of Florida Press, 1957), p. 86; H. E. Markley and J. Brauntuch, "How Home Care Works in a City of 48,000," *Hospitals*, Vol. 32, p. 35 (June 1, 1958).

[17] Hospital Council of Greater New York, *Organized Home Medical Care in New York City*, (Cambridge, Mass.: Harvard University Press, 1956), p. 41.

[18] P. Rogatz and G. M. Crocetti, "Home Care Programs—Their Impact on the Hospital's Role in Medical Care," *American Journal of Public Health*, Vol. 48, p. 1125 (September, 1958).

[19] *Report of a Study Concerning the Feasibility of Providing Visiting Nurse Service Following Hospitalization for Blue Cross Subscribers*, Associated Hospital Service of New York, 1957.

costs. By this procedure, the hospital increases the availability of its facilities for the more urgent cases.[20]

*Nursing Homes.* The rapidly evolving system of medical care in the United States has recently brought to the fore nursing homes and allied facilities that cater primarily to the aged. Also contributing to the development of these institutions is the increasing availability of cash incomes to the aged, principally from social insurance and related programs, public assistance, and private pensions.

The nursing home provides a measure of medical and nursing care to the long-term patient who, while not needing or perhaps not having access to the intensive and costly care of the hospital, does require more care than can be had in his home. Although precise lines of distinction may sometimes be hard to draw, nursing homes are distinguished from the custodial or domiciliary care homes for the aged on the basis of the level of care provided. Thus skilled nursing homes provide not only residential and personal care, but more particularly services for the chronically ill, convalescent, infirm, or disabled, by professional or practical nurses who can administer treatment ordered by a physician.[21]

Nursing homes are operated under public, proprietary, and nonprofit voluntary auspices.[22] Although every state licenses and regulates its nursing homes, their variation in quality from excellent to poor has led to proposed standards of care.[23] It is generally required that each patient in a

---

[20] A proposal for home care for those who "neither require hospitalization, nor are . . . at the same time capable of the minimal ambulation necessary for continuing care as outpatients" is described by A. Feigenbaum and B. Kutner, "Hospital Based Pre-Hospitalization Home Care," *Journal of Chronic Diseases,* Vol. 9, p. 405 (April, 1959).

[21] J. Solon and A. M. Baney, "Inventory of Nursing Homes and Related Facilities," *Public Health Reports,* Vol. 69, p. 1121 (December, 1954).

[22] F. R. Brown, "Nursing Homes: Public and Private Financing of Care Today," *Social Security Bulletin,* May, 1958.

[23] *Standards of Care for Older People in Institutions,* National Committee on the Aging of the National Social Welfare Assembly, New York, Sections I and II, 1953; Section III, 1954. See also *The Aged and Aging in the United States: A National Problem* (Hearings before the Subcommittee on Problems of the Aged and Aging, U.S. Senate, 86th Cong., 2d sess., 1960), p. 131.

nursing home be under the supervision of a physician and highly desirable that one be available on emergency call. The Commission on Chronic Illness "believes that development of these institutions as elements of general hospitals is one of the best ways of raising standards, and recommends this arrangement. When outright affiliation is impossible, a close and active working relationship should be maintained."[24] Either of these connections would bring the patients of the nursing home within easy reach of the specialized facilities of the general hospital.[25]

The statement of the Commission on Chronic Illness was included, in substance, among the recommendations of the first National Conference on Nursing Homes and Homes for the Aged.[26] Regarding the medical care of the patient, the Conference recommended that each patient be under continuous supervision of a personal physician, that he receive a medical evaluation near the time of his admission, that the personal physician ascertain the frequency of his visits, and that the home maintain a definite program for providing medical care to its patients. The latter would include arrangements for transfer to hospitals.[27] It was also recommended that each nursing home appoint a principal medical adviser on its problems who could also act in emergencies in the absence of the personal physician.

On the basis of a survey made in 1954, the Public Health Service estimated that there were then about 7,000 skilled nursing homes with about 180,000 beds.[28] In addition, there

[24] Commission on Chronic Illness, Vol. II, *op. cit.*, p. 198.

[25] J. Solon and A. M. Baney, *General Hospitals and Nursing Homes,* Public Health Monograph No. 44, Public Health Service, Washington, D.C., 1956, p. 10.

[26] *National Conference on Nursing Homes and Homes for the Aged, February 25–28, 1958, Washington, D.C.,* Public Health Service Publication No. 625, Washington, D.C., 1958.

[27] See *Guides for Medical Care in Nursing Homes and Related Facilities,* prepared jointly by the American Nursing Home Association and the Council on Medical Service of the American Medical Association, June, 1959.

[28] As of January, 1959, there were 245,831 skilled nursing home beds, of which almost half were regarded as unsatisfactory; a need was expressed for

are about 2,000 custodial or domiciliary homes with 80,000 beds and providing skilled nursing only as an adjunct to its personal care.[29] These are exclusive of another 16,000 homes with 190,000 beds that provide only personal care or shelter with a minimum of medical care. The average age of those living in these various types of homes is 80 years, and two thirds are women. It has been estimated that the nursing home care provided averages four days per aged person annually in the general population.[30]

Although the need for more nursing homes is generally recognized, the only estimate of the volume of possible referrals was made from a survey of physicians in Pennsylvania.[31] Encouragement for the construction of nursing homes was given in the 1954 amendment to the Hill-Burton program, which made provision for nonprofit institutions, and by the Small Business Administration for financing proprietary institutions.

*Homes for the Aged.* Private boarding homes, voluntary homes, and public homes for the aged, commonly classed as custodial or domiciliary care homes, vary widely in the medical care they provide. Although some may provide only a minimum of care, if any at all, the high incidence of morbidity among the aged has led to the establishment of infirmaries in an increasing number of such homes for the treatment of minor and temporary conditions.[32] Arrangements are

---

an additional 252,000 by L. M. Abbe, "Hospitals and Nursing Homes in the United States, 1959," *Public Health Reports,* Vol. 74, p. 1089 (December, 1959).

[29] J. Solon, D. W. Roberts, D. E. Krueger, and A. M. Baney, *Nursing Homes, Their Patients and Their Care,* Public Health Monograph No. 46, Public Health Service, Washington, D.C., 1957, p. 53.

[30] A. W. Brewster, "Care in Nursing Homes Through Prepayment Hospital Plans," *Research and Statistics Note No. 41,* Division of Program Research, Social Security Administration, November 25, 1958.

[31] I. Altman, "The Need for Certain Types of Medical Facilities in Pennsylvania as Estimated by Physicians," *The Pennsylvania Medical Journal,* Vol. 60, p. 1346 (October, 1957).

[32] E. E. Nicholson, *Planning New Institutional Facilities for Long-Term Care* (New York: G. P. Putnam's Sons, 1956), p. 64.

usually made to have a physician ready to call when needed.[33]

**Mental Hospitals.** Although about half of all hospital beds in the country are in mental and allied institutions (largely under state or local government control), the need for more such beds is evidenced by large waiting lists and by the rate at which new hospitals are being filled. This pressure upon available facilities is created not only by the aging of the population, but also by a greater readiness to accept the services of the mental hospital. Notwithstanding problems created by crowding and a shortage of trained personnel, the trend in the mental hospital is increasingly toward rehabilitation of the patient rather than custodial care, so that he can take his place in society. This trend is being facilitated by the introduction of tranquilizing drugs, which has made it possible to release patients to the care of private physicians or for treatment in outpatient clinics. Another important consequence, from the point of view of cost, has been to reduce the average length of hospital stay.

The mental hospitals are also adapting their services to suit the needs of their patients by experimenting with both "day" and "night" hospitals. In the former, the patient requiring something between full-time hospital care and outpatient clinic care goes home every night. The night hospital patient sleeps and receives treatment there each night, but enters community life during the day.

Although the mental hospital has by far the largest burden in caring for the mentally ill of the country, there are many other provisions for their institutional care.[34] Thus, the Commission on Chronic Illness states that, "Not all mental patients needing institutional care require care in a spe-

---

[33] *Standards of Care for Older People in Institutions, op. cit.,* Section I, pp. 33–35, and Section III, pp. 84–86. See also *Guides for Medical Care in Nursing Homes and Related Facilities, op. cit.*

[34] *State Programs for the Aging, A Review of the Problem and of Recent Action in the States,* Council of State Governments, Chicago, December, 1956, pp. 22, 23.

cial mental institution. For many of these patients the general hospital offering psychiatric services represents the appropriate source of care."[35] Furthermore, "Some long-term mental patients—the patients whose behavior has reached a safe social level—can be adequately cared for in a carefully selected protective setting at home, in foster homes, or in public or private nursing homes provided psychiatric supervision is available." There is also the advantage of more economic care.

*Other Services.*   Although, at any one time, most aged persons are not receiving any of the forms of care just described, a great many are using the services of the private physician either at home or in his office no differently than younger persons.[36] The aged ambulatory person may also be using, as the occasion calls for, any of the diagnostic, treatment, or rehabilitation clinics in the community available to the rest of the population. Within recent years, a few hospitals have established geriatric clinics as outpatient services primarily for the aged medically indigent person.[37] In these clinics, a team of medical and allied specialists acts as a unit in assessing the psychological, social, and economic needs of the aged person, in addition to studying his medical problems. This co-ordinated approach has as its purpose the rehabilitation of the aged person with a medical problem to his greatest potential. The advantage claimed for the geriatric clinic over the general medical clinic is twofold. First, the team in the geriatric clinic gains a special experience in handling the problems of the aged. Second, the aged person is not faced with the possibility of preferential attention given the younger patients in the general medical clinic. There is,

---

[35] Commission on Chronic Illness, Vol. II, *op. cit.,* p. 216.

[36] The problems involved in making dental services available to institutionalized and homebound aged persons are being studied in two local areas in cooperation with the Division of Dental Public Health, United States Public Health Service; see *Proceedings of the First National Conference of the Joint Council to Improve the Health Care of the Aged,* Chicago, 1959, pp. 115 and 158.

[37] S. Gertman, "The Geriatric Clinic as a New Form of Medical Service," *Services for the Aging, op. cit.,* p. 37.

further, a likelihood that ambulatory care in a geriatric clinic may reduce the need for hospital bed care. However, the role of the geriatric clinic has been questioned on the grounds that it produces an unnecessary specialization in the care of the older person and that older persons generally prefer not to attend centers identified only with the aged.[38]

With the rapid development of the many kinds of medical care programs for those with chronic illness, a need has grown in the larger communities for a central referral agency to which physicians and patients may turn for information regarding the services and facilities that may be available. To meet this need, chronic-illness information centers have been established in several communities. These also act as consultants to the operators of such facilities on matters of standards of care, procedures, and costs. Some of these centers act as co-ordinators on chronic-illness problems within the community.[39]

## UTILIZATION OF MEDICAL CARE SERVICES

Data describing the utilization of medical care services by the aged are even more fragmentary than data regarding their morbidity. For the most part, the available data are concerned with hospital utilization. There are some data regarding the use of physicians' services, a little on surgery, very little on dental care and on nursing home care, and practically none on home care. Such data as do exist must be interpreted with regard to the populations to which they relate and the circumstances under which they were collected.

---

[38] R. T. Monroe, "The Mechanisms of the Geriatric Clinic and Its Place in the Community," *The New England Journal of Medicine,* Vol. 258, p. 882 (May 1, 1958). The issues involved in creating geriatric clinics are discussed further by J. T. Freeman in a letter to the editor of *The New England Journal of Medicine,* Vol. 259, p. 197 (July 24, 1958).

[39] Council on Medical Service, "Chronic Illness Information Centers," *Journal of the American Medical Association,* Vol. 169, p. 1763 (April 11, 1959). Liaison activities are also emphasized in the "Guide for State and Local Committees of Hospital Associations on Care of Chronically Ill and Aged," approved by the Board of Trustees of the American Hospital Association, February, 1959.

In particular, these data by themselves give little, if any, direct evidence of the extent to which medical care services are over- or underutilized. On this score, evidence must be sought from other sources. Thus, there are indications that hospital stay may be prolonged because of an inadequate housing situation.[40]

*The Hospital Population.* According to a hospital census taken by the American Medical Association in 1953, on the day of reporting there were 1,267,600 patients of which 259,100, or one fifth, were at ages 65 and over (Table 4.1). The rate at which the general population was then hospitalized was 20 per 1,000 at ages 65 and over, compared with 8 per 1,000 at all ages. The heavy burden of this hospital load is borne by the mental institutions, these accounting for half of the aged patients. On the day of the census, almost three eighths of the aged patients were in general hospitals and one eighth in various other types of hospitals.

The findings of the American Medical Association with regard to confinement in nervous and mental institutions is borne out by the 1950 census of population (Table 2.2). At that time, the aged population institutionalized in mental hospitals constituted a little over 1 per cent of the total aged; the percentage was greater at ages 75 and over than at ages 65–74 years. The total number of persons at ages 65 and over in institutions then constituted 3.1 per cent of the total population in that period of life. Of those institutionalized, 56 per cent were in homes for the aged and nursing homes, 37 per cent in mental hospitals (principally under state or local support), and the rest in chronic-disease hospitals, tuberculosis hospitals, and correctional and other institutions.[41]

*Hospitalization—Population Experience.* Data regarding the hospitalization experience of the general population are usually gathered by surveys. As such, they have most of the limitations found in morbidity survey data, particularly

---

[40] H. A. Rusk, J. E. Silson, J. Novey, and M. M. Dacso, *op. cit.*

[41] J. Fisher, "Trends in Institutional Care of the Aged," *Social Security Bulletin,* October, 1953.

TABLE 4.1

HOSPITAL PATIENTS AT ALL AGES AND AT AGES 65 AND OVER ON "DAY OF REPORTING" TO THE AMERICAN MEDICAL ASSOCIATION,* UNITED STATES,1953

| Status | All Ages | | | Ages 65 and Over | | |
|---|---|---|---|---|---|---|
| | Both Sexes | Males | Fe-males | Both Sexes | Males | Fe-males |
| | Basic Data, Thousands | | | | | |
| Number of patients†... | 1,267.6 | 674.6 | 593.0 | 259.1 | 130.6 | 128.5 |
| U.S. population, 1953.. | 159,629 | 79,354 | 80,274 | 13,324 | 6,236 | 7,088 |
| Patients per 1,000 population............. | 7.94 | 8.50 | 7.39 | 19.45 | 20.94 | 18.13 |
| | Hospitals Classified by Type of Service, Per Cent | | | | | |
| All types............. | 100.0 | 100.0 | 100.0 | 100.0 | 100.0 | 100.0 |
| General............ | 41.0 | 39.6 | 42.7 | 36.5 | 37.7 | 35.3 |
| Nervous and mental. | 48.2 | 48.2 | 48.3 | 50.9 | 47.9 | 54.1 |
| Tuberculosis........ | 5.7 | 7.0 | 4.3 | 3.0 | 4.3 | 1.7 |
| Convalescent and rest | .7 | .7 | .7 | 1.8 | 1.6 | 2.0 |
| Institutions......... | 1.2 | 1.6 | .7 | 3.1 | 3.9 | 2.4 |
| All other........... | 3.2 | 2.9 | 3.3 | 4.6 | 4.6 | 4.5 |
| | Hospitals Classified by Type of Control, Per Cent | | | | | |
| All types............. | 100.0 | 100.0 | 100.0 | 100.0 | 100.0 | 100.0 |
| Veterans Administration............. | 8.4 | 15.6 | .3 | 3.5 | 6.9 | .1 |
| Other federal....... | 4.2 | 6.8 | 1.4 | .6 | 1.0 | .1 |
| State.............. | 46.0 | 43.2 | 49.1 | 49.3 | 46.4 | 52.2 |
| County........... | 6.5 | 6.5 | 6.5 | 9.5 | 10.7 | 8.3 |
| City.............. | 3.9 | 3.9 | 3.9 | 5.3 | 6.0 | 4.6 |
| City—County...... | .7 | .7 | .8 | 1.1 | 1.4 | .9 |
| Church............. | 12.7 | 9.6 | 16.1 | 11.8 | 10.7 | 12.8 |
| Nonprofit......... | 14.6 | 11.5 | 18.1 | 15.1 | 13.8 | 16.4 |
| Other nongovernmental.............. | 3.0 | 2.2 | 3.8 | 3.8 | 3.1 | 4.6 |

* Based on data for the "day of reporting" of 6,539 of the 6,840 registered hospitals by the American Medical Association. Maternity cases are included.
  † Includes an estimate for 301 nonreplying hospitals.
  Source: F. G. Dickinson, "Age and Sex Distribution of Hospital Patients," Bulletin 97, Bureau of Medical Economic Research, American Medical Association, Chicago, 1955.

the difficulties due to the memory factor.[42] Secondly, they miss persons living alone who were hospitalized at the time of the survey. Lastly, they systematically understate the actual situation because they generally exclude persons who were hospitalized during the survey period but died before the survey date.[43] The understatement becomes of increasing significance with advance in age because of the rise in mortality. Adjustments for this understatement were made in reporting on a survey conducted in March, 1952 for the calendar year 1951. Such adjustments have not yet been made in reports on a hospitalization survey for the year ending September, 1956, and reports by the National Health Survey program for July, 1957–June, 1958; the results of these are presented in Tables 4.2 and 4.3.[44]

The data from the National Health Survey program in Table 4.2 relate to members in interviewed households who were discharged from the hospital during the year prior to the time of interview, which fell within the period July, 1957–June, 1958. This survey covers only the noninstitutional population and therefore relates only to the experience, in general, of short-stay hospitals; it therefore excludes patients discharged from psychiatric, tuberculosis and other long-stay institutions. The unit of count is the number of hospital discharges, which is greater than the number of persons discharged since one person may have several episodes of hospital stay during the year.

---

[42] B. S. Sanders, "How Good Are Hospital Data from a Household Survey?" *American Journal of Public Health,* Vol. 49, p. 1596 (December, 1959).

[43] I. S. Falk and A. W. Brewster, "Hospitalization Insurance and Hospital Utilization Among Aged Persons: March 1952 Survey," *Social Security Bulletin,* November, 1952; B. M. Siegel, N. B. Belloc, and F. E. Hesse, "Household Surveys for Hospital Planning: Adjustments for Decedents Missed," *Public Health Reports,* Vol. 72, p. 989 (November, 1957); *Health in California,* Department of Public Health, State of California, Berkeley, 1957, p. 30; and *Hospitalization Insurance for OASDI Beneficiaries,* Report submitted to the Committee on Ways and Means by the Secretary of Health, Education, and Welfare, Washington, D.C., April 3, 1959, pp. 20, 78, and 101.

[44] For sake of comparability, the data for 1951 in Table 4.3 are not adjusted for understatement.

# TABLE 4.2

GENERAL HOSPITAL EXPERIENCE OF NONINSTITUTIONAL POPULATION AC-
CORDING TO RACE, FAMILY INCOME, RESIDENCE, AND GEOGRAPHIC LOCATION,
BY SEX. ALL AGES AND AGES 65 AND OVER, UNITED STATES; PATIENTS DIS-
CHARGED WITHIN YEAR PRIOR TO HOUSEHOLD INTERVIEW DURING
JULY, 1957–JUNE, 1958

| Characteristic | All Ages | | | Ages 65 and Over | | |
|---|---|---|---|---|---|---|
| | Both Sexes | Males | Females | Both Sexes | Males | Females |
| **All persons** | | | | | | |
| Discharges per 1,000 population per year. | 99. | 74. | 123. | 121. | 122. | 120. |
| Ages 65–74 | — | — | — | 119. | 121. | 118. |
| Ages 75 and over | — | — | — | 124. | 123. | 125. |
| Average days stay per case | 8.6 | 11. | 7.2 | 14.7 | 15.8 | 13.8 |
| Ages 65–74 | — | — | — | 14.3 | 15.8 | 12.8 |
| Ages 75 and over | — | — | — | 15.6 | 15.8 | 15.5 |
| Average days stay per person per year.... | .85 | .81 | .89 | 1.78 | 1.93 | 1.65 |
| Ages 65–74 | — | — | — | 1.7 | 1.92 | 1.5 |
| Ages 75 and over | — | — | — | 1.93 | 1.95 | 1.92 |
| **Race** | | | | | | |
| Discharges per 1,000 population per year | | | | | | |
| White | 103. | 79. | 128. | 126. | 127. | 125. |
| Nonwhite | 68. | 46. | 83. | 56. | 63. | 50. |
| Average days stay per case | | | | | | |
| White | 8.4 | 10.6 | 7.2 | 14.8 | 15.9 | 13.8 |
| Nonwhite | 10.2 | 16.5 | 7.2 | 12.2 | 12.4 | 12. |
| **Family income** | | | | | | |
| Discharges per 1,000 population per year | | | | | | |
| Under $2,000 | 93. | — | — | 110. | — | — |
| $2,000–$3,999 | 104. | — | — | 135. | — | — |
| $4,000–$6,999 | 101. | — | — | 114. | — | — |
| $7,000 and over | 98. | — | — | 162. | — | — |
| Unknown | 95. | — | — | 103. | — | — |
| Average days stay per case | | | | | | |
| Under $2,000 | 11.7 | — | — | 14.8 | — | — |
| $2,000–$3,999 | 8.5 | — | — | 13.4 | — | — |
| $4,000–$6,999 | 7.2 | — | — | 15.2 | — | — |
| $7,000 and over | 7.9 | — | — | 15.7 | — | — |
| Unknown | 12.2 | — | — | 15.8 | — | — |
| **Residence** | | | | | | |
| Discharges per 1,000 population per year | | | | | | |
| Urban | 101. | 76. | 124. | 121. | 123. | 120. |
| Rural nonfarm | 104. | 77. | 131. | 131. | 134. | 127. |
| Rural farm | 81. | 63. | 101. | 102. | 96. | 110. |
| Average days stay per case | | | | | | |
| Urban | 8.9 | 11.1 | 7.7 | 15.9 | 17.1 | 14.9 |
| Rural nonfarm | 7.7 | 10.4 | 6.2 | 12.3 | 13.2 | 11.4 |
| Rural farm | 8.7 | 11.6 | 6.8 | 13.3 | 15.2 | 11.5 |
| **Region** | | | | | | |
| Discharges per 1,000 population per year | | | | | | |
| Northeast | 97. | — | — | 107. | — | — |
| North Central | 105. | — | — | 128. | — | — |
| South | 96. | — | — | 125. | — | — |
| West | 100. | — | — | 121. | — | — |
| Average days stay per case | | | | | | |
| Northeast | 9.4 | — | — | 16.5 | — | — |
| North Central | 9.0 | — | — | 16.4 | — | — |
| South | 7.8 | — | — | 11.1 | — | — |
| West | 7.5 | — | — | 15. | — | — |

Source: U.S. National Health Survey, *Hospitalization: Patients Discharged from Short-Stay Hospitals, United States, July 1957–June 1958*, Public Health Service, Washington, D.C., December, 1958.

TABLE 4.3

GENERAL HOSPITAL EXPERIENCE OF NONINSTITUTIONAL POPULATION BY AGE AND SEX, UNITED STATES; YEAR ENDING SEPTEMBER, 1956 AND CALENDAR YEAR 1951

| Age | Persons Hospital-ized per 1,000 Popula-tion per Year | Annual Hospital Admissions per Person Hospitalized | Average Days Stay per Hos-pitalized Per-son per Year | | Average Days Stay per Person per Year | |
|---|---|---|---|---|---|---|
| | | | Total | Exclud-ing Days after 60th | Total | Exclud-ing Days after 60th |
| Males: Year Ending September, 1956 | | | | | | |
| All ages............ | 65 | 1.17 | — | — | — | — |
| Under 14........ | 54 | 1.11 | 6.1 | — | .33 | — |
| 14–64............ | 64 | 1.17 | 12.5 | 11.5 | .80 | .74 |
| 65 and over...... | 108 | 1.30 | 20.5 | 15.0 | 2.21 | 1.72 |
| 65–69.......... | 79 | 1.67 | 30.6 | — | 2.41 | — |
| 70–74.......... | 102 | 1.30 | 15.2 | — | 1.55 | — |
| 75 and over.... | 122 | 1.30 | 21.2 | — | 2.58 | — |
| Females: Year Ending September, 1956 | | | | | | |
| All ages............ | 107 | 1.16 | — | — | — | — |
| Under 14........ | 43 | 1.12 | 5.3 | — | .23 | — |
| 14–64............ | 137 | 1.16 | 7.7 | 7.4 | 1.05 | 1.02 |
| 65 and over...... | 92 | 1.21 | 14.6 | 14.1 | 1.35 | 1.30 |
| 65–69.......... | 85 | 1.14 | 13.7 | — | 1.17 | — |
| 70–74.......... | 88 | 1.22 | 13.7 | — | 1.20 | — |
| 75 and over.... | 102 | 1.27 | 16.3 | — | 1.66 | — |
| Ages 65 and Over: Calendar Year 1951 | | | | | | |
| Males............ | 73 | — | 25.2 | 18.4 | 1.84 | 1.34 |
| Females.......... | 61 | — | 24.3 | 19.4 | 1.48 | 1.18 |

Source: A. W. Brewster, "Hospital Utilization by Persons Insured and Uninsured in September 1956," *Research and Statistics Note No. 19,* Division of Program Research, Social Security Administration, June 23, 1958.

At ages 65 and over, the annual rate of hospital discharge was 121 per 1,000 persons, compared with 99 per 1,000 at all ages. The discharge rates tend to rise with advance in age in the terminal years, but are not much different for the two sexes. The duration of hospital stay averaged 14.7 days for the aged and 8.6 days for all persons. For aged males, the average stay was two days longer than for aged females, being 15.8 and 13.8 days respectively. At ages 75 and over, the average stay was 15.6 days, more than one day greater than for ages 65–74 years. When the days of hospital stay are related to all persons in the population, and not only those discharged, the average length of stay per person 65 and over is 1.78 days, over twice the average of .85 days for all ages. Within the later years, the average length of hospital stay per person tends to rise with advance in age. This aspect of hospitalization will be referred to in greater detail in a later section.

Among the aged, the rate of hospital utilization by the nonwhite population is far below that for the white population. Thus, the hospital discharge rates at ages 65 and over were only 56 per 1,000 for nonwhite persons, less than half the rate for white persons. Also, the average duration of hospital stay was only 12.2 days for the nonwhites, compared with 14.8 days for the whites. These differences between the races may reflect, in considerable degree, not only the effect of the lower income level of the nonwhites and their high concentration in the rural South, but also such significant social factors as level of education, traditions, and culture. With improvement in the social-economic status of the nonwhites, their hospital utilization may approach that of the white population.

According to the findings of the National Health Survey program, the rate of hospital utilization among the aged was greatest in the highest income bracket, namely $7,000 and over. For this category, the annual discharge rate was 162 per 1,000 and the average stay 15.7 days; it will be recalled that for all aged persons the rate was 121 per 1,000 and the average stay was 14.7 days. Income variations may also be reflected in the pattern according to place of residence. The hospital discharge rate for the aged was lowest in rural farm areas, namely 102 per 1,000 persons and their average days of stay per case, 13.3 days, was 2.6 days under that for the urban aged. Although the aged of the Northeast had the lowest hospital discharge rate, only 107 per 1,000 persons, their hospital stay was longest, averaging 16.5 days. On the other hand, the aged of the South had a discharge rate of 125 per 1,000 and an average stay of 11.1 days.

The hospitalization data gathered by the Bureau of the Census in connection with its monthly Current Population Survey of September, 1956 yielded results summarized in Table 4.3. These data relate to hospital admissions, instead of discharges, and also present findings with regard to numbers of persons hospitalized in addition to cases of admission. On the whole, the pattern according to age and sex with regard to persons admitted in this survey is similar to that with regard to cases discharged in the later National Health Survey program study. In the survey of September, 1956, the average reporting aged male who was hospitalized was admitted 1.30 times during the year; for females, there were 1.21 admissions per hospitalized person.[45]

Compared with an annual survey of the general population for 1951, the survey for the year ending September, 1956 showed, for persons 65 and over, a rise in the hospitalization rate amounting to 50 per cent. On the other hand, the annual average stay per hospitalized person decreased by about five days for males and ten days for females. However, the decrease in stay for persons hospitalized was offset by the increase in the rate of hospitalization, so that the length of stay related to all aged persons in the general population showed little change during the five years.

*Hospitalization—Insurance Experience.* There are several features of interest in the 1951 survey among the aged. In urban places, the days of hospital stay per person were the greater for the noninsured, but in farm areas the insured lives had the greater stay. Also, for insured lives, the average hospital days per person exposed was longer in farm areas than in urban places, but the noninsured had a contrary experi-

---

[45] The frequency of hospital repeaters among the aged is high; see M. I. Roemer and G. W. Myers, "Multiple Admissions to Hospital," *Canadian Journal of Public Health,* Vol. 47, p. 469 (November, 1956).

ence. As expected, those in the labor force had a shorter average hospital stay than those outside of it, whether insured or not.[46]

The 1956 survey of the general population also inquired into insurance status; the results of the data collected in this regard for persons 65 and over are shown in Table 4.4, with some comparable data for 1951.[47] For the insured of each sex, the more recent survey showed 125 persons hospitalized per 1,000 population. These rates are substantially in excess of those for the uninsured, namely by 28 per cent for males and by 65 per cent for females. The length of stay for insured males who were hospitalized averaged 14.8 days annually; this was ten days less than for the uninsured. However, the stay for insured females, 15 days, was little different from that for the uninsured who were hospitalized. On the other hand, there are wide gaps between the insured and uninsured when days of stay are related to all aged persons in the population. In the case of males, the annual days of hospital stay per person are fewer for the insured than the uninsured; for females, there is a contrary situation.[48]

Both the insured and uninsured of each sex among the aged experienced large increases in hospital admissions dur-

---

[46] I. S. Falk and A. W. Brewster, "Hospitalization and Insurance Among Aged Persons," *Bureau Report No. 18,* Division of Research and Statistics, Social Security Administration, Washington, D.C., April, 1953.

[47] In addition to the source cited in Table 4.4, see M. E. Odoroff and L. M. Abbe, "Use of General Hospitals. Variation with Methods of Payment," *Public Health Reports,* Vol. 74, p. 316 (April, 1959).

[48] These findings do not shed light on the contention sometimes made that insured persons are frequently hospitalized for diagnostic tests that could just as well have been made elsewhere, or that the presence of insurance may occasion hospitalization or lengthen hospital stay merely as a convenience to the doctor or his patient. A study of the chain of events leading to hospital admission and discharge has been undertaken on a sample of admissions to hospitals in Massachusetts; this study is being conducted jointly by the National Opinion Research Center of the University of Chicago and the Health Information Foundation. The study is expected to indicate the relative importance of personal, social, and medical factors in hospitalization. See also M. I. Roemer and M. Shain, *Hospital Utilization Under Insurance,* Hospital Monograph Series No. 6 (Chicago: American Hospital Association, 1959).

TABLE 4.4

General Hospital Experience of Noninstitutional Population
According to Insurance Status,* by Age and Sex, United States;
Year Ending September, 1956 and Calendar Year 1951

| Insurance Status; Age | Persons Hospitalized per 1,000 Population per Year | Annual Hospital Admissions per Person Hospitalized | Average Days Stay per Hospitalized Person per Year | | Average Days Stay per Person per Year | |
|---|---|---|---|---|---|---|
| | | | Total | Excluding Days after 60th | Total | Excluding Days after 60th |
| **Males: Year Ending September, 1956** | | | | | | |
| Insured | | | | | | |
| Ages 65 and over.. | 125 | 1.24 | 14.8 | 14.3 | 1.85 | 1.77 |
| 65–69......... | 115 | 1.24 | 14.3 | — | 1.65 | — |
| 70–74......... | 113 | 1.21 | 16.4 | — | 1.85 | — |
| 75 and over.... | 164 | 1.31 | 14.3 | — | 2.35 | — |
| Uninsured | | | | | | |
| Ages 65 and over.. | 98 | 1.34 | 24.9 | 17.3 | 2.44 | 1.70 |
| 65–69......... | 90 | 1.37 | 35.3 | — | 3.17 | — |
| 70–74......... | 94 | 1.38 | 14.4 | — | 1.35 | — |
| 75 and over.... | 108 | 1.28 | 24.6 | — | 2.66 | — |
| **Females: Year Ending September, 1956** | | | | | | |
| Insured | | | | | | |
| Ages 65 and over.. | 124 | 1.23 | 15.0 | 14.2 | 1.86 | 1.80 |
| 65–69......... | 108 | 1.18 | 15.0 | — | 1.62 | — |
| 70–74......... | 130 | 1.22 | 15.8 | — | 2.06 | — |
| 75 and over.... | 150 | 1.31 | 14.3 | — | 2.15 | — |
| Uninsured | | | | | | |
| Ages 65 and over.. | 75 | 1.20 | 14.4 | 13.7 | 1.08 | 1.03 |
| 65–69......... | 66 | 1.09 | 12.0 | — | .79 | — |
| 70–74......... | 66 | 1.23 | 11.7 | — | .77 | — |
| 75 and over.... | 88 | 1.25 | 17.3 | — | 1.52 | — |
| **Ages 65 and Over: Calendar Year 1951** | | | | | | |
| Males   —Insured... | 106 | — | 16.0 | 15.9 | 1.69 | 1.69 |
| Uninsured | 59 | — | 32.2 | 20.4 | 1.90 | 1.20 |
| Females—Insured... | 76 | — | 17.1 | 16.6 | 1.30 | 1.26 |
| Uninsured | 57 | — | 27.1 | 20.5 | 1.55 | 1.17 |

* Insurance status as of survey month, September, 1956.

Source: A. W. Brewster, "Hospital Utilization by Persons Insured and Uninsured in September 1956," *Research and Statistics Note No. 19*, Division of Research Program, Social Security Administration, June 23, 1958.

ing the five years from 1951 to 1956, but shortened days of stay for persons hospitalized, particularly in the case of the uninsured.

The limitations and understatements typical in hospitalization data gathered by population surveys are not present in records derived from insurance experience. On the other hand, the results derived from insurance experiences reflect the characteristics of the plans (particularly the maximum period for which benefits are paid), the areas of the country in which the plans are operating, and the categories of the population covered by them. Moreover, insurance plans to cover the medical care expenses of the aged have had only a recent growth and the experiences developed under them are fragmentary. Piecing together whatever material was available, and with extrapolation toward the extreme ages of life, the actuarial subcommittee working with the New York State Insurance Department produced a Basic Table for Hospital Expense Coverage, Excluding Maternity Confinements. Figures for specimen ages are shown in the upper tier of Table 4.5.[49]

According to the source, "The scope of hospital coverage in the New York 1957 Study's cost data includes care for all sickness and injury, including such long-term disabilities as tuberculosis and mental or nervous disorders whether in a general or special hospital." In order to test the extent to which this Basic Table conforms with actual experience, the average annual numbers of days of hospitalization per person covered for a 120-day benefit, shown in the last column of Table 4.5, were multiplied by the corresponding population of New York State in 1956 distributed by sex and age. The resulting total of patient days of hospital confinement, excluding maternity confinements, agreed very closely with an independent estimate from another source. However, this

---

[49] *Voluntary Health Insurance and the Senior Citizen; A Report on the Problem of Continuation of Medical Care Benefits for the Aged in New York State,* Insurance Department, State of New York, February 26, 1958.

## TABLE 4.5

DATA FOR SPECIMEN AGES FROM BASIC TABLE FOR HOSPITAL EXPENSE COVERAGE (EXCLUDING MATERNITY CONFINEMENTS), NEW YORK 1957 STUDY AND FROM EXPERIENCE OF ASSOCIATED HOSPITAL SERVICE OF PHILADELPHIA

| Age; Sex | Cases Hospitalized per Year per 1,000 Covered Persons | Average Annual Number of Days of Covered Hospitalization | | Average Annual Number of Days of Hospitalization per Covered Person | |
|---|---|---|---|---|---|
| | | 31-Day Benefit | 120-Day Benefit | 31-Day Benefit | 120-Day Benefit |
| New York 1957 Study | | | | | |
| Males | | | | | |
| 25 | 73 | 6.4 | 7.2 | .47 | .53 |
| 35 | 70 | 7.6 | 8.5 | .53 | .60 |
| 45 | 91 | 8.7 | 9.7 | .79 | .88 |
| 55 | 121 | 10.2 | 12.4 | 1.23 | 1.50 |
| 65 | 154 | 11.8 | 15.8 | 1.82 | 2.43 |
| 75 | 181 | 13.9 | 20.2 | 2.52 | 3.66 |
| 85 | 241 | 16.5 | 26.0 | 3.98 | 6.27 |
| Females | | | | | |
| 25 | 102 | 6.4 | 7.2 | .65 | .73 |
| 35 | 119 | 7.6 | 8.5 | .90 | 1.01 |
| 45 | 135 | 8.7 | 9.7 | 1.17 | 1.31 |
| 55 | 143 | 10.2 | 12.4 | 1.46 | 1.77 |
| 65 | 158 | 11.8 | 15.8 | 1.86 | 2.50 |
| 75 | 181 | 13.9 | 20.2 | 2.52 | ·3.66 |
| 85 | 241 | 16.5 | 26.0 | 3.98 | 6.27 |
| Associated Hospital Service of Philadelphia* | | | | | |
| Both sexes | | | | | |
| Under 20 | 110 | 7.1 | | .78 | |
| 20–29 | 75 | 6.7 | | .50 | |
| 30–39 | 81 | 7.8 | | .64 | |
| 40–49 | 108 | 9.3 | | 1.00 | |
| 50–59 | 117 | 10.8 | | 1.26 | |
| 60–64 | 148 | 12.4 | | 1.83 | |
| 65–69 | 170 | 13.1 | | 2.23 | |
| 70–79 | 201 | 13.5 | | 2.72 | |
| 80–89 | 215 | 13.7 | | 2.95 | |
| 90–99 | 128 | 26.6 | | 3.42 | |

* In 1954, there were 39,712 subscribers at ages 70–79 years; 5,315 at ages 80–89 years; and 234 at ages 90–99 years. Conditions of pregnancy and days used by children are excluded. Successive periods of hospitalization were considered as a single period if discharge and readmission occurred within a 90-day period. No separation was made between cases discharged dead and those living. The days of hospital benefit covered run from 21 to 70, according to year of coverage and whether a group or individual subscriber.

Source: *Voluntary Health Insurance and the Senior Citizen: A Report on the Problem of Continuation of Medical Care Benefits for the Aged in New York State*, Insurance Department, State of New York, February 26, 1958, p. 60, and personal communication to the author from E. A. van Steenwyk, Executive Vice-President, Associated Hospital Service of Philadelphia, May 22 and August 5, 1958.

agreement in aggregate does not necessarily ensure close agreement for each sex and for successive age groups. On the other hand, the Basic Table is not intended primarily to represent experience, but rather to form a background for setting equitable rates for participants in an insurance plan providing hospital coverage and also for establishing reserves for the payment of future benefits. Any insurer may modify the Basic Table to suit its particular circumstances and needs.

A comparison of some interest may be made between the Basic Table for Hospital Expense Coverage from the New York 1957 Study, representing a composite of heterogeneous experiences and containing an extrapolation for the extreme ages, with an actual experience from the Associated Hospital Service of Philadelphia.[50] The data for the latter, presented in the lower tier of Table 4.5, show the experience of Blue Cross subscribers enrolled on both a group and individual basis under contracts paying benefits for various specified periods of hospital confinement.[51] Both series of data show rising rates of hospital admissions and days of stay up to very high ages. At the older ages, from 65 to 79 years, the hospital admission rates from the New York 1957 Study fall appreciably below those of the Associated Hospital Service of Philadelphia, which has a limited provision for hospitalization in tuberculosis and in mental and nervous institutions. Above age 80, the New York 1957 Study has the higher rates of admission. The days of hospital stay per person covered at ages 65 to 79 years are somewhat higher in the Philadelphia experience than those for the 31 day benefit in the New York

---

[50] Personal communication from E. A. van Steenwyk, Executive Vice-President, Associated Hospital Service of Philadelphia, May 22 and August 5, 1958.

[51] In 1954, the Associated Hospital Service of Philadelphia had a graduated scale of days of hospital benefit covered, running from 30 days during the first year of coverage to 70 days in the fifth year for group subscribers and 21 to 30 days for nongroup subscribers. Successive periods of hospitalization were considered as a single period if discharge and readmission occurred within a 90-day period.

1957 Study, but after age 80 they are substantially lower. Some special aspects of hospitalization insurance experience are described in Chapter 6.

*Hospitalization—Duration of Stay.* It has been noted previously that the average length of hospital stay for the aged is appreciably greater than that for the rest of the popu-

TABLE 4.6

GENERAL HOSPITAL EXPERIENCE OF NONINSTITUTIONAL POPULATION ACCORDING TO LENGTH OF HOSPITAL STAY, BY SEX, ALL AGES AND AGES 65 AND OVER, UNITED STATES; PATIENTS DISCHARGED WITHIN YEAR PRIOR TO HOUSEHOLD INTERVIEW DURING JULY, 1957–JUNE, 1958

| Days of Hospital Stay | All Ages | | | Ages 65 and Over | | |
|---|---|---|---|---|---|---|
| | Both Sexes | Males | Females | Both Sexes | Males | Females |
| | Per Cent Distribution of Discharged Patients | | | | | |
| All patients | 100.0 | 100.0 | 100.0 | 100.0 | 100.0 | 100.0 |
| 1 | 10.4 | 13.7 | 8.5 | 3.8 | 4.2 | 3.5 |
| 2–7 | 60.0 | 48.2 | 66.8 | 37.4 | 31.7 | 42.3 |
| 8–14 | 18.0 | 20.8 | 16.4 | 29.7 | 31.6 | 28.1 |
| 15–30 | 7.9 | 11.4 | 5.9 | 18.7 | 21.6 | 16.2 |
| 31 and over | 3.5 | 5.6 | 2.3 | 9.8 | 10.0 | 9.6 |
| Unknown | .2 | .3 | .2 | .6 | .9 | .4 |
| | Per Cent Distribution of Hospital Days | | | | | |
| All hospital days | 100.0 | 100.0 | 100.0 | 100.0 | 100.0 | 100.0 |
| 1 | 1.2 | 1.2 | 1.2 | .3 | .3 | .3 |
| 2–7 | 29.7 | 18.9 | 39.1 | 11.6 | 9.5 | 13.6 |
| 8–14 | 22.5 | 20.8 | 23.9 | 22.0 | 22.0 | 22.0 |
| 15–30 | 19.5 | 22.4 | 17.0 | 27.4 | 30.1 | 24.6 |
| 31 and over | 27.1 | 36.7 | 18.8 | 38.8 | 38.0 | 39.5 |

Source: U.S. National Health Survey, *Hospitalization: Patients Discharged from Short-Stay Hospitals, United States, July 1957–June 1958*, Public Health Service, Washington, D.C., December, 1958.

lation. The distribution according to length of stay is shown in Table 4.6, taken from the National Health Survey interview of households from July, 1957 through June, 1958. Among the aged discharged from a hospital during the year prior to interview within this period, 41.2 per cent had a stay of less than eight days, compared with 70.4 per cent for those of all ages. On the other hand, 9.8 per cent of the aged stayed

31 days or more, these accounting for 38.8 per cent of the total days of hospital stay. For all ages, only 3.5 per cent had a stay of 31 or more days; these cases included 27.1 per cent of all days of hospital stay.

Some aspects in the pattern of hospital utilization lacking in data for the United States can be inferred from Canadian experiences in Saskatchewan and British Columbia, where comprehensive hospital programs have been generally available to the population for several years.[52] The data relating to British Columbia in Table 4.7 are unique, because they show, for detailed age groups in the later years, the distribution of cases according to the length of their hospital stay and also the distribution of days of stay among these cases.[53] The pattern is generally one of increasing average length of stay per case at ages after 65 years, with a relatively small proportion of cases with long stay accounting for a disproportionately large share of the total days of stay. For example, among males at ages 65 and over admitted during 1954, 15.8 per cent of the cases stayed 31 days or more, but these accounted for 50.5 per cent of the total days of stay. At ages 85 and over, the comparable figures are 19.7 per cent and 60.8 per cent respectively. On the other hand, only 6.1 per cent of the males at ages 20–64 years had a stay of 31 or more days. The record for average days of stay per case discharged during 1955 shows a steady rise with advance in age for males after 65 years, from 16.1 at ages 65–69 to 20.3 at ages 85 and over; at ages 20–64 years, the average is only 10.8 days. The pattern for females is very much like that for males.

---

[52] The Saskatchewan Hospital Services Plan had its start in 1947. Hospital care is available to beneficiaries of the Plan without limit, subject only to medical necessities. The British Columbia Hospital Insurance Service, established in 1949, provides general hospital services to residents for acute conditions and the acute phases of chronic conditions. In both provinces the principal exceptions are persons provided with hospital care by federal or other provincial governmental programs. Details regarding the plans are described in the Annual Reports of the Services.

[53] Tables 4.7, 4.8 and 4.11 were computed by the author from tabulations made available by the Hospital Insurance Service, Department of Health and Welfare, British Columbia, to whom thanks are due.

TABLE 4.7

PER CENT OF CASES AND OF DAYS OF HOSPITAL STAY AMONG THEM OF
DURATION *t* OR MORE DAYS, ACCORDING TO AGE AND SEX; CASES ADMITTED TO
BRITISH COLUMBIA HOSPITALS DURING 1954 AND DISCHARGED
BEFORE APRIL 1, 1955*

| Length of Stay, *t* Days or More | Ages under 20 | Ages 20–64 | Ages 65 and Over | | | | | |
|---|---|---|---|---|---|---|---|---|
| | | | Total | 65–69 | 70–74 | 75–79 | 80–84 | 85 and Over |
| *Males—Cases* | | | | | | | | |
| 8 | 27.3 | 42.2 | 67.1 | 64.7 | 67.7 | 69.1 | 68.6 | 66.4 |
| 14 | 11.5 | 21.2 | 43.4 | 39.8 | 43.8 | 45.3 | 47.1 | 46.5 |
| 31 | 3.1 | 6.1 | 15.8 | 14.0 | 15.5 | 16.4 | 18.2 | 19.7 |
| 60 | 1.0 | 1.6 | 4.5 | 3.4 | 4.1 | 4.8 | 5.9 | 7.8 |
| 100 | .3 | .5 | 1.5 | 1.1 | 1.4 | 1.6 | 1.6 | 3.2 |
| *Males—Days of Stay* | | | | | | | | |
| 8 | 68.9 | 80.3 | 93.2 | 91.9 | 93.2 | 94.0 | 94.0 | 94.5 |
| 14 | 48.1 | 60.4 | 80.3 | 76.9 | 79.9 | 81.7 | 83.4 | 85.6 |
| 31 | 25.8 | 32.0 | 50.5 | 46.1 | 48.5 | 52.8 | 54.9 | 60.8 |
| 60 | 14.4 | 14.8 | 26.0 | 21.1 | 23.4 | 29.3 | 30.2 | 38.8 |
| 100 | 7.9 | 7.1 | 14.3 | 11.1 | 12.5 | 17.3 | 14.7 | 23.8 |
| *Females—Cases* | | | | | | | | |
| 8 | 26.0 | 40.8 | 69.7 | 66.9 | 71.1 | 69.9 | 71.0 | 72.3 |
| 14 | 9.5 | 12.5 | 45.9 | 42.3 | 46.4 | 46.6 | 49.9 | 51.6 |
| 31 | 2.4 | 2.7 | 16.5 | 13.8 | 15.6 | 17.4 | 20.0 | 23.4 |
| 60 | .7 | .6 | 4.9 | 3.2 | 4.5 | 5.6 | 6.6 | 9.0 |
| 100 | .3 | .2 | 1.4 | .6 | 1.5 | 1.8 | 1.8 | 2.9 |
| *Females—Days of Stay* | | | | | | | | |
| 8 | 64.1 | 69.8 | 93.7 | 92.1 | 93.8 | 94.1 | 94.6 | 95.4 |
| 14 | 41.5 | 38.6 | 80.9 | 76.7 | 80.7 | 82.2 | 84.2 | 86.8 |
| 31 | 22.1 | 16.9 | 50.2 | 42.5 | 49.0 | 53.0 | 55.4 | 63.4 |
| 60 | 12.6 | 7.2 | 25.6 | 16.4 | 25.5 | 29.2 | 29.5 | 38.9 |
| 100 | 8.4 | 3.5 | 12.2 | 4.9 | 13.7 | 15.3 | 12.2 | 20.5 |
| *Average Days of Stay per Case†* | | | | | | | | |
| Males | 7.6 | 10.8 | 17.9 | 16.1 | 17.8 | 18.7 | 19.6 | 20.3 |
| Females | 7.0 | 8.5 | 18.4 | 16.7 | 18.5 | 18.4 | 20.5 | 22.3 |

* For lengths of stay of 150 days or more, the observed numbers of cases were multiplied by 1.85 and the observed numbers of days of stay by 2.50 to approximate an allowance for cases discharged after March 31, 1955. These ratios were derived from a comparison with durations of stay for all cases discharged during 1955.

† These averages relate to all cases discharged during 1955 irrespective of year of admission.

Source: Computed from basic data supplied by the Hospital Insurance Service, Department of Health and Welfare, British Columbia.

A frequent source of comment is the appreciably greater rate of general hospital utilization in Saskatchewan than in the United States. For example, the annual days of hospitalization per person of all ages were 1.9 for males in Saskatchewan in 1951, as compared with 1.2 for the United States in 1953; for females, the respective averages were 2.6 and 1.1.[54] The differentials are even more marked at the older ages. Thus, at ages 65 and over, the average days of hospitalization per male were 7.4 in Saskatchewan in 1951, but only 2.8 in the United States in 1953; the corresponding averages for females were 7.6 and 2.3.

A number of contributing factors have been cited for the lengthier average stays in Saskatchewan general hospitals as compared with the United States. Thus, the program of hospital insurance in Saskatchewan is practically universal and provides no limit to the duration of stay. In the United States in 1953, on the other hand, only a fraction of the aged were protected by hospital expense insurance and the plans then available provided benefits for a limited period.[55] Within this frame is also to be considered the rural nature of the population of Saskatchewan and its wide dispersal, as a result of which physicians find it a convenience to hospitalize patients rather than treat them at home or in their office. It has been stated, further, that the high utilization record for the Province reflects the general availability of the large number of hospital beds.[56] Another influencing factor in the lengthier average stay for Saskatchewan is that the small general hospitals of the Province assume the kind of care usually given in nursing homes in the United States.

*Hospitalization—Causes.* The British Columbia experience is also informative for its detail regarding the diagnos-

---

[54] M. S. Goldstein, *Morbidity Experience of Saskatchewan General Hospitals, 1951, Frequency and Duration of Hospitalization by Primary Diagnosis,* Division of Public Health Methods, Public Health Service, Washington, D.C., October, 1958, pp. 2 and 3.

[55] See page 211 of Chapter 7.

[56] F. B. Roth, M. S. Acker, M. I. Roemer, and G. W. Myers, "Some Factors Influencing Hospital Utilization in Saskatchewan," *Canadian Journal of Public Health,* Vol. 46, p. 303 (August, 1955).

TABLE 4.8

Average Duration of Hospital Stay for Major Diagnostic Groups, According to Age and Sex; Cases Discharged from British Columbia Hospitals During 1955

| Major Diagnostic Group | Average Days of Stay per Case | | Per Cent Distribution | | | |
|---|---|---|---|---|---|---|
| | | | Cases | | Days of Stay | |
| | Ages 20–64 | Ages 65 and Over | Ages 20–64 | Ages 65 and Over | Ages 20–64 | Ages 65 and Over |
| | | | Males | | | |
| All Causes.................................... | 10.8 | 17.9 | 100.0 | 100.0 | 100.0 | 100.0 |
| Infective and parasitic diseases................. | 22.2 | 19.1 | 2.0 | 1.1 | 4.1 | 1.2 |
| Neoplasms.................................... | 18.2 | 23.0 | 4.5 | 11.3 | 7.6 | 14.6 |
| Allergic, endocrine, metabolic, and nutritional diseases................................... | 11.7 | 18.4 | 3.0 | 4.1 | 3.3 | 4.2 |
| Diseases of the blood and blood-forming organs.. | 12.9 | 15.8 | .2 | .8 | .3 | .8 |
| Mental, psychoneurotic, and personality disorders. | 7.9 | 18.7 | 3.7 | 1.1 | 2.7 | 1.1 |
| Diseases of the nervous system and sense organs... | 13.1 | 18.7 | 4.0 | 8.3 | 4.9 | 8.7 |
| Diseases of the circulatory system............. | 15.5 | 18.2 | 9.0 | 22.2 | 12.9 | 22.7 |
| Diseases of the respiratory system............. | 6.9 | 14.1 | 12.6 | 10.0 | 8.1 | 7.9 |
| Diseases of the digestive system................ | 9.8 | 14.5 | 18.0 | 13.8 | 16.4 | 11.3 |
| Diseases of the genito-urinary system.......... | 9.8 | 20.0 | 5.9 | 12.8 | 5.4 | 14.3 |
| Diseases of the skin and cellular tissue.......... | 8.3 | 20.0 | 4.0 | 1.9 | 3.0 | 2.2 |
| Diseases of the bones and organs of movement... | 12.9 | 17.6 | 6.4 | 2.7 | 7.6 | 2.7 |
| Symptoms, senility and ill-defined conditions.... | 6.1 | 9.4 | 2.6 | 2.5 | 1.5 | 1.3 |
| Accidents, poisonings, and violence............. | 10.0 | 17.9 | 23.4 | 6.8 | 21.7 | 6.9 |
| Other conditions............................. | 9.1 | 11.9 | .7 | .6 | .5 | .1 |
| | | | Females | | | |
| All Causes.................................... | 8.5 | 18.4 | 100.0 | 100.0 | 100.0 | 100.0 |
| Infective and parasitic diseases................. | 22.6 | 18.7 | .8 | .8 | 2.1 | .9 |
| Neoplasms.................................... | 11.9 | 21.8 | 6.8 | 11.3 | 9.5 | 13.4 |
| Allergic, endocrine, metabolic, and nutritional diseases................................... | 10.8 | 18.5 | 2.7 | 5.6 | 3.4 | 5.6 |
| Diseases of the blood and blood-forming organs.. | 13.8 | 15.9 | .3 | 1.3 | .4 | 1.1 |
| Mental, psychoneurotic, and personality disorders. | 10.0 | 15.0 | 2.3 | 1.3 | 2.8 | 1.1 |
| Diseases of the nervous system and sense organs... | 12.1 | 17.9 | 1.9 | 10.7 | 2.7 | 10.4 |
| Diseases of the circulatory system............. | 12.7 | 19.2 | 4.7 | 22.5 | 7.1 | 23.5 |
| Diseases of the respiratory system............. | 7.0 | 13.5 | 5.9 | 7.8 | 4.9 | 5.7 |
| Diseases of the digestive system................ | 9.7 | 15.4 | 8.4 | 13.3 | 9.7 | 11.1 |
| Diseases of the genito-urinary system.......... | 7.3 | 13.2 | 10.8 | 5.9 | 9.4 | 4.3 |
| Deliveries and complications of pregnancy, childbirth, and puerperium...................... | 6.8 | — | 46.3 | — | 37.2 | — |
| Diseases of the skin and cellular tissue.......... | 8.7 | 18.0 | 1.5 | 1.9 | 1.5 | 1.9 |
| Diseases of the bones and organs of movement... | 13.4 | 19.5 | 2.2 | 4.3 | 3.5 | 4.5 |
| Symptoms, senility, and ill-defined conditions.... | 6.9 | 10.6 | 1.3 | 1.9 | 1.0 | 1.1 |
| Accidents, poisonings, and violence............. | 9.7 | 25.8 | 3.8 | 10.9 | 4.3 | 15.3 |
| Other conditions............................. | 9.8 | 13.5 | .3 | .5 | .5 | .1 |

Source: Computed from basic data supplied by the Hospital Insurance Service, Department of Health and Welfare, British Columbia.

tic classification of the aged admitted for hospital care; this is summarized in Table 4.8.[57] Three diagnostic categories— diseases of the circulatory system, diseases of the digestive system, and the neoplasms—account for almost half of the cases hospitalized at ages 65 and over. The proportions for each category, practically identical for the two sexes, are respectively about 22 per cent, 13 per cent, and 11 per cent. About one eighth of the aged males are hospitalized for diseases of the genitourinary system and one tenth for respiratory conditions. Among aged females, about one tenth were hospitalized for diseases of the nervous system and sense organs, and a like proportion for accidents, poisonings, and violence.

The average duration of hospital stay was longest for females at ages 65 and over admitted for accidents, poisonings, and violence. Also long was the average stay for neoplasms, 23.0 days for males and 21.8 days for females. Aged males had protracted stays for diseases of the genito-urinary system and of the skin and cellular tissue, averaging 20.0 days for each category. For diseases of the circulatory system, the average stay among the aged was 18.2 days for males and 19.2 days for females.

According to the National Health Survey for the period July, 1957–June, 1958, among the aged discharged from hospitals, 37.5 per cent of the males and 43.3 of the females were surgical cases. Lower proportions were found in the sample survey made in the United States in September, 1956, where operations were given as the reason for hospital admission by 32 per cent of the reporting males at ages 65 and over, and by 28 per cent of the aged females.[58] However, an

---

[57] In this connection, pertinent data are also presented by M. S. Goldstein, *op. cit.*, and by T. D. Woolsey, *Patient-Load Profile of an Average Day in General Hospitals Based on Discharges from Saskatchewan General Hospitals, 1951,* Division of Public Health Methods, Public Health Service, Washington, D.C., October, 1958.

[58] A. W. Brewster, "The Relationship of Marital Status to Hospital Utilization and of Insurance Ownership to Methods of Paying for Hospital Care, Year Ending September 1956," *Research and Statistics Note No. 25,* Division of Program Research, Social Security Administration, July 23, 1958.

TABLE 4.9

Per Cent of Population at Ages 65 and Over Living in Institutions, According to Sex and Marital Status, United States Census of April, 1950

| Institution | Marital Status | | | | |
|---|---|---|---|---|---|
| | Total | Single | Married | Widowed | Divorced |
| | Males | | | | |
| Total population........ | 100.0 | 100.0 | 100.0 | 100.0 | 100.0 |
| In institutions.......... | 3.0 | 12.5 | 1.0 | 4.9 | 7.2 |
| Mental hospitals...... | 1.1 | 5.2 | .5 | 1.1 | 2.7 |
| Homes for aged....... | 1.6 | 6.0 | .4 | 3.4 | 3.6 |
| All others........... | .3 | 1.3 | .1 | .4 | .9 |
| | Females | | | | |
| Total population........ | 100.0 | 100.0 | 100.0 | 100.0 | 100.0 |
| In institutions.......... | 3.2 | 8.8 | 1.4 | 3.4 | 5.7 |
| Mental hospitals...... | 1.1 | 3.3 | 1.0 | .8 | 4.0 |
| Homes for aged....... | 1.9 | 4.9 | .4 | 2.4 | 1.6 |
| All others........... | .2 | .6 | * | .2 | .1 |

\* Less than .05.

Source of basic data: Bureau of the Census, *U.S. Census of Population: 1950, Special Reports* Vol. IV, Part 2, Chapter C, pp. 21, 26 and 34, and Chapter D, p. 15, Washington, D.C., 1953'

appreciable proportion of the admissions of the aged was a result of accidents and injuries, 8.6 per cent for males and 14.5 per cent for females. Although the annual rate of hospital admission because of accidents and injuries among aged males was about the same for the insured and the uninsured, in the case of aged females the insured had the much higher rate. Also, for each sex among the aged, the insured had an appreciably greater rate of hospital admission because of operations than the uninsured.[59]

*Hospitalization—Marital Status.* Considerable stress on the role of social factors in the utilization of medical services is given in reports on the National Health Service of Eng-

---

[59] For a more detailed picture of the leading surgical and nonsurgical conditions in hospital admissions among a body of aged insured persons, see "Hospitalization at the Older Ages," *Statistical Bulletin,* Metropolitan Life Insurance Company, October, 1959.

land and Wales.[60] In this regard, the living arrangements of
the aged may be of particular significance, as mentioned
earlier.[61] A clue in this direction may be obtained from data
on hospital utilization with respect to marital status since
this has some relationship to living arrangement.

The United States census of 1950 showed that the proportion of population at ages 65 and over living in institutions (mental hospitals, homes for the aged and the like) was
much greater for the unmarried, particularly the single, than
for the married. For example, among aged males, 12.5 per
cent of the single were living in institutions, as compared
with only 1.0 of the married (Table 4.9). Also, the proportions of the single and divorced aged persons in mental institutions were well above those for the married and widowed, apparently reflecting a tendency for persons with
mental disturbances to remain single and for people to seek a
divorce when a marital partner is so disturbed.[62] However, it
is also likely that many of the married or widowed aged with
a mental condition are kept at home in the care of the spouse
or children. The very small proportions of the married in
homes for the aged, as compared with the unmarried, is un-
derstandable. In the case of the unmarried—whether single,
widowed, or divorced—the absence of close family ties brings
many to homes for the aged.

According to experience in England and Wales, "With ad-
vancing age among both sexes the proportion in hospital rises
most sharply for the single, less so for the widowed and divorced, and even less so for the married."[63] With regard to
sex, "At all ages, the proportion of single, widowed and di-

---

[60] B. Abel-Smith and R. M. Titmuss, *The Cost of the National Health
Service in England and Wales* (Cambridge, England: Cambridge University
Press, 1956); *Report of the Committee of Enquiry Into the Cost of the
National Health Service,* (London: H. M. Stationery Office, 1956).

[61] See p. 6 of Chapter 2.

[62] S. S. Bellin and R. H. Hardt, "Marital Status and Mental Disorders
Among the Aged," *American Sociological Review,* Vol. 23, p. 155 (April,
1958).

[63] B. Abel-Smith and R. M. Titmuss, *op. cit.,* p. 140.

vorced men in hospital is higher, and rises more sharply, than the corresponding rates for women." In the United States, the pattern for males is similar to that in England and Wales, but for females it is somewhat different according to the results from the sample survey of September, 1956, shown in Table

TABLE 4.10

GENERAL HOSPITAL EXPERIENCE OF NONINSTITUTIONAL POPULATION ACCORDING TO MARITAL STATUS, BY AGE AND SEX, UNITED STATES; YEAR ENDING SEPTEMBER, 1956

| Age | Annual Admissions per 1,000 Population | | Average Days of Stay per Admission | | Average Days of Stay per Person per Year | |
|---|---|---|---|---|---|---|
| | Married | Not Married | Married | Not Married | Married | Not Married |
| Males | | | | | | |
| Ages 14 and over.. | 89 | 67 | 10.8 | 14.6 | .96 | .98 |
| 14–64.......... | 84 | 54 | 10.4 | 11.4 | .88 | .62 |
| 65 and over..... | 132 | 158 | 12.5 | 22.1 | 1.65 | 3.49 |
| 65–69........ | 131 | 137 | 12.7 | 36.0 | 1.66 | 4.94 |
| 70–74........ | 130 | 139 | 9.4 | 17.3 | 1.22 | 2.41 |
| 75 and over... | 137 | 185 | 15.7 | 17.1 | 2.15 | 3.16 |
| Females | | | | | | |
| Ages 14 and over.. | 190 | 80 | 6.3 | 10.8 | 1.20 | .87 |
| 14–64.......... | 196 | 71 | 6.1 | 9.9 | 1.20 | .70 |
| 65 and over..... | 110 | 112 | 11.3 | 12.5 | 1.25 | 1.40 |
| 65–69........ | 102 | 93 | 11.4 | 12.6 | 1.16 | 1.17 |
| 70–74........ | 107 | 108 | 10.7 | 11.5 | 1.15 | 1.24 |
| 75 and over... | 139 | 127 | 11.7 | 13.2 | 1.62 | 1.67 |

Source: A. W. Brewster, "The Relationship of Marital Status to Hospital Utilization and of Insurance Ownership to Methods of Paying for Hospital Care, Year Ending September, 1956," *Research and Statistics Note No. 25*, Division of Program Research, Social Security Administration, July 23, 1958.

4.10. Here it is found that among aged males the unmarried have not only higher admission rates than the married, but also a more rapid rise in rates with advance in age. Also, for both the married and the unmarried, the admission rates for aged males are generally above those for females. On the other hand, among aged females the admission rates for the unmarried are little different from those for the married.

However, it should be noted that the United States data relate to admission rates, whereas those for England and Wales relate to the proportions in hospital.

When the duration of hospital stay is taken into account, the record of the unmarried aged in the United States is less favorable than that of the married. According to Table 4.10, the average length of stay per admission for males at ages 65 and over is 22.1 days for the unmarried and 12.5 days for the married; for aged females, the respective stays are 12.5 days and 11.3 days. When the length of hospital stay is related to all aged persons, the average days are 3.49 for unmarried males and 1.65 for married males; the like figures for aged females are 1.40 and 1.25 days, respectively.

A more detailed picture of hospital stay with regard to marital status is provided by the British Columbia experience shown in Table 4.11. This shows, for example, that 21.1 per cent of the single hospitalized males at ages 65 and over had a stay of 31 or more days and that these cases accounted for 61.8 per cent of the total days of stay. For married males in this age period, only 13.5 per cent of the cases had the same length of stay and their days were 44.3 per cent of the total. The lowest tier of the table shows that single males aged 70 and over have a greater average stay than the married at each age period, while those of other marital status fall between the two. In the case of aged females, the advantage in length of stay of the married is not as great as among males; also, the differential between the single and those of other marital status for females is generally smaller than for males.

The uniform record of greater hospital utilization on the part of the unmarried in the United States, England and Wales, and Canada is noteworthy. Although morbidity and mortality data indicate a poorer health status for the unmarried,[64] their record is undoubtedly also influenced by

---

[64] D. E. Hailman, *The Prevalence of Disabling Illness Among Male and Female Workers and Housewives,* Public Health Bulletin No. 260, Public Health Service, Washington, D.C., 1941; D. Shurtleff, "Mortality and Marital Status," *Public Health Reports,* Vol. 70, p. 248 (March, 1955).

their living arrangements. Without close family ties, an aged person in need of medical care is the more likely to be sent to a hospital for attention, more likely to be sent at an earlier stage in his illness, and more likely to be kept there longer.

TABLE 4.11

PER CENT OF CASES AND OF DAYS OF HOSPITAL STAY AMONG THEM OF DURATION $t$ OR MORE DAYS, ACCORDING TO MARITAL STATUS AND SEX; CASES ADMITTED TO BRITISH COLUMBIA HOSPITALS DURING 1954 AND DISCHARGED BEFORE APRIL 1, 1955*

| Length of Stay, $t$ Days or More | Males | | | Females | | |
|---|---|---|---|---|---|---|
| | Single | Married | Other | Single | Married | Other |
| | Cases at Ages 65 and Over | | | | | |
| 8 | 70.6 | 65.4 | 68.6 | 71.9 | 67.8 | 71.0 |
| 14 | 48.5 | 40.7 | 46.3 | 51.4 | 43.1 | 47.9 |
| 31 | 21.1 | 13.5 | 17.4 | 22.7 | 14.8 | 17.3 |
| 60 | 7.6 | 3.2 | 5.5 | 7.7 | 4.3 | 5.2 |
| 100 | 2.7 | 1.0 | 2.0 | 1.7 | 1.2 | 1.6 |
| | Days of Stay for Cases at Ages 65 and Over | | | | | |
| 8 | 95.1 | 92.0 | 94.0 | 94.9 | 92.9 | 94.2 |
| 14 | 85.5 | 77.0 | 82.7 | 85.0 | 78.6 | 82.3 |
| 31 | 61.8 | 44.3 | 53.7 | 58.3 | 47.2 | 51.6 |
| 60 | 38.3 | 19.5 | 29.3 | 30.1 | 23.1 | 27.0 |
| 100 | 22.6 | 9.8 | 16.6 | 8.9 | 10.6 | 13.7 |
| Age | Average Days of Stay per Case† | | | | | |
| All ages | 9.3 | 12.1 | 17.7 | 7.8 | 8.7 | 16.0 |
| Under 20 | 7.6 | 5.7 | — | 7.1 | 6.2 | 6.2 |
| 20–49 | 9.5 | 9.1 | 11.5 | 8.5 | 7.5 | 9.4 |
| 50–59 | 14.5 | 12.4 | 16.4 | 13.9 | 12.0 | 13.5 |
| 60–64 | 16.9 | 14.5 | 16.0 | 17.1 | 14.4 | 15.9 |
| 65–69 | 16.3 | 15.8 | 16.9 | 20.3 | 16.3 | 16.9 |
| 70–74 | 22.7 | 16.2 | 18.6 | 19.2 | 17.6 | 19.2 |
| 75–79 | 22.3 | 16.9 | 20.2 | 18.7 | 18.0 | 18.7 |
| 80–84 | 23.5 | 17.5 | 20.5 | 22.0 | 17.3 | 21.4 |
| 85 and over | 22.3 | 18.5 | 20.8 | 30.5 | 20.0 | 22.0 |
| Not stated | 11.9 | 9.3 | 39.5 | 2.7 | 5.6 | 22.7 |

* For lengths of stay of 150 days or more, the observed numbers of cases were multiplied by 1.85 and the observed numbers of days of stay by 2.50 to approximate an allowance for cases discharged after March 31, 1955. These ratios were derived from a comparison with durations of stay for all cases discharged during 1955.

† These averages relate to all cases discharged during 1955 irrespective of year of admission.

Source: Computed from basic data supplied by the Hospital Insurance Service, Department o Health and Welfare, British Columbia.

In some measure, the situation might be alleviated by better housing provisions for the unmarried aged, provision for home care and housekeeper services, and facility for transfer to nursing homes.

*Hospitalization—Trends.* The comparison of the hospitalization experiences for the United States in 1951 and 1956 made previously referred only to ages 65 and over as a whole.[65] A more detailed insight into recent hospitalization trends is provided by the experience of Saskatchewan, where a provincial government program providing practically unlimited care has been operating since 1947. This plan covers 94 per cent of the population of the province. The trend data according to age and sex are shown in Table 4.12.

In the early years of the provincial program, all ages experienced a sharp rise in hospital utilization, as evidenced in the rates for discharged cases per 1,000 beneficiaries from 1947 through 1950. On the other hand, only the aged showed a rise in the average days of stay per case. These early rises were due, most likely, to an accumulation of remedial medical care needs. After 1950, the hospitalization rates for persons under age 65 maintained a relatively constant level, those for ages 65–69 years moved slowly upward, and those for ages 70 and over rose rapidly. Meanwhile, the average days of stay per case tended downward, due in part to administrative measures. The stability of the hospitalization rates for ages under 65 reflects, to a large extent, the success of new therapies for the control of the infectious and many chronic diseases by treatment at home or in the physician's office.

A number of influences may have contributed to the rise in hospitalization rates for the aged in the United States and Saskatchewan. Thus, more beds may be becoming available either through hospital construction or a relatively lesser utilization by younger people; the aged may be losing their

[65] A detailed discussion for the population of all ages will be found in *Progress in Health Services,* Vol. 8 (October, 1959), Health Information Foundation, New York.

fear of the hospital, which was once regarded as a place for terminal illness; the medical practitioner may see, increasingly, advantages to his aged patient and himself in hospitalization for purposes of diagnosis; many new medical advances require the equipment of the hospital; and lastly, there are the shifts in family and living arrangements already referred to. The increasing numbers and proportion of the

TABLE 4.12

HOSPITAL EXPERIENCE OF BENEFICIARIES OF THE SASKATCHEWAN HOSPITAL SERVICES PLAN, BY AGE AND SEX, FROM 1947 TO 1957

| Year | Males | | | Females | | |
|---|---|---|---|---|---|---|
| | Ages under 65* | Ages 65–69 | Ages 70 and Over | Ages under 65* | Ages 65–69 | Ages 70 and Over |
| | Discharged Hospital Cases per 1,000 Beneficiaries | | | | | |
| 1947 | 104 | 182 | 266 | 195 | 201 | 241 |
| 1948 | 123 | 215 | 302 | 216 | 242 | 286 |
| 1949 | 145 | 240 | 328 | 239 | 260 | 311 |
| 1950 | 145 | 250 | 352 | 241 | 281 | 345 |
| 1951 | 136 | 260 | 382 | 235 | 287 | 376 |
| 1952 | 142 | 251 | 392 | 243 | 285 | 387 |
| 1953 | 141 | 265 | 397 | 243 | 280 | 394 |
| 1954 | 135 | 255 | 405 | 243 | 286 | 407 |
| 1955 | 131 | 259 | 417 | 237 | 308 | 421 |
| 1956 | 131 | 272 | 440 | 238 | 307 | 440 |
| 1957 | 139 | 292 | 447 | 246 | 313 | 454 |
| | Average Days of Stay for Discharged Cases | | | | | |
| 1947 | 8.7 | 17.4 | 19.8 | 8.7 | 16.8 | 20.3 |
| 1948 | 9.0 | 18.6 | 21.6 | 8.8 | 18.2 | 21.3 |
| 1949 | 8.9 | 18.5 | 21.2 | 8.5 | 17.4 | 22.0 |
| 1950 | 9.2 | 18.3 | 22.7 | 8.9 | 18.1 | 24.3 |
| 1951 | 9.3 | 19.5 | 24.1 | 8.9 | 17.4 | 24.9 |
| 1952 | 9.0 | 18.2 | 21.8 | 8.6 | 17.9 | 22.0 |
| 1953 | 8.8 | 16.7 | 20.9 | 8.4 | 18.8 | 22.8 |
| 1954 | 8.8 | 16.9 | 21.4 | 8.1 | 17.4 | 20.4 |
| 1955 | 8.8 | 16.6 | 19.7 | 8.2 | 15.8 | 19.7 |
| 1956 | 8.9 | 16.1 | 19.3 | 8.2 | 16.3 | 20.3 |
| 1957 | 8.5 | 16.0 | 19.4 | 7.8 | 15.6 | 19.6 |

* Age-adjusted by author on the basis of the age distribution for both sexes combined of the beneficiaries in 1956.

Source: 1947–1952 from G. W. Myers, "Hospitalization Experience of a Government Hospital Care Insurance Plan," *Canadian Journal of Public Health*, Vol. 45, p. 372 (September, 1954); 1953–1957, *Annual Reports of the Saskatchewan Hospital Services Plan*.

aged in the population, their greater rate of hospitalization, and their longer stay will produce a rapidly growing demand for hospital accommodations.

*Hospitalization—Aged Beneficiaries of Old-Age and Survivors Insurance.* Although the aged beneficiaries under the national Old-Age and Survivors Insurance program constitute a large proportion of the total aged in the general population, they are by no means a representative sample. Nevertheless, their hospital utilization experience is particularly pertinent since it relates to the aged who have retired from the labor force, and their aged spouses. The principal results of a survey of such aged beneficiaries are summarized in Table 4.13. This survey was conducted in the fall of 1957 among a sample of aged persons who were receiving benefits from Old-Age and Survivors Insurance in December, 1956 and relates to their experience during the year prior to interview. The data exclude persons who died during the survey year. However, beneficiaries hospitalized in institutions are included, a feature not usual in general population surveys. Also included are beneficiaries hospitalized for the whole year covered by the survey. It should be noted, in Table 4.13, that the category of widowed females relates only to those who are receiving widow's benefits; widows receiving benefits as a result of their own employment are included among the single.

Confirming general population experience, the married males among the OASI beneficiaries have a better record than the unmarried with regard to both the annual rate of admission to general hospitals and the annual average duration of stay per beneficiary. A corresponding comparison cannot be made for females because of the manner in which widows are classified.

Among all aged beneficiaries, for each sex and marital status category, the hospital admission rate is higher for those with health insurance than for those without it, but the reverse situation is found with regard to the average days of stay per hospitalized beneficiary. However, when the days of

## TABLE 4.13

GENERAL HOSPITAL EXPERIENCE OF AGED BENEFICIARIES UNDER OLD-AGE
AND SURVIVORS INSURANCE, FOR SURVEY YEAR ENDING WITH INTERVIEW
IN THE FALL OF 1957*

| Age; Insurance Status | Males† | | Females† | | |
|---|---|---|---|---|---|
| | Single | Married | Single | Married | Widowed |
| Beneficiaries Hospitalized per 1,000 Beneficiaries per Year | | | | | |
| 65 and over, total............ | 126 | 107 | 119 | 109 | 99 |
| Insured.................. | 135 | 144 | 158 | 128 | 145 |
| Not insured.............. | 122 | 76 | 81 | 92 | 70 |
| Hospital Admissions per 1,000 Beneficiaries per Year | | | | | |
| 65 and over, total............ | 150 | 134 | 144 | 135 | 111 |
| Insured.................. | 166 | 185 | 198 | 151 | 161 |
| Not insured.............. | 142 | 91 | 91 | 121 | 80 |
| Average Days Stay per Hospitalized Beneficiary per Year | | | | | |
| 65 and over, total............ | 21.9 | 21.9 | 19.8 | 21.3 | 19.2 |
| Insured.................. | 18.2 | 16.1 | 19.5 | 19.3 | 14.1 |
| Not insured.............. | 23.7 | 31.1 | 20.2 | 23.8 | 25.8 |
| Average Days Stay per Beneficiary per Year´ | | | | | |
| 65 and over, total............ | 2.76 | 2.34 | 2.36 | 2.32 | 1.90 |
| Insured.................. | 2.46 | 2.32 | 3.08 | 2.48 | 2.05 |
| Not insured.............. | 2.89 | 2.36 | 1.63 | 2.19 | 1.81 |
| 65–69, total.............. | 3.65 | 2.79 | 1.24 | 2.17 | 1.55 |
| Insured.................. | .52 | 1.72 | 1.79 | 1.76 | 1.15 |
| Not insured.............. | 5.17 | 4.04 | .48 | 2.57 | 1.86 |
| 70–74, total.............. | 2.53 | 1.33 | 2.61 | 2.35 | 1.23 |
| Insured.................. | 4.02 | 2.02 | 3.91 | 2.90 | 1.56 |
| Not insured.............. | 1.79 | .78 | 1.10 | 1.89 | .97 |
| 75–79, total.............. | 3.25 | 2.71 | 2.26 | 2.69 | 2.65 |
| Insured.................. | 2.58 | 4.28 | 3.00 | 4.75 | 3.26 |
| Not insured.............. | 3.58 | 1.55 | 1.84 | 1.51 | 2.38 |
| 80 and over, total........... | 1.37 | 1.92 | 5.86 | 2.56 | 2.97 |
| Insured.................. | 1.26 | 1.45 | 5.85 | 1.24 | 4.57 |
| Not insured.............. | 1.40 | 2.16 | 5.86 | 3.13 | 2.39 |

\* Data on age and marital status of beneficiary, as well as ownership of health insurance, are as of the end of the survey year.

† Divorced, separated, or widowed beneficiaries are classified as single persons, except that women entitled to widow's benefits are shown separately. Widows entitled to benefits on their own employment record are included with other "single" women.

Source: "Aged Beneficiaries of Old-Age and Survivors Insurance: Highlights on Health Insurance and Hospitalization Utilization, 1957 Survey," *Social Security Bulletin*, December, 1958, p. 3.

stay are related to all aged beneficiaries and studied in detail with regard to age, no definite picture of hospital utilization emerges (lowest tier of Table 4.13). Thus, at ages 70–74 and 75–79, in all but one sex-marital status category, hospital utilization among the insured was greater than among those not insured. On the other hand, at ages 65–69 those not insured made the greater use of the hospital, except for single females. The record for males at ages 65–69 without health insurance was particularly poor, not only compared with others of that age group but also with the higher ages. It is possible that these uninsured males have many among them who retired at the first opportunity because of their state of health.

On the whole, the duration of general hospital stay was greater for the insured than the uninsured among the aged beneficiaries, the annual days of stay per person being 2.48 and 2.26 respectively.[66] However, 83 per cent of the days of stay among the insured were accounted for by individual stays lasting less than 31 days, compared with 54 per cent for the uninsured. For all aged beneficiaries, the annual days of stay per person averaged 2.36 for general hospitals, 1.72 for mental, tuberculosis, and other chronic-disease institutions, and 2.76 in nursing homes. About seven eighths of these aged were in the nursing home for 30 or more days during the survey year, and two thirds for over 60 days. The numbers admitted within the year of survey, per 100 aged beneficiaries, were 11 for general hospitals, 1.0 for mental, tuberculosis, and other chronic-disease institutions, and 1.3 for nursing homes.

**Surgical Services.** Only a very limited body of data is available to describe the utilization of surgical services at the older ages. The more recent data, summarized in Table 4.14, indicate a higher rate of surgery for the aged than for younger persons. Other sources show that the aged also have a longer period of convalescence after surgery, both inside

---

[66] *Hospitalization Insurance for OASDI Beneficiaries, op. cit.,* p. 20, 22, and 23.

TABLE 4.14

ANNUAL RATE OF SURGICAL PROCEDURES IN SEVERAL EXPERIENCES, BY SEX,
ALL AGES AND AGES 65 AND OVER

| | Annual Rate of Surgery per 100 Persons | | | | | |
|---|---|---|---|---|---|---|
| | Both Sexes | | Males | | Females | |
| Experience | All Ages | Ages 65 and Over | All Ages | Ages 65 and Over | All Ages | Ages 65 and Over |
| United States, 1953[a] | 7.0 | 6.0 | 6.0 | 5.0 | 8.0 | 8.0 |
| Surgically insured persons | 9.0 | 6.0 | 7.0 | 4.0 | 10.0 | 8.0 |
| Not surgically insured | 5.0 | 7.0 | 4.0 | 5.0 | 6.0 | 8.0 |
| Health Insurance Plan, 1956[b] (hospitalized surgery only) | 3.5 | 4.5 | 2.9 | 5.0 | 3.4 | 3.6 |
| Eye, ear, nose, and throat | .7 | .5 | .7 | .5 | .6 | .5 |
| Gastrointestinal and abdominal | .8 | 1.3 | 1.0 | 1.4 | .5 | 1.1 |
| Genito-urinary | .6 | 1.3 | .4 | 1.9 | .1 | .3 |
| Gynecological-obstetrical | .6 | .2 | — | — | 1.3 | .5 |
| Orthopedic | .2 | .3 | .2 | .2 | .2 | .4 |
| Other | .6 | .9 | .6 | .9 | .7 | .8 |
| Metropolitan Life Insurance Company[c] personnel (hospitalized surgery only) | — | — | — | 7.2† | — | 4.9† |
| Ages 60–64 | — | — | — | 7.2 | — | 4.5 |
| Ages 65–74 | — | — | — | 6.9 | — | 4.9 |
| Ages 75 and over | — | — | — | 7.9 | — | 5.7 |
| Herniotomy | — | — | — | .9† | — | — |
| Gallbladder | — | — | — | .3† | — | — |
| Prostatectomy | — | — | — | .8† | — | — |
| Cystoscopy | — | — | — | .7† | — | — |
| Benign tumor | — | — | — | .5† | — | — |
| Hemorrhoid | — | — | — | .3† | — | — |
| Cataract | — | — | — | .3† | — | — |
| Fracture | — | — | — | .3† | — | — |
| Thoracic surgery | — | — | — | .2† | — | — |
| Cancer | — | — | — | .2† | — | — |
| Birmingham Blue Cross–Blue Shield[d] | 8.3 | 5.1* | 7.4 | 7.5* | 9.2 | 3.0* |
| Hospitalized surgery | 5.0 | 2.2* | 4.0 | 3.3* | 6.0 | 1.1* |
| Nonhospitalized surgery | 3.3 | 2.9* | 3.4 | 4.2* | 3.2 | 1.9* |
| Boston Blue Cross–Blue Shield[d] | 11.1 | 11.5* | 10.4 | 12.0* | 11.6 | 11.0* |
| Hospitalized surgery | 7.9 | 9.3* | 7.3 | 10.0* | 8.4 | 8.8* |
| Nonhospitalized surgery | 3.2 | 2.1* | 3.2 | 2.1* | 3.3 | 2.2* |
| Boston, Aetna Life Insurance Company[d] | 9.9 | 10.3* | — | — | — | — |
| Hospitalized surgery | 6.1 | 6.9* | — | — | — | — |
| Nonhospitalized surgery | 3.8 | 3.4* | — | — | — | — |
| Basic Surgical Expense Table[e] | — | 10.8 | — | 10.8 | — | 10.8 |
| Composite of 5 illness surveys, 1928 to 1943[f] | | | | | | |
| All operations | 6.4 | 4.3 | 6.1 | 4.1 | 6.7 | 4.5 |
| Hospital operations | 3.9 | 2.5 | 3.2 | 2.5 | 4.5 | 2.5 |

\* Ages 55 and over.  † Ages 60 and over.

Sources:

[a] O. W. Anderson and J. J. Feldman, *Family Medical Costs and Voluntary Health Insurance: A Nationwide Survey* (New York: McGraw-Hill Book Co., Inc., 1956), p. 193. Data exclude circumcision of newborn and suturing of wounds.

[b] S. Shapiro and M. Einhorn, "Experience With Older Members in a Prepaid Medical Care Plan," *Public Health Reports*, Vol. 73, p. 687 (August, 1958). Data exclude circumcision of newborn.

[c] "Hospitalization at the Older Ages," *Statistical Bulletin*, Metropolitan Life Insurance Company, October, 1959. Data relate to persons actively at work, the retired, and those on total and permanent disability.

[d] O. W. Anderson, *Voluntary Health Insurance in Two Cities* (Cambridge, Mass.: Harvard University Press, 1957), pp. 82–84. Data exclude circumcision of newborn and suturing of wounds.

[e] *Voluntary Health Insurance and the Senior Citizen: A Report on the Problem of Continuation of Medical Care Benefits for the Aged in New York State*, Insurance Department, State of New York, February 26, 1958, p. 144.

[f] S. D. Collins, J. L. Lehmann, and K. S. Trantham, *Surgical Experience in Selected Areas of the United States*, Public Health Monograph No. 38, Public Health Service, Washington, D.C., 1956.

and outside the hospital.[67] According to a sample survey conducted in the United States in 1953, the annual rate of surgical procedures at ages 65 and over was 5 per 100 for males and 8 per 100 for females; this includes surgery inside and outside the hospital. Counting hospitalized surgery only, aged persons in the Health Insurance Plan of Greater New York had a rate of 5.0 per 100 for males and 3.6 per 100 for females. The rate for males for cases with hospital surgery in the experience of personnel of the Metropolitan Life Insurance Company was higher, namely 7.2 per 100 at ages 60 and over. Rather wide variations in the frequency of surgery among persons at ages 55 and over were recorded in the insurance experiences of Birmingham and Boston, with rates of 5.1 per 100 persons of both sexes in the former city and of 11.5 in the latter. The level for Boston is practically the same as the rate, 10.8 per 100 persons, estimated for insurance purposes from various sources by the actuarial subcommittee working with the New York State Insurance Department.

Variations in rates of surgery reflect variations in medical practice and also differences in expression of medical care needs. Medical progress can also introduce changes. Thus, with modern techniques many cases are brought to surgery which would have been considered too great a risk in earlier years.[68] Also, a number of conditions formerly operated are now treated by other means. There is, further, the possibility that the growth of insurance for the costs of surgery permits increasing numbers to have operations which they could not otherwise afford; some of these operations may be elective.[69]

---

[67] H. J. Saffeir, "The Duration of Surgical Convalescence as Indicated by Insurance Statistics," and K. G. Bartels and C. G. Johnston, "A Study of the Complications of the Posthospitalization Period of Surgical Convalescence," *Annals of the New York Academy of Sciences*, Vol. 73, pp. 444 and 500 (September 10, 1958).

[68] "Surgery Much Safer," *Statistical Bulletin*, August, 1959, Metropolitan Life Insurance Co., New York.

[69] H. le Riche, *A Sample Study on the Participants of a Canadian Prepayment Medical Care Plan*, Physicians' Services Incorporated, Toronto, Ontario, 1957, p. 31.

The experience of the Health Insurance Plan of Greater New York shows that two fifths of the hospitalized surgical cases among aged males involve the genito-urinary system. For each sex, the rates for the aged are also high for gastrointestinal and abdominal surgeries. About two thirds of the operations for the eye, ear, nose, and throat among the aged are for cataract and glaucoma. The hospitalized surgical experience of the personnel of the Metropolitan Life Insurance Company at ages 60 and over (including those actively at work, those on total and permanent disability, and the retired) relates to a group insured under a liberal program. Among males, hospital admissions for surgery during 1957 and 1958 occurred at an annual rate of about 7 per 100 at ages 60–74 and 8 per 100 at ages 75 and over; for females, the rates were lower but rose steadily with advance in age. Among males at ages 60 and over, the leading causes of hospitalized surgery were herniotomy, prostatectomy, cystoscopy, and benign tumor. Abdominal surgery, benign tumor, eye conditions (principally cataract), and fracture led the causes of hospitalized surgery among aged women.

*Physicians' Services.* The first report of the United States National Health Survey program is concerned with the volume of physician visits. Since the report, which is preliminary, covers July–September, 1957, the results reflect the seasonally low rates of utilization of physicians' services. Selected data from this and other sources are shown in Table 4.15.

The greater need of the aged for medical attention is reflected in the observation that 24 per cent of those 65 and over contacted a physician within the month before interview, as compared with 18 per cent for those of all ages. Although the proportion of older persons who contacted a physician within the year prior to the interview is about the same as that for persons of all ages, in each instance it was greater for females than for males, namely 69 per cent and 58 per cent at ages 65 and over. The number of physician visits per person per year was also greater for aged females

TABLE 4.15

INCIDENCE AND CHARACTERISTICS OF PHYSICIANS' SERVICES IN SEVERAL
EXPERIENCES, BY SEX, ALL AGES AND AGES 65 AND OVER

| Experience and Service | All Ages | | | Ages 65 and Over | | |
|---|---|---|---|---|---|---|
| | Both Sexes | Males | Females | Both Sexes | Males | Females |
| United States, July–September, 1957[a] | | | | | | |
| Per cent having last physician visit | | | | | | |
| Within one month | 18.0 | 15.0 | 21.0 | 24.0 | 22.0 | 26.0 |
| Within one year | 63.0 | 59.0 | 67.0 | 64.0 | 58.0 | 69.0 |
| Within five years | 91.0 | 89.0 | 93.0 | 88.0 | 85.0 | 91.0 |
| United States, May–June, 1957[b] | | | | | | |
| Per cent having last physician visit | | | | | | |
| Within one month | — | — | — | 29.0 | 26.0 | 32.0 |
| Within one year | — | — | — | 63.0 | 59.0 | 67.0 |
| Within five years | — | — | — | 85.0 | 83.0 | 87.0 |
| Five or more years ago | — | — | — | 10.0 | 12.0 | 8.0 |
| Never and not stated | — | — | — | 5.0 | 5.0 | 5.0 |
| United States, July, 1957–June, 1958[a] | | | | | | |
| Physician visits per person per year | | | | | | |
| All visits | 5.3 | 4.5 | 6.0 | 6.8 | 6.1 | 7.4 |
| Office | 3.4 | 2.9 | 3.9 | 4.2 | 3.9 | 4.5 |
| Home | .5 | .4 | .6 | 1.5 | 1.2 | 1.8 |
| Hospital clinic | .5 | .5 | .6 | .5 | .4 | .5 |
| Other | .8 | .7 | .9 | .6 | .5 | .7 |
| Type of service | | | | | | |
| Diagnosis and treatment | 4.0 | 3.6 | 4.4 | 5.6 | 5.2 | 6.1 |
| All other | 1.4 | 1.0 | 1.7 | 1.3 | 1.0 | 1.5 |
| United States, May–June, 1957[b] | | | | | | |
| Physician visits per person per year | | | | | | |
| All visits | — | — | — | 7.6 | 6.7 | 8.4 |
| Office | — | — | — | 5.2 | 4.6 | 5.8 |
| Home | — | — | — | 1.7 | 1.3 | 2.0 |
| Clinic | — | — | — | .6 | .7 | .4 |
| Telephone | — | — | — | .1 | .1 | .2 |
| United States, 1952–53[c] | | | | | | |
| Estimated per cent with 15 or more out-of-hospital physicians' calls | 7 | 4 | 9 | 13 | 9 | 17 |
| California Health Survey, May, 1954–April, 1955[d] | | | | | | |
| Physician visits per person per year | 5.2 | 4.5 | 5.8 | 8.0 | 5.5 | 10.3 |
| Office | 4.1 | 3.7 | 4.4 | 5.4 | 4.0 | 6.7 |
| Home | .5 | .3 | .6 | 2.3 | 1.1 | 3.4 |
| Hospital and other clinic | .6 | .5 | .8 | .3 | .4 | .2 |
| New York City Sample, 1951[e] | | | | | | |
| Per cent who saw a doctor during the year | — | 55.3 | 61.2 | — | 61.2 | 65.9 |

TABLE 4.15—*Continued*

| Experience and Service | All Ages | | | Ages 65 and Over | | |
|---|---|---|---|---|---|---|
| | Both Sexes | Males | Fe-males | Both Sexes | Males | Fe-males |
| Health Insurance Plan, New York, 1951[e] | | | | | | |
| Per cent who saw a doctor during the year | — | 68.9 | 71.8 | — | 82.0 | 75.0 |
| Health Insurance Plan, New York, 1955–56[f] | | | | | | |
| Per cent of enrollees seen by HIP doctor during the year | 74.0 | 72.5 | 75.5 | 69.7 | 68.6 | 72.0 |
| Physician services per enrollee per year, total | 5.2 | 4.8 | 5.5 | 7.3 | 7.6 | 6.8 |
| Place of service: Office | 4.1 | 3.8 | 4.4 | 5.3 | 5.4 | 5.2 |
| Home | .5 | .5 | .5 | .5 | .4 | .6 |
| Hospital | .6 | .5 | .6 | 1.5 | 1.8 | 1.0 |
| Physician specialty: | | | | | | |
| Family physician | 3.0 | 2.9 | 3.0 | 4.1 | 4.1 | 4.0 |
| Internist | .2 | .2 | .2 | .6 | .7 | .6 |
| Ophthalmology, otolaryngology | .3 | .3 | .3 | .6 | .6 | .6 |
| Radiology | .4 | .4 | .4 | .6 | .6 | .5 |
| Surgery | .2 | .3 | .2 | .5 | .5 | .3 |
| Urology | .1 | .1 | * | .5 | .7 | .1 |
| Orthopedy | .2 | .2 | .2 | .2 | .2 | .4 |
| Gynecology, obstetrics | .4 | — | .8 | .1 | — | .2 |
| Other | .4 | .4 | .4 | .1 | .2 | .1 |
| Canadian Sickness Survey, 1950–51[g] | | | | | | |
| Per cent of persons with doctors' calls and clinic visits | 43.2 | 38.9 | 47.6 | 49.6 | 44.8 | 54.7 |
| Low income | 40.0 | 35.2 | 44.0 | 51.7 | 47.2 | 55.5 |
| Medium income | 44.2 | 39.3 | 49.2 | 43.1 | 36.2 | 51.9 |
| High income | 44.0 | 40.2 | 48.1 | 52.5 | 51.1 | 54.8 |
| Doctors' calls or clinic visits per person per year, total | 1.8 | 1.5 | 2.1 | 2.8 | 2.4 | 3.1 |
| Doctors' calls, total | 1.6 | 1.3 | 2.0 | 2.6 | 2.3 | 2.8 |
| Office | 1.1 | .9 | 1.4 | 1.3 | 1.1 | 1.4 |
| Home | .5 | .4 | .6 | 1.3 | 1.1 | 1.4 |
| Clinic visits | .1 | .2 | .1 | .2 | — | — |

* Less than .05.

Sources:

[a] U.S. National Health Survey, *Preliminary Report on Volume of Physician Visits, United States, July–September 1957,* and *Selected Survey Topics, United States, July 1957–June 1958,* Public Health Service, Washington, D.C., 1958.

[b] Unpublished data from the 1957 survey by the National Opinion Research Center sponsored by the Health Information Foundation.

[c] O. W. Anderson and J. J. Feldman, *Family Medical Costs and Voluntary Health Insurance: A Nationwide Survey* (New York: McGraw-Hill Book Co., Inc., 1956), p. 196.

[d] *Health in California,* Department of Public Health, State of California, Berkeley, 1957, pp. 33 and 96.

[e] *Health and Medical Care in New York City* (Cambridge, Mass.: Harvard University Press, 1957), p. 49.

[f] S. Shapiro and M. Einhorn, "Experience With Older Members in a Prepaid Medical Care Plan," *Public Health Reports,* Vol. 73, p. 687 (August, 1958).

[g] Dominion Bureau of Statistics and Department of National Health and Welfare, *Canadian Sickness Survey, 1950–51,* No. 8, *Volume of Health Care,* Table 6D, and No. 9, *Volume of Health Care for Selected Income Groups,* Table 4D, Ottawa, October, 1955 and February, 1956.

than for aged males. Most contacts with the physician by the aged were at his office. Moreover, home visits were relatively more frequent for aged females than for aged males. Less than one tenth of the contacts with a physician were at a hospital clinic. Four fifths of the physicians' visits by the aged were for diagnosis and treatment and only one tenth for a general check-up. These findings by the National Health Survey corroborate those from the survey made by the National Opinion Research Center during May–June, 1957, as evident in Table 4.15.

The relatively greater use of physicians' services by the aged, as compared with the population as a whole is seen also in several other experiences, notably the California Health Survey conducted from May, 1954 to April, 1955, nationwide sample surveys of the United States, and the Canadian Sickness Survey of 1950–51. In particular, it was estimated from the United States survey of 1952–53 that 13 per cent of the aged had 15 or more out-of-hospital physician calls annually—practically twice the rate for persons of all ages. Also, aged women made this intensive use of physicians' services much more frequently than aged men.

In the experience of enrollees in the Health Insurance Plan of Greater New York in 1955–56, it was found that over half of the visits by the aged were to the family physician, at a rate of 4.1 per person per year out of a total of 7.3 for all physician visits. However, these figures relate only to visits made to physicians on the panels of the Plan; no record is available of visits to physicians outside the Plan. Less than one tenth of the visits by the aged were to physicians in each of a number of specialties, as internal medicine, ophthalmology, or otolaryngology, radiology, surgery, and urology.

A feature of some interest, in the Canadian Sickness Survey of 1950–51, is that the category of aged population there classified as with medium income had a smaller proportion with doctors' calls than those with low or high incomes. This was not evident in the proportions for persons of all ages.

The leading role of the cardiovascular diseases among the

morbid conditions of the aged, as reported in sickness surveys, is reflected in the reasons given by physicians for the visits of their patients, as shown in Table 4.16. The data, which relate to the state of Washington in 1953, were obtained from a sample of about one third of the physicians

TABLE 4.16

DISTRIBUTION OF REASONS FOR VISIT OF PATIENTS AGED 65 AND OVER BY SEX, AS REPORTED BY PHYSICIANS ACCORDING TO BROAD ILLNESS CATEGORIES, STATE OF WASHINGTON, 1953

| Rank | Reason for Visit | Per Cent | | |
|---|---|---|---|---|
| | | Both Sexes | Males | Females |
| | Total | 100.0 | 100.0 | 100.0 |
| 1 | Cardiovascular | 24.5 | 23.0 | 25.9 |
| 2 | Nervous system and special senses | 11.2 | 11.1 | 11.3 |
| 3 | Musculoskeletal | 8.0 | 6.5 | 9.4 |
| 4 | Digestive | 7.3 | 8.3 | 6.4 |
| 5 | Neoplasms | 7.0 | 7.8 | 6.4 |
| 6 | Genito-urinary | 6.8 | 9.1 | 4.7 |
| 7 | Respiratory | 6.8 | 7.8 | 5.9 |
| 8 | Accidents | 6.6 | 5.7 | 7.4 |
| 9 | Symptoms and ill-defined | 4.8 | 5.1 | 4.5 |
| 10 | Metabolic and nutritive | 4.1 | 3.4 | 4.6 |
| 11 | Skin and subcutaneous tissues | 3.3 | 3.5 | 3.2 |
| 12 | Blood diseases | 3.2 | 2.4 | 4.0 |
| 13 | Allergies | 2.0 | 2.1 | 1.9 |
| 14 | Health supervision | 1.5 | 1.6 | 1.4 |
| 15 | Mental | 1.4 | 1.0 | 1.8 |
| 16 | Infectious and parasitic | 1.3 | 1.6 | 1.0 |
| 17 | Malformations | .1 | .1 | .2 |

Source: S. Standish, Jr., B. M. Bennett, K. White, and L. E. Powers, *Why Patients See Doctors* (Seattle: University of Washington Press, 1955), p. 15.

of the state using the records of all patients seen on four Tuesdays spaced at three-month intervals. The cardiovascular conditions accounted for one quarter of the visits at ages 65 and over and conditions of the nervous system and special senses for one ninth.[70] Third place was taken by conditions

---

[70] The May–June, 1957 survey of the National Opinion Research Center also found that about one fourth of the aged saw a doctor in the home, office, or clinic because of diseases of the circulatory system, as reported in *Progress in Health Services*, Vol. 8 (April, 1959), Health Information Foundation, New York.

of the genito-urinary system among aged males and of the musculoskeletal system by aged females. Only 1.5 per cent of the visits by the aged were for health supervision.

The list of diagnoses reported for the aged by physicians were also led by cardiovascular conditions, as shown in Table

TABLE 4.17

DIAGNOSES MOST FREQUENTLY REPORTED BY PHYSICIANS FOR PATIENTS AGED 65 AND OVER, STATE OF WASHINGTON, 1953

| Diagnosis of Physician | Per Cent of All Visits |
|---|---|
| All diagnoses | 100.0 |
| Arteriosclerotic heart disease, including coronary disease | 6.1 |
| Essential benign hypertension without mention of heart | 4.2 |
| Other and unspecified diseases of heart | 4.0 |
| Arthritis, unspecified | 3.3 |
| Diabetes mellitus | 3.0 |
| Other and unspecified hypertensive heart disease | 2.6 |
| Hyperplasia of prostate | 2.1 |
| Osteoarthritis (arthrosis) and allied conditions | 1.8 |
| Anaemia of unspecified type | 1.7 |
| Cerebral haemorrhage | 1.6 |
| General arteriosclerosis | 1.4 |
| Pernicious and other hyperchronic anaemias | 1.4 |
| Asthma | 1.4 |
| Cystitis | 1.3 |
| Other myocardial degeneration | 1.2 |
| Fracture of neck of femur | 1.2 |
| Cataract | 1.2 |
| Other and ill-defined vascular lesions affecting central nervous system | 1.1 |
| Refractive errors | 1.1 |
| Hernia of abdominal cavity without mention of obstruction | 1.0 |
| Examinations | 1.0 |
| All other | 56.3 |

Source: P. 21 of source in Table 4.16.

4.17. The three leading specific conditions—arteriosclerotic heart disease (including coronary disease), essential benign hypertension without mention of heart, and other and unspecified diseases of the heart—jointly accounted for 14.3 per cent of all visits at ages 65 and over. The two conditions with mention of heart disease, together with the categories consisting of other and unspecified hypertensive heart disease and of other myocardial degeneration make up 13.9 per cent of the total diagnoses. It is interesting to note in this connection that in the Baltimore survey 14.2 per cent of the diagnoses found on clinical evaluation among the aged were for heart disease.[71]

**Dental Services.** The United States National Health Survey for July–September, 1957, showed that 60 per cent of the population at ages 65 and over had lost all their teeth; among those at ages 75 and over, 67 per cent were edentulous. The proportion edentulous among the aged in rural areas, 64 per cent, was higher than in urban places, 57 per cent (Table 4.18). With such high proportions of the aged without any teeth, the proportion who last visited their dentist within the year prior to interview was understandably low, only 15.8 per cent, as compared with 35.9 per cent for persons of all ages. About the same proportion was found in a nationwide sample survey of the United States in 1953 (13 per cent).[72] Whereas only 14.8 per cent of the population of all ages in the 1957 survey last saw a dentist five or more years ago, for the aged the proportion was 54.8 per cent. Corresponding to these differentials between the entire population and older persons, the number of dental visits per person per year was only .6 at ages 65 and over, compared with 1.6 at all ages. The data relate only to the noninstitutional population of the country. The dental care of the aged in institutions or confined to the home requires the development of special techniques since office visits are not possible.

Although the Health Insurance Plan of Greater New York does not provide for dental services, the situation regarding dental care among its enrollees was included in a survey of medical care made in 1951; at the same time a corresponding survey was made of the general population in New York City for comparative purposes. The inferences were that persons

---

[71] See Table 3.6.

[72] The nationwide survey on a sample of the population of the United States in 1955 by the National Opinion Research Center showed that 84 per cent of the aged did not make it a practice to see a dentist at least once a year (see p. 79 of Chapter 3).

## TABLE 4.18

INCIDENCE AND CHARACTERISTICS OF DENTAL SERVICES IN SEVERAL
EXPERIENCES, BY SEX, ALL AGES AND AGES 65 AND OVER

| Experience | All Ages | | | Ages 65 and Over | | |
|---|---|---|---|---|---|---|
| | Both Sexes | Males | Fe-males | Both Sexes | Males | Fe-males |
| **United States, July–September, 1957[a]** | | | | | | |
| Per cent of persons who are edentulous | | | | | | |
| Total......................... | 13.0 | — | — | 60.0 | — | — |
| Urban................... | 13.0 | — | — | 57.0 | — | — |
| Rural..................... | 13.0 | — | — | 64.0 | — | — |
| Per cent having last visit to dentist | | | | | | |
| Within one year............... | 35.9 | 33.8 | 37.9 | 15.8 | 16.4 | 15.2 |
| 1–2 years ago................. | 22.2 | 22.4 | 22.0 | 14.2 | 13.8 | 14.4 |
| 3–4 years ago................. | 6.4 | 6.5 | 6.4 | 7.8 | 6.9 | 8.7 |
| 5 or more years ago............ | 14.8 | 14.8 | 14.8 | 54.8 | 54.4 | 55.1 |
| Never or unknown............. | 20.6 | 22.5 | 18.9 | 7.5 | 8.5 | 6.5 |
| Dental visits per person per year... | | | | | | |
| Total......................... | 1.6 | — | — | .6 | — | — |
| Urban.................... | 1.9 | — | — | .8 | — | — |
| Rural..................... | 1.2 | — | — | .4 | — | — |
| **United States, July, 1957–June, 1958[a]** | | | | | | |
| Dental visits per person per year | | | | | | |
| Total......................... | 1.6 | 1.4 | 1.8 | .8 | .8 | .7 |
| Fillings..................... | .7 | .6 | .8 | .1 | .1 | .1 |
| Extractions................. | .3 | .3 | .3 | .2 | .2 | .1 |
| Cleanings................... | .2 | .2 | .2 | .0 | .0 | .1 |
| Other...................... | .5 | .4 | .6 | .4 | .5 | .4 |
| **United States, 1953[b]** | | | | | | |
| Per cent of persons receiving dental services...................... | 34.0 | 31.0 | 36.0 | 13.0 | 13.0 | 12.0 |
| **New York City Sample, 1951[c]** (data relate to 8-week period preceding interview) | | | | | | |
| Dental visits per 100 persons...... | 31.3 | — | — | 8.5 | — | — |
| Attended dental conditions per 100 persons, total................ | 9.9 | 9.0 | 10.7 | 3.5 | 4.8 | 2.4 |
| Dental conditions only.......... | 6.1 | 5.9 | 6.2 | 1.4 | 1.9 | 1.0 |
| Dental and medical conditions... | 3.8 | 3.1 | 4.5 | 2.1 | 2.9 | 1.4 |
| Dental and medical conditions still present on day preceding interview per 100 persons.......... | 1.3 | .8 | 1.7 | .7 | 1.0 | .4 |
| **Health Insurance Plan, New York, 1951[c]** (data relate to 8-week period preceding interview) | | | | | | |
| Dental visits per 100 persons...... | 38.6 | — | — | 24.1 | — | — |
| Attended dental conditions per 100 persons, total................ | 12.0 | 10.9 | 13.2 | 8.7 | 9.8 | 5.8 |
| Dental conditions only.......... | 6.8 | 6.2 | 7.5 | 3.1 | 4.2 | — |
| Dental and medical conditions... | 5.2 | 4.7 | 5.7 | 5.6 | 5.6 | 5.8 |
| Dental and medical conditions still present on day preceding interview per 100 persons............ | 1.5 | 1.3 | 1.7 | 2.6 | 2.1 | 3.9 |

Sources:
[a] U.S. National Health Survey, *Preliminary Report on Volume of Dental Care, United States, July–September 1957*, and *Selected Survey Topics, United States, July 1957–June 1958*, Public Health Service, Washington, D.C., 1958.
[b] O. W. Anderson and J. J. Feldman, *Family Medical Costs and Voluntary Health Insurance: A Nationwide Survey* (New York: McGraw-Hill Book Co., Inc., 1956), p. 198.
[c] *Health and Medical Care in New York City* (Cambridge, Mass.: Harvard University Press 1957), pp. 173, 176, 178.

insured for physicians' services would be more frequently referred for dental care and that, with medical care prepaid, more of the enrollees would be able to pay for dental care. In support of these inferences, it was found that the rate of dental visits within the eight weeks preceding the interview was greater for the enrollees than for the comparable general population; at ages 65 and over, the rates per 100 persons were 24.1 and 8.5 respectively. The aged enrollees also had a greater frequency of attended dental conditions within the period, namely 8.7 per 100 persons, whereas the general population had a rate of 3.5 per 100. Moreover, two thirds of these aged enrollees with dental conditions also had some medical condition (the two not necessarily being related), compared with three fifths for the population.[73]

An insight into the services provided by dentists to their patients was obtained from a sample survey conducted by the American Dental Association in May, 1954; a summary of some results is shown in Table 4.19. These data are not representative of the population since they reflect the situation among persons sufficiently aware of their needs to visit a dentist and generally with incomes well above average. Although many of the aged were edentulous, about one third of the patients were in need of fillings.[74] Also, close to one third of the aged patients required extractions, about the same proportion as for patients of all ages. However, for the aged the average number of teeth needing extraction was high, namely 2.83 for white males at ages 70 and over and 1.55 for white females of the same ages. At these ages, 19.7 per cent of the males and 27.6 per cent of the females required partial dentures. Complete upper and lower dentures

---

[73] For another study of dental health care utilization, but with data for ages 65 and over based upon a very limited number of cases, see *Comprehensive Dental Care in a Group Practice*, Public Health Service Publication No. 395, Washington, D.C., November, 1954.

[74] Pertinent to the content of this paragraph is the article by D. J. Galagan, "Development of Dental Health Care Programs for Persons with Chronic Illness," *Journal of the American Dental Association*, Vol. 53, p. 686 (December, 1956).

TABLE 4.19

DENTAL NEEDS IN A SAMPLE OF PATIENTS AGED 65 AND OVER, BY SEX, 1954

| Dental Service | White Males | | | White Females | | |
|---|---|---|---|---|---|---|
| | All Ages | Ages 65–69 | Ages 70 and Over | All Ages | Ages 65–69 | Ages 70 and Over |
| | Per Cent of Cases Needing Specified Service | | | | | |
| Teeth needing fillings | 65.4 | 31.8 | 23.9 | 68.7 | 33.6 | 36.9 |
| Extractions.......... | 34.1 | 35.4 | 38.9 | 30.7 | 30.0 | 29.7 |
| Crowns.............. | 5.3 | 5.0 | 7.4 | 4.7 | 2.9 | 3.9 |
| Fixed bridges | | | | | | |
| First.............. | 14.9 | 6.8 | 4.0 | 15.5 | 8.1 | 4.2 |
| Second............ | 5.8 | 2.1 | 3.1 | 6.0 | 3.1 | .8 |
| Third............. | 1.5 | .6 | .9 | 1.6 | 1.6 | .3 |
| Removable bridges | | | | | | |
| First.............. | 4.6 | 4.2 | 4.9 | 5.3 | 5.1 | 4.5 |
| Second............ | 1.3 | .9 | .9 | 1.4 | .9 | 1.1 |
| Partial dentures | | | | | | |
| First.............. | 12.0 | 16.8 | 14.8 | 13.8 | 13.8 | 22.3 |
| Second............ | 4.0 | 6.0 | 4.9 | 4.3 | 3.4 | 5.3 |
| Complete dentures | | | | | | |
| Lower only........ | 1.0 | 5.3 | 4.3 | 1.1 | 5.6 | 5.0 |
| Upper only........ | 3.3 | 9.2 | 5.8 | 3.5 | 5.8 | 8.1 |
| Upper and lower... | 8.0 | 24.6 | 28.5 | 5.7 | 25.1 | 19.2 |
| Periodontal treatment | 7.5 | 10.9 | 7.4 | 8.1 | 8.2 | 12.7 |
| No dental needs*..... | 8.2 | 7.1 | 8.6 | 8.2 | 9.2 | 8.4 |
| Permanent teeth missing.............. | 56.0 | 96.6 | 88.6 | 55.0 | 74.1 | 95.2 |
| Permanent teeth previously replaced.... | 19.1 | 46.3 | 48.9 | 21.8 | 53.0 | 51.5 |
| | Average Number of Teeth Needing Service per Case | | | | | |
| Teeth needing fillings. | 3.00 | .88 | .52 | 3.07 | .79 | .94 |
| Extractions.......... | 1.66 | 2.65 | 2.83 | 1.41 | 2.36 | 1.55 |
| Crowns.............. | .10 | .07 | .18 | .09 | .06 | .05 |
| Fixed bridges | | | | | | |
| First.............. | .21 | .13 | .06 | .21 | .16 | .06 |
| Second............ | .08 | .04 | .05 | .08 | .06 | .02 |
| Third............. | .02 | .01 | .02 | .02 | .02 | .01 |
| Removable bridges | | | | | | |
| First.............. | .12 | .12 | .17 | .14 | .14 | .14 |
| Second............ | .03 | .03 | .06 | .03 | .05 | .03 |
| Partial dentures | | | | | | |
| First.............. | .58 | .95 | .83 | .66 | .77 | 1.33 |
| Second............ | .19 | .32 | .25 | .20 | .20 | .28 |
| Periodontal treatment | 1.03 | 1.26 | .80 | 1.10 | .76 | 1.46 |
| Permanent teeth missing.............. | 5.43 | 18.21 | 15.66 | 4.27 | 11.50 | 16.61 |
| Permanent teeth previously replaced.... | 1.70 | 6.33 | 7.30 | 1.79 | 7.93 | 8.33 |

* Other than prophylaxis.

Source: *Survey of Needs for Dental Care*, American Dental Association, Chicago, 1954.

were needed by 28.5 per cent of the aged males and 19.2 per cent of the aged females. All but a small fraction of the aged were missing some permanent teeth, averaging near 16 per person, and about half had permanent teeth replaced. Only a little more than 8 per cent of those aged 70 and over had no dental needs.

*Other Services.* Very few data are available to describe the utilization of other medical care services by the aged. The September, 1956 sample survey showed that outpatient care in general hospitals was received annually by 41 persons per 1,000 population at ages 65 and over outside institutions, compared with 47 per 1,000 at all ages. These rates relate to care received in the hospital, such as in a clinic, emergency room, outpatient department, and similar facilities, in which an overnight stay was not involved.[75] Outpatient visits were made at an annual rate of 193 per 1,000 population at ages 65 and over, and 161 per 1,000 at all ages. Since the reporting in the survey depended upon recall, it is likely that these findings understate the actual use of outpatient hospital facilities.

The survey conducted during May–June, 1957 by the National Opinion Research Center on a sample of persons at ages 65 and over showed that 7.4 per cent had some nursing care during the four weeks preceding the interview; for males it was 5.5 per cent and for females 9.1 per cent.[76] Four fifths of this nursing care was given by a relative, one seventh by a friend, only 5 per cent by a nurse, and the rest by some other person or no reply was given. Males received a larger proportion of their nursing care from relatives than did females, but females were helped in a larger proportion of cases by friends. As part of the California Health Survey, an inquiry was made into home nursing care received from January through April, 1955.[77] Because chronic conditions are usually involved

[75] M. E. Odoroff and L. M. Abbe, "Use of General Hospitals: Factors in Outpatient Visits," *Public Health Reports,* Vol. 72, p. 478 (June, 1957).

[76] *Progress in Health Services,* Vol. 8 (April, 1959), Health Information Foundation, New York.

[77] *Health in California, op. cit.,* p. 34.

HV
1461
.S6
1160

HIS
232 02   Afr

MUS
232 01   Afr

REL
230 02   Sur

https://campuswe

in home nursing care, it was believed that the seasonal influence was not great. During the survey months, home nursing care was received at a rate of 65 per 1,000 population at ages 65 and over and at a rate of 5 per 1,000 by younger persons; about two fifths of the home nursing was for full time care. Home nursing care is very likely to grow in importance as a result of the rising income of the aged and of those upon whom they are dependent, the development of home care programs, and the increasing awareness of the benefits of medical supervision in the home environment.

Earlier in this chapter, reference was made to a survey of nursing homes and like facilities conducted by the Public Health Service in 1954. For the 13 states included in this survey, the number of patients in proprietary nursing homes at ages 65 and over per 1,000 population was 7.3 for males and 13.7 for females. For both sexes, the rates per 1,000 rose from 3.7 at ages 65–74 years to 18.7 at ages 75–84 and then to 63.8 at ages 85 and over. Nearly 90 per cent of the patients in proprietary nursing homes and in domiciliary care homes were at ages 65 and over; for voluntary and public nursing homes, nearly 80 per cent were at these ages.

*Veteran Experience.* It is estimated that as of November, 1956 about 2.5 per cent of the veterans at ages 65 and over were hospitalized under the hospital program of the Veterans Administration.[78] These aged veterans then constituted 16.0 per cent of all veterans hospitalized under the V.A. program. Psychotic and other psychiatric conditions accounted for 46 per cent of the aged patients, general medical and surgical conditions (principally heart diseases, cancer and tumors, and diseases of the digestive system) for over 40 per cent, tuberculosis for 7 per cent, and neurological conditions for 6 per cent.

---

[78] This estimate is derived from the table on p. 11 of the Annual Report of the Administrator of Veterans Affairs for Fiscal Year Ending June 30, 1957, and an estimate of 700,000 veterans at ages 65 and over in 1955. See also p. 228 of Chapter 7.

# Medical Care Expenditures of the Aged

5

MOST DATA used to describe medical care expenditures in this section relate to 1950 and the years immediately following. Medical expenditures during this period have been affected by a number of factors. Thus, the rise in income of the aged has given them more funds for their medical care needs. Then, advances in medicine have introduced new therapies and services to be paid for; at the same time, the costs of medical and hospital care have risen more rapidly than the general cost of living.[1] Lastly, the rapid growth of health insurance has increased the flow of funds available for medical and hospital care costs.

## INDIVIDUAL EXPENDITURES

*Distribution.* The consumer expenditure survey conducted on a sample of the urban population of the United States by the Bureau of Labor Statistics in 1950 yielded medical care data summarized, in part, in Table 5.1. In this survey, the annual out-of-pocket medical care expenditures averaged $65 per person of all ages, $87 at ages 65–74 years, and $76 at ages 75 and over. These expenditures include health insurance premiums paid by family members, medical expenses incurred during illness exclusive of those paid by

---

[1] *The Story in Charts of the Economic Position of Medical Care, 1929–1953,* Bulletin 99A, Bureau of Medical Economic Research (Chicago: American Medical Association, 1955).

TABLE 5.1

SELECTED CHARACTERISTICS OF MEDICAL CARE EXPENDITURES OF PERSONS AT
ALL AGES AND AGES 65 AND OVER
Urban Population of the United States, 1950

| Characteristics | All Ages | Ages 65 and Over | | |
|---|---|---|---|---|
| | | Total | 65–74 | 75 and over |
| Average out-of-pocket medical care expenditures per person......... | $65 | — | $87 | $76 |
| Per cent distribution of persons by amount of out-of-pocket medical care expenditures, total......... | 100.0 | — | 100.0 | 100.0 |
| None...................... | 17.4 | — | 19.2 | 30.7 |
| $1–$49.99.................. | 47.9 | — | 41.3 | 37.2 |
| $50–$99.99................. | 17.5 | — | 12.9 | 11.6 |
| $100–$199.99............... | 10.2 | — | 16.7 | 11.4 |
| $200 and over.............. | 7.0 | — | 9.9 | 9.1 |
| Per cent distribution of medical care expenditures by amount of out-of-pocket medical care expenditures, total......................... | 100.0 | — | 100.0 | 100.0 |
| $1–$49.99.................. | 17.4 | — | 11.2 | 11.5 |
| $50–$99.99................. | 19.1 | — | 10.6 | 10.8 |
| $100–$199.99............... | 22.2 | — | 27.2 | 21.2 |
| $200 and over.............. | 41.3 | — | 51.0 | 56.5 |
| Per cent distribution of persons in families spending $1,000 or more for medical care............... | 100.0 | 14.2 | — | — |
| Per cent of persons reporting free medical care.................. | 7.2 | — | 6.1 | 7.5 |
| Per cent of persons with some health insurance coverage............ | | | | |
| All persons.................. | 60.7 | 36.6 | 41.8 | 25.7 |
| Persons in families with medical care expenditures of $1,000 or more.................... | 60.9 | 41.3 | — | — |
| Per cent distribution of population | | | | |
| United States................ | 100.0 | 8.1 | 5.6 | 2.5 |
| Sample survey............... | 100.0 | 8.6 | 5.8 | 2.8 |

Source: S. Mushkin, "Age Differential in Medical Spending" and "Characteristics of Large Medical Expenses," *Public Health Reports*, Vol. 72, pp. 115 and 697 (February and August, 1957); S. Mushkin and B. Crowther, "Free Medical Care in Cities," *Public Health Reports*, Vol. 73, p. 1107 (December, 1958).

an insurance coverage, and miscellaneous expenses for routine physical and dental examinations, nonprescription drugs, and the like.

At all ages, the burden of heavy medical expenditures fell upon relatively few, the 7.0 per cent of persons with out-of-pocket expenditures of $200 or more accounting for 41.3 per cent of the total expenditures. However, among the aged, almost one tenth had annual medical expenses of $200 or more, and these bore well over half of all such expenditures at that stage of life. Furthermore, the aged, who were only 8.6 per cent of the total population in the survey, accounted for 14.2 per cent of the persons in families with medical expenditures of $1,000 or more. Free medical care was received by 6.1 per cent of those at ages 65–74 and 7.5 per cent at ages 75 and over, compared with 7.2 per cent for all ages.[2] At that time, among the urban aged in families incurring medical care expenditures of $1,000 or more, 41.3 per cent had the protection of health insurance.

Although the nationwide survey supported by the Health Information Foundation during 1952–53 was later than that of the Bureau of Labor Statistics and the two had differences in definition, both yielded an average annual expenditure of $65 per person of all ages. The principal difference is that the later study excludes health insurance premiums from expenditures, but does include the cost of services received which are paid in full or in part by an insurance plan; the earlier study, as already indicated, allocated premiums to current expenditures and excluded any benefits received by health insurance coverage. At ages 65 and over, there was

---

[2] Free medical care, in the 1950 survey, includes not only free services in public and private clinics, but also "(a) automobile and other casualty insurance received as a result of an accident, (b) workmen's compensation medical services and inplant medical services, and (c) medical services in union health facilities and in special railroad hospitals," and "free care . . . in public hospitals or financed under public programs, . . . , care financed by private welfare, health, and religious agencies and hospitals, and care provided without charge by members of a health profession as a matter of professional courtesy or as charity."

an average annual medical care expenditure of $83 per person in 1950, compared with $102 in 1952–53.

The 1952–53 survey showed an average annual medical care charge of $77 per aged male and $124 per aged female (Table 5.2). The higher average charge for females was evident for each type of service except dental care, which is only a minor item. Of the total annual medical care charge of $102 per aged person, one fourth was for hospital services, over one third for the physician, over one fifth for medicines, and one sixth for other medical services. The principal difference in the charges between persons with hospital insurance and those not so protected lies in the higher hospital charges for the latter. The bottom tier of Table 5.2 shows that the aged person with a hospital bill incurred an average charge of $203 if insured and $254 if not insured.

Whereas the annual medical care charge for the aged averaged $102 in the 1952–53 survey, in a corresponding survey for 1957–58 made jointly by the Health Information Foundation and the National Opinion Research Center the average was $177, an increase of 73.5 per cent.[3] However, for persons of all ages combined the average annual medical care charge in 1957–58 was $94, the increase since 1952–53 amounting to 42.4 per cent. Between the two periods, the average charges for the aged almost doubled for hospital expenditures—rising to $49 per person—and for drugs and medications, which rose to $42 per person. Dental costs increased even more rapidly, from $4 to $10. For physician's charges, the average annual expenditure per aged person was $55 in 1957–58, about 1½ times that in 1952–53. As a result of these shifts, a smaller proportion of the medical care expenditures of the aged is going to physicians and a larger proportion for hospital care, drugs and medications,

---

[3] *Progress in Health Services,* Vol. 9 (February, 1960), Health Information Foundation, New York. This source notes that some of this increase, particularly for the older ages, may be due to the epidemic of Asian influenza during the later survey period.

TABLE 5.2

AVERAGE GROSS CHARGES PER PERSON FOR SPECIFIC TYPES OF PERSONAL
HEALTH SERVICES AT ALL AGES AND AGES 65 AND OVER, BY SEX,
UNITED STATES, 1952–53

| Insurance Status and Service | All Ages | | | Ages 65 and Over | | |
|---|---|---|---|---|---|---|
| | Both Sexes | Males | Fe-males | Both Sexes | Males | Fe-males |
| | All Persons | | | | | |
| **Total sample** | | | | | | |
| All charges............ | $ 65 | $ 51 | $ 80 | $102 | $ 77 | $124 |
| Hospital............ | 13 | 9 | 17 | 25 | 16 | 32 |
| Physician............ | 25 | 19 | 31 | 36 | 30 | 41 |
| Medicines............ | 10 | 7 | 12 | 22 | 17 | 26 |
| "Other" medical..... | 8 | 7 | 9 | 17 | 11 | 23 |
| Dental............ | 10 | 9 | 12 | 4 | 5 | 3 |
| **Insured persons*** | | | | | | |
| All charges............ | 74 | 60 | 88 | 111 | 70 | 158 |
| Hospital............ | 16 | 12 | 20 | 31 | 16 | 50 |
| Physician............ | 38 | 22 | 33 | 36 | 27 | 47 |
| Medicines............ | 10 | 8 | 12 | 23 | 17 | 29 |
| "Other" medical..... | 9 | 7 | 10 | 19 | 8 | 32 |
| Dental............ | 12 | 11 | 13 | 3 | 3 | 2 |
| **Uninsured persons** | | | | | | |
| All charges............ | 55 | 39 | 70 | 98 | 80 | 112 |
| Hospital............ | 9 | 6 | 13 | 22 | 17 | 26 |
| Physician............ | 21 | 15 | 28 | 36 | 32 | 39 |
| Medicines............ | 9 | 6 | 12 | 21 | 16 | 25 |
| "Other" medical..... | 7 | 6 | 9 | 16 | 12 | 19 |
| Dental............ | 8 | 6 | 9 | 5 | 6 | 4 |
| | Persons Incurring Specified Service | | | | | |
| **Total sample** | | | | | | |
| All charges............ | $ 94 | $ 78 | $106 | $140 | $115 | $161 |
| Hospital............ | 140 | 143 | 139 | 233 | 176 | 275 |
| Physician............ | 57 | 51 | 62 | 74 | 68 | 78 |
| Medicines............ | 26 | 23 | 28 | 42 | 37 | 45 |
| "Other" medical..... | 38 | 37 | 39 | 61 | 46 | 71 |
| Dental............ | 32 | 31 | 33 | 37 | 43 | 31 |
| **Insured persons*** | | | | | | |
| All charges............ | 98 | 84 | 110 | 140 | 98 | 181 |
| Hospital............ | 140 | 142 | 138 | 203 | 131 | 261 |
| Physician............ | 58 | 51 | 62 | 65 | 54 | 77 |
| Medicines............ | 25 | 23 | 26 | 40 | 38 | 43 |
| "Other" medical..... | 38 | 36 | 39 | 64 | 34 | 87 |
| Dental............ | 32 | 32 | 33 | 24 | 36 | 12 |
| **Uninsured persons** | | | | | | |
| All charges............ | 87 | 69 | 100 | 141 | 124 | 152 |
| Hospital............ | 142 | 145 | 140 | 254 | 211 | 285 |
| Physician............ | 57 | 49 | 62 | 78 | 77 | 79 |
| Medicines............ | 27 | 23 | 29 | 42 | 36 | 46 |
| "Other" medical..... | 40 | 40 | 39 | 59 | 52 | 63 |
| Dental............ | 32 | 29 | 34 | 43 | 47 | 39 |

Note: In many instances, the component charges in the source do not add to the total.
* Insured persons are those with hospital insurance at end of survey year.

Source: O. W. Anderson and J. J. Feldman, *Family Medical Costs and Voluntary Health Insurance: A Nationwide Survey* (New York: McGraw-Hill Book Co., Inc., 1956), pp. 126–31.

and dental care. This change in pattern is very much like that for persons of all ages.

*Sources of Payment.* The sample survey inquiring into the economic status of the aged conducted by the Bureau of the Census in April, 1952, yielded the data regarding the patterns of medical care expenditures summarized in Table 5.3;[4] the data relate to 1951. During that year, medical services were received by 55.2 per cent of the aged unrelated males, 63.1 per cent of the aged unrelated females, and 69.2 per cent of one or both members of the couples in which the husband was 65 years or older. These figures for 1951, which relate to all services, are of the same magnitude as those cited in Table 4.15 for persons receiving physicians' services within the year prior to interview in the survey of July–September, 1957.

Of those aged persons who received medical services during 1951, no cash outlay was paid by these persons or their families in the case of 10.1 per cent of the unrelated males, 8.1 per cent of the unrelated females, and 5.5 per cent of the couples. In 1951, the proportion of aged couples who had their medical services paid for by hospital or medical insurance averaged only 12.9 per cent; for unrelated persons, it was about half that figure. Free medical services were then received by 6 to 8 per cent of the aged, and a variety of other sources by about 9 per cent of the unrelated persons and 4.5 per cent of the couples. Some of the aged used more than one of these sources. About 96 per cent of the aged incurred no medical debts during 1951 and only 1 per cent had debts of $200 or more.[5]

---

[4] See p. 30 of Chapter 2. Steiner and Dorfman define "medical expenses" to encompass "all the expenses associated with ill health, including hospital expenses, drugs, nursing, as well as strictly medical expenses."

[5] A study of patients at ages 65 and over discharged from two community hospitals in Genesee County, New York, during October, 1955 showed that 53.0 per cent paid their entire bill, 31.3 per cent paid by insurance, and 15.7 per cent had their bill paid by some agency (compared with 7.8 per cent at ages under 65); see A. W. Brewster, *Research and Statistics Note No. 6,* Division of Program Research, Social Security Administration, February 24, 1958.

A later picture of the sources of payment for medical care, but relating only to general hospital charges, was obtained in the September, 1956 survey cited earlier; the data, summarized in Table 5.4, relate to the 12 months preceding the interview.[6] Among the aged receiving hospital services, 43

TABLE 5.3

SOME FINANCIAL ASPECTS IN THE MEDICAL CARE EXPENDITURES OF AGED COUPLES AND OF UNRELATED MALES AND FEMALES, UNITED STATES, 1951

| Financing Aspect | Couples[a] | Unrelated Males[b] | Unrelated Females[b] |
|---|---|---|---|
| Medical services, per cent | 100.0 | 100.0 | 100.0 |
| None | 30.8 | 44.8 | 36.9 |
| Received services | 69.2 | 55.2 | 63.1 |
| Made medical payments[e] | 65.5 | 49.6 | 58.1 |
| No medical payments | 3.7 | 5.6 | 5.0 |
| Size of annual medical payment, per cent | 100.0 | 100.0 | 100.0 |
| None | 5.5 | 10.1 | 8.1 |
| $1–$49 | 30.6 | 42.8 | 40.3 |
| $50–$149 | 34.0 | 26.9 | 31.7 |
| $150–$299 | 15.2 | 6.7 | 10.8 |
| $300 or more | 14.7 | 13.4 | 9.2 |
| Median size | $91.0 | $47.0 | $57.0 |
| Per cent receiving noncash medical services[d] | | | |
| Hospital or medical insurance[e] | 12.9 | 6.4 | 6.8 |
| Free services[f] | 5.6 | 7.7 | 6.1 |
| Other[g] | 4.5 | 8.9 | 9.2 |
| Size of medical debts, per cent | 100.0 | 100.0 | 100.0 |
| None | 95.6 | 97.2 | 95.8 |
| $1–$199 | 3.3 | 2.0 | 3.5 |
| $200 or more | 1.1 | .8 | .7 |

[a] In an aged couple, the husband is 65 years or over, irrespective of the age of the wife.
[b] Ages 65 and over.
[c] Payments made by aged person or family; in case of couples, payments were made for either member.
[d] Payments not paid for by aged persons or relations; percentages for specific services are not exclusive. In case of couples, data relate to either member.
[e] Includes all prepayment or insurance plans, irrespective of payor for the cost.
[f] Services without charge by physician, hospital, sanatorium, clinic, etc.
[g] Medical expenses paid by nonrelatives, by a charitable organization, or by a union or employer (except through a prepaid plan). Does not include amounts later reimbursed.
Source: P. O. Steiner and R. Dorfman, *The Economic Status of the Aged* (Berkeley and Los Angeles: University of California Press, 1957), pp. 143–45.

[6] The charges include "all charges made by the hospital and charges by surgeons, anesthetists, special nurses, or others engaged by the patient for service in the hospital."

per cent then had their bill paid in full or in part by a prepaid plan, 38 per cent paid their bill completely out-of-pocket or with the help of relatives, 8 per cent received free care, and the rest used other methods.[7] The free cases involved lengthy stays, averaging 32.4 days per case compared with 14.0 days for all aged persons. However, the aged who

TABLE 5.4

GENERAL HOSPITAL EXPERIENCE OF NONINSTITUTIONAL POPULATION ACCORDING TO METHOD OF PAYMENT FOR CARE FOR ALL AGES AND FOR AGES 65 AND OVER, UNITED STATES, YEAR ENDING SEPTEMBER, 1956

| Method of Payment for Care | Annual Admission per 1,000 Population | | Average Days of Stay per Admission | | Average Days of Stay per Person per Year | |
|---|---|---|---|---|---|---|
| | All Ages | Ages 65 and Over | All Ages | Ages 65 and Over | All Ages | Ages 65 and Over |
| All methods............ | 101 | 125 | 8.1 | 14.0 | .81 | 1.74 |
| Prepayment plan only | 29 | 18 | 6.5 | 11.2 | .19 | .20 |
| Prepayment plan plus self or relatives..... | 36 | 36 | 7.5 | 12.5 | .27 | .45 |
| Self or relatives, or both.............. | 23 | 48 | 7.0 | 11.9 | .16 | .57 |
| No charge........... | 6 | 10 | 20.1 | 32.4 | .12 | .31 |
| Other methods....... | 5 | 13 | 14.2 | 16.7 | .07 | .22 |

Source: M. E. Odoroff and L. M. Abbe, "Use of General Hospitals: Variation with Methods of Payment," *Public Health Reports*, Vol. 74, p. 316 (April, 1959).

had their hospital bill paid in full by a prepayment plan had an average stay of only 11.2 days.

The recent situation with regard to sources of payments for physicians' services outside the hospital is shown in Table 5.5. These data are derived from a survey of a nationwide sample of aged persons conducted during May–June, 1957 by the National Opinion Research Center with the support of the Health Information Foundation; they refer to the four

---

[7] In this connection, see W. Polner, "Voluntary Health Insurance Payments for Short-Term General Hospital Stays of Aged Persons," *Journal of the American Medical Association*, Vol. 171, p. 1113 (October 24, 1959).

weeks preceding the interview.[8] In this sample, 71 per cent stated they made out-of-pocket payments to the physician, over 20 per cent made no such payments (this includes bills covered by insurance), and over 8 per cent did not answer. Among those reporting on the amount, the average payment during the four weeks was $12.26.

TABLE 5.5

SOURCES AND AMOUNT OF PAYMENT FOR PHYSICIAN CHARGES OUTSIDE THE HOSPITAL BY PERSONS AT AGES 65 AND OVER DURING FOUR WEEKS PRIOR TO INTERVIEW, SURVEY OF MAY–JUNE, 1957

| Payment Item | Per Cent |
|---|---|
| Payment for services of physician | 100.0 |
| Did pay out-of-pocket | 71.0 |
| Did not pay out-of-pocket | 20.5 |
| No answer | 8.5 |
| Amount of payment reported | 100.0 |
| $ 1–$ 4 | 25.6 |
| 5– 9 | 31.8 |
| 10– 29 | 35.4 |
| 30– 49 | 5.2 |
| 50 and over | 2.0 |
| Average | $12.26 |
| Source of payments* | |
| Own resources | |
| Income | 67.6 |
| Savings | 21.1 |
| Other | 2.4 |
| Child or relative | 8.3 |
| Someone else | 1.5 |
| No answer | 2.4 |
| Reasons for not paying | 100.0 |
| Welfare or charitable agency paid | 36.1 |
| Bills covered by insurance | 14.4 |
| All others | 49.5 |

* Per cents total to more than 100 since the doctor may have been paid from several sources by an individual.

Source: "Use of Health Services by the Aged," *Progress in Health Services*, Vol. 8 (April, 1959), Health Information Foundation, New York. The detailed data corresponding to those in the charts of this report were supplied by the Health Information Foundation.

---

[8] *Progress in Health Services,* Vol. 8 (April, 1959), Health Information Foundation, New York.

The aged relied very largely upon their own resources in paying for physicians' services outside the hospital. Among these aged persons, 68 per cent reported paying from current income, 21 per cent from savings, and over 2 per cent from other resources. On the other hand, a child or relative paid in over 8 per cent of the cases and someone else for 1½ per cent.

In the case of the aged who made no out-of-pocket payment for their physicians' services during the four weeks, 36 per cent had their bill paid by a welfare or charitable agency, over 14 per cent by insurance, and the rest by other sources.[9]

**Aged Beneficiaries of Old-Age and Survivors Insurance.** The 1957 survey of aged beneficiaries under OASI, already referred to, included among its medical cost items not only payments to physicians, hospitals, and for prescribed medication, but also expenditures for the incidental items that go into the family medicine chest.[10] Accordingly, it is not surprising to find that among the beneficiary couples, one of whom might be under 65 years of age, only 3 per cent incurred no medical costs and almost half had an annual cost of less than $200; free care was reported in 6 per cent of these cases. For these couples, the proportion of persons with medical costs per person of less than $100 (including no costs) ranged from 70 per cent where the money income was less than $1,200 to 50 per cent where it was $5,000 or more. The items included in these costs are not indicated. One possibility is that those with the higher income may devote a larger share of their medical expenditures to so-called "luxury" items. On the other hand, where income is low, large medical expenditures are obviously impossible. Among the unmarried beneficiaries, half had costs of less than $100,

---

[9] Other aspects of the sources of payment for individual medical care expenditures are described in *The Aging of Three Parishes,* National Conference of Catholic Charities, Washington, D.C., and the detailed report for each parish.

[10] *Hospitalization Insurance for OASDI Beneficiaries, op. cit.,* pp. 24–31; "Medical Care Costs of Aged OASI Beneficiaries: Highlights from Preliminary Data, 1957 Survey," *Social Security Bulletin,* April, 1959.

including 8 per cent with no such costs; 8 per cent had some free care.

When all medical care expenditures are considered, including the trivial items, the proportion having insurance cover some of these costs is naturally low. For aged beneficiary couples it amounted to 14 per cent and for the unmarried it was 9 per cent. These proportions become appreciably greater in cases with large medical expenditures. Costs of $800 or more during the year were incurred by 9 per cent of the beneficiary couples. These high costs were met by various means, often by more than one. Thus, 53 per cent had insurance cover some of their costs, 84 per cent used some of their own resources (assets or current income or both), 15 per cent had their relatives assume some responsibility, 25 per cent increased their medical debt, and 2 per cent had at least some of it paid by a health or welfare agency.

In the case of unmarried beneficiaries, 8 per cent incurred annual medical care expenditures of $500 or more. In this instance, 38 per cent had some of their costs covered by insurance, 61 per cent relied in whole or in part upon their own resources, 31 per cent were helped by relatives, 10 per cent increased their medical debt, and 12 per cent received some aid from a health or welfare agency.

Among the aged beneficiaries in the 1957 study of the OASI, 30.0 per cent were at ages 75 and over. The proportion was 37.1 per cent for those aged beneficiaries who were also recipients of Old-Age Assistance.[11] This age differential is reflected in a comparison of the medical care utilization and costs of the two groups. Whereas 9.8 per cent of all aged beneficiaries incurred no medical costs during the survey year, for those who were also OAA recipients the proportion was only 5.7 per cent. Excluding those with no such costs and those for whom they were not known, the median costs amounted to $87 for all OASI beneficiaries and $100 for

---

[11] S. Ossman, "Characteristics of Aged Old-Age and Survivors Insurance Beneficiaries Who Receive Public Assistance," *Social Security Bulletin,* October, 1959.

beneficiaries also in receipt of OAA. It was also found that the proportions hospitalized during the survey year were 12.9 per cent and 22.6 per cent, respectively. The relation between the OASI and the OAA programs is discussed further in Chapter 7.

*Relation to Income and Savings.* It will be recalled that the prevalence of disability from chronic conditions among the aged was high where family income was very small and also where it was rather large. Since low income is frequently a consequence of disability, often lasting over a protracted period, there is an obvious need for the study of medical care expenditures in relation to resources over a closely corresponding period.[12] For example, a family whose breadwinner experiences costly and protracted illness during one year will consequently have a low income, but its income in the years preceding and following the illness might have been moderate or even appreciable. However, studies as that summarized in Table 5.6 generally describe the situation during one calendar year. These data, which relate to 1951, show that the aged without medical services during the year had greater proportions in the higher-income brackets and with larger assets than those who used such services.[13] For example, among aged couples who had no medical services, 9.2 per cent had annual receipts of $5,000 or more, compared with 7.0 per cent for those using medical services. Also, the respective proportions with assets of $3,000 or more are 69.8 and 66.2 per cent.

The major medical care charges—physicians' and hospital services—are usually related to income; the physician may set his fee accordingly and the wealthier patient will ask for the better hospital accommodation. Most other medical care services or goods have fixed unit prices. The data for aged couples in Table 5.6 reflect the situation. Thus, the propor-

---

[12] M. Spiegelman, "New Frontiers in Medical Statistics," *The Milbank Memorial Fund Quarterly,* Vol. 35, p. 48 (January, 1957).

[13] Receipts, in Table 5.6, include income, occasional cash gifts, lump-sum receipts such as insurance payments on inheritance, and the use of savings.

# TABLE 5.6

## RELATION OF ANNUAL RECEIPTS AND NET VALUE OF ASSETS TO SIZE OF MEDICAL CARE EXPENDITURES OF AGED COUPLES AND OF UNRELATED MALES AND FEMALES, UNITED STATES, 1951

| Total Unit Receipts and Net Value of Assets | Total | No Medical Service in 1951 | Units with Medical Service in 1951 | | | | |
|---|---|---|---|---|---|---|---|
| | | | Total | Amount Paid by Family | | | |
| | | | | None | $1 to $49 | $50 to $299 | $300 and Over |
| **Couples[a]** | | | | | | | |
| Number of sample cases......... | 1,010[d] | 305 | 695[e] | 36 | 218 | 336 | 101 |
| Total unit receipts, per cent....... | 100.0 | 100.0 | 100.0 | 100.0 | 100.0 | 100.0 | 100.0 |
| Less than $500[c]............... | 14.9 | 14.7 | 14.7 | *13.9* | 13.7 | 15.2 | 15.8 |
| $500–$1,499................. | 35.4 | 31.5 | 37.6 | 38.9 | 43.6 | 38.4 | 20.8 |
| $1,500–$4,999............... | 41.9 | 44.6 | 40.7 | 44.4 | 38.1 | 39.3 | 49.5 |
| $5,000 and over.............. | 7.8 | 9.2 | 7.0 | *2.8* | 4.6 | 7.1 | 13.9 |
| Amount of net value of assets, per cent................... | 100.0 | 100.0 | 100.0 | 100.0 | 100.0 | 100.0 | 100.0 |
| None....................... | 13.1 | 11.2 | 14.1 | *25.0* | 13.8 | 14.6 | *8.9* |
| $1–$2,999.................. | 16.0 | 15.4 | 16.5 | *11.1* | 19.3 | 16.9 | 11.9 |
| $3,000 and over.............. | 66.6 | 69.8 | 66.2 | 61.1 | 63.7 | 65.8 | 74.3 |
| Not reported................ | 4.3 | 3.6 | 3.2 | *2.8* | *3.2* | 2.7 | *4.9* |
| **Unrelated Males[b]** | | | | | | | |
| Number of sample cases......... | 488[d] | 219 | 266[e] | 26 | 113 | 88 | 37 |
| Total unit receipts, per cent....... | 100.0 | 100.0 | 100.0 | 100.0 | 100.0 | 100.0 | 100.0 |
| Less than $500[c]............... | 36.7 | 37.5 | 35.7 | 42.3 | 40.7 | 36.4 | *16.2* |
| $500–$1,499................. | 41.8 | 35.6 | 47.0 | 57.7 | 40.7 | 47.7 | 54.1 |
| $1,500 and over.............. | 21.5 | 26.9 | 17.3 | — | 18.6 | 15.9 | 29.7 |
| Amount of net value of assets, per cent................... | 100.0 | 100.0 | 100.0 | 100.0 | 100.0 | 100.0 | 100.0 |
| None....................... | 33.6 | 37.9 | 30.5 | 46.2 | 26.5 | 37.5 | *10.8* |
| $1–$2,999.................. | 23.8 | 17.8 | 28.9 | *34.6* | 30.1 | 27.3 | 27.0 |
| $3,000 and over.............. | 38.7 | 40.6 | 37.6 | *19.2* | 40.7 | 29.5 | 62.2 |
| Not reported................ | 3.9 | *3.7* | *3.0* | — | *2.7* | *5.7* | — |
| **Unrelated Females[b]** | | | | | | | |
| Number of sample cases......... | 1,064[d] | 386 | 666[e] | 49 | 264 | 287 | 60 |
| Total unit receipts, per cent....... | 100.0 | 100.0 | 100.0 | 100.0 | 100.0 | 100.0 | 100.0 |
| Less than $500[c]............... | 58.0 | 59.1 | 57.1 | 53.0 | 57.6 | 59.2 | 53.3 |
| $500–$1,499................. | 31.3 | 29.3 | 32.7 | 38.8 | 34.5 | 30.3 | 30.0 |
| $1,500 and over.............. | 10.7 | 11.6 | 10.2 | *8.2* | 7.9 | 10.5 | 16.7 |
| Amount of net value of assets,.... per cent................... | 100.0 | 100.0 | 100.0 | 100.0 | 100.0 | 100.0 | 100.0 |
| None....................... | 25.4 | 25.1 | 26.0 | 38.8 | 26.1 | 22.0 | 35.0 |
| $1–$2,999.................. | 31.1 | 27.2 | 33.9 | 46.9 | 29.5 | 38.3 | 20.0 |
| $3,000 and over.............. | 37.8 | 42.0 | 36.0 | *8.2* | 40.2 | 36.9 | 36.7 |
| Not reported................ | 5.7 | 5.7 | 4.1 | *6.1* | 4.2 | *2.8* | *8.3* |

[a] In an aged couple, the husband is 65 years or over, irrespective of the age of the wife.
[b] Ages 65 and over.
[c] Includes no receipts.
[d] Includes cases with data not available regarding medical services.
[e] Includes cases with data not available regarding amount paid.

Note: Italicized figures based upon less than 10 cases.

Source: Unpublished data tabulated by the Bureau of the Census from the April, 1952, Follow-up Survey of Persons 65 Years of Age and Over.

tion with annual receipts of $5,000 or more rose from 4.6 per cent among those with medical care expenditures of less than $50 to 13.9 per cent where they amounted to $300 or more; the proportions with assets of $3,000 or more rose from 63.7 to 74.3 per cent. The data for unrelated males and females show a corresponding tendency, although the numbers involved are too small for reliable inference in most instances.

## NATIONAL EXPENDITURES

*Source and Distribution.* The Social Security Administration has estimated that the total private and public outlay for medical care for those aged 65 years and over in 1955–56 amounted to $2.34 billion, or nearly 16 per cent out of an outlay of $14.95 billion for all ages (Table 5.7). Of the outlay for the aged, private expenditures accounted for $1.44 billion, or somewhat over three fifths of the total, and expenditures under public medical care programs for $.78 billion, or one third of the total; only 5 per cent was represented by federal income tax subsidies for medical care deductions in tax returns or by employer contributions to health plans. For persons of all ages, larger shares of the total outlay were made through private expenditures and federal tax-saving subsidies, and an appreciably smaller share through public medical care programs. As a result, about one fourth of the public medical care outlays were on behalf of the aged.

Nearly two thirds ($500 million) of the expenditures through public medical care programs for the aged were for hospital care—chiefly state and local. Nursing home care accounted for over one fifth ($165 million) of this total, other public assistance for over one eighth ($100 million), and various social insurance benefits for a very small proportion.

The estimates of the total private expenditures for medical care among the aged shown in Table 5.8 were obtained on the basis of averages from the nationwide survey for the fiscal year 1952–53 supported by the Health Information Foundation. During that period, the private expenditures amounted to $.5 billion for aged males and $.9 billion for aged females.

The aged accounted for one sixth of the total private outlay for hospitals, one eighth for physicians, and one fifth for prescriptions and other medical goods and services.

*The Impact of Trends in Costs of Medical Care.* The general consumer price index rose by 20.2 per cent from

TABLE 5.7

APPROXIMATE PRIVATE AND PUBLIC OUTLAYS FOR MEDICAL CARE OF CIVILIANS OF ALL AGES AND AT AGES 65 AND OVER, UNITED STATES, 1955–56
(Amounts in Billions)

| Source | All Ages | | Ages 65 and Over | | Amount for Ages 65 and Over as Per Cent of All Ages |
|---|---|---|---|---|---|
| | Amount | Per Cent | Amount | Per Cent | |
| Total..................... | $14.95 | 100.0 | $2.34 | 100.0 | 15.7 |
| Private expenditures[a]....... | 10.50 | 70.2 | 1.44 | 61.6 | 13.7 |
| Federal tax-saving subsidies.. | 1.10 | 7.4 | .12 | 5.1 | 10.9 |
| Individual income tax[b].... | .60 | 4.0 | .10 | 4.3 | 16.7 |
| Corporate income tax[c]..... | .50 | 3.4 | .02 | .8 | 4.0 |
| Public medical care programs. | 3.35 | 22.4 | .78 | 33.3 | 23.3 |
| Social insurance[d]........ | .36 | 2.5 | .02 | .6 | 4.1 |
| General revenue | | | | | |
| Hospital care.......... | 2.50 | 16.7 | .50 | 21.4 | 20.0 |
| Federal[e]............. | .75 | 5.0 | .15 | 6.4 | 20.1 |
| State and local....... | 1.75 | 11.7 | .35 | 15.0 | 19.9 |
| Nursing home care...... | .20 | 1.3 | .16 | 7.0 | 84.6 |
| Other public assistance[f].. | .17 | 1.1 | .10 | 4.3 | 58.8 |
| Other[g]................ | .12 | .8 | — | — | — |

[a] Excludes amounts subsidized through Federal tax savings.
[b] Based on medical care deductions in income tax returns.
[c] Based on employer contributions to health plans.
[d] Medical benefits under workmen's compensation and temporary disability insurance.
[e] Including about $90 million spent for in-patient care for persons 65 and over in medical institutions of the Veterans Administration.
[f] Including physicians' services, drugs, dentists, appliances, etc.
[g] Maternal and child health programs; medical rehabilitation.

Source: F. R. Brown, "Governmental Expenditures and Other Public Financial Support for Personal Medical Care of Persons Aged 65 and Over, 1955–56," *Research and Statistics Note No. 3,* Division of Program Research, Social Security Administration, February 4, 1958.

1947–49 to 1957. However, this general price index does not reflect the consumption pattern of older persons, particularly their relatively high expenditures for medical care, of which hospital costs, physicians' charges, and medicines are the

major components.[14] Except for the last, the prices for these
items have risen more rapidly than the general price index
since 1947–49, the increases by 1957 amounting to 38.0 per
cent for all medical care items, 87.3 per cent for hospital

TABLE 5.8

TOTAL GROSS CHARGES FOR SPECIFIC TYPES OF PERSONAL HEALTH SERVICES
AT ALL AGES AND AT AGES 65 AND OVER, BY SEX, UNITED STATES, 1952–53

| Service or Goods | All Ages | | | Ages 65 and Over | | |
|---|---|---|---|---|---|---|
| | Both Sexes | Males | Fe-males | Both Sexes | Males | Fe-males |
| | Billions of Dollars* | | | | | |
| Total................ | $10.2 | $3.8 | $6.4 | $1.4 | $.5 | $.9 |
| Hospitals.......... | 2.0 | .7 | 1.3 | .3 | .1 | .2 |
| Physicians......... | 3.9 | 1.4 | 2.5 | .5 | .2 | .3 |
| Prescriptions and other medicines... | 1.5 | .5 | 1.0 | .3 | .1 | .2 |
| Other medical goods and services...... | 1.2 | .5 | .7 | .2 | .1 | .1 |
| Dentists........... | 1.6 | .7 | .9 | .1 | † | † |
| | Per Cent Distribution According to Age and Sex | | | | | |
| Total................ | 100 | 37 | 63 | 13 | 5 | 8 |
| Hospitals.......... | 100 | 33 | 67 | 16 | 5 | 11 |
| Physicians......... | 100 | 37 | 63 | 12 | 5 | 7 |
| Prescriptions and other medicines... | 100 | 36 | 64 | 19 | 7 | 12 |
| Other medical goods and services...... | 100 | 42 | 58 | 18 | 5 | 13 |
| Dentists........... | 100 | 42 | 58 | 3 | 2 | 1 |

* The figures for all ages, both sexes, differ slightly from those shown by O. W. Anderson and
J. J. Feldman, *Family Medical Costs and Voluntary Health Insurance: A Nationwide Survey*
(New York: McGraw-Hill Book Co., Inc., 1956), p. 109.

† Less than .05.

Source: Computed by the author on the basis of the data by Anderson and Feldman in
Table 5.2 and on an estimate of population by age and sex for the civilian population for January 1, 1953, derived from Bureau of the Census, *Current Population Reports*, Series P-25, No.
146, November 12, 1956.

[14] Z. Campbell, "Spending Patterns of Older Persons," *Management
Record*, Vol. 21, p. 85 (March, 1959); S. Goldstein, "Consumer Patterns
of Aged Spending Units," *Journal of Gerontology*, Vol. 14, p. 328 (July,
1959).

rates, 32.5 per cent for physicians' fees, and 16.7 per cent for prescriptions and drugs.[15] At the same time, the relative importance of medical care among the total of personal consumption expenditures has risen, from 4.1 per cent in 1947 to 5.3 per cent in 1957.[16] The course of the consumer price index and of its components for the aged, as well as the trend in the distribution of their personal consumption expenditures, is yet to be studied. In any event, there is an obvious need to stabilize the costs of medical care.[17]

## ATTITUDES TOWARD THE FINANCING OF HEALTH SERVICES

In view of the relatively high costs of medical care of the aged, their attitudes on this matter, as expressed in the 1955 survey of the National Opinion Research Center, are particularly pertinent. Almost half of the aged agreed that there are "people around here who don't get as much medical care as they need because they don't have the money"; however, nearly one third disagreed and one fifth stated they did not know (Table 5.9).[18] Nevertheless, practically three fifths of the aged recognized that, "If someone around here got sick and didn't have any money to pay," there was a "place he could go that would take care of him." Also, a like proportion of the aged thought that the quality of care given in such a

---

[15] *Medical Care Prices: Long Run versus Short Run,* Miscellaneous Publication M-116, Bureau of Medical Economic Research, American Medical Association, September, 1958; H. I. Greenfield and O. W. Anderson, *The Medical Care Price Index,* Research Series 7 (New York: Health Information Foundation, 1959). In this connection, see also A. W. Brewster, "Per Capita Expenditures for Medical Care and Health Insurance in Relation to Disposable Personal Income, 1948, 1952, and 1955," *Research and Statistics Note No. 21,* Division of Program Research, Social Security Administration, June 13, 1957.

[16] L. W. Martin, "Personal Consumption Expenditures, 1947–1957—New Series Versus Old Series," *Journal of the American Medical Association,* Vol. 169, p. 608 (February 7, 1959).

[17] I. Altman, *Principles and Recommendations for the Planning of Medical Facilities in Pennsylvania,* Department of Welfare, Commonwealth of Pennsylvania, Harrisburg, January, 1958.

[18] The quotes here and later in this section are excerpted from the questionnaire of the survey by the National Opinion Research Center.

TABLE 5.9

ATTITUDES TOWARD THE FINANCING OF HEALTH SERVICES;
UNITED STATES, 1955

| Attitude Question | Age | | |
|---|---|---|---|
| | 21 and Over | 21 to 64 | 65 and Over |
| There are people around here who don't get as much medical care as they need because they don't have the money | 100% | 100% | 100% |
| Agree | 55 | 56 | 47 |
| Don't agree | 33 | 33 | 32 |
| Don't know | 12 | 11 | 21 |
| If some one around here got sick and didn't have any money to pay, there is a place to go that would take care of him | 100% | 100% | 100% |
| Agree | 68 | 69 | 58 |
| Don't agree | 13 | 13 | 17 |
| Don't know | 19 | 18 | 25 |
| Compared with the care a private doctor would give, the quality of care given in the place for people who cannot pay is | 100% | 100% | 100% |
| Better | 6 | 5 | 12 |
| About the same | 58 | 59 | 49 |
| Not as good | 27 | 27 | 25 |
| Don't know | 9 | 9 | 14 |
| In general, the costs of medical care are | 100% | 100% | 100% |
| Much too high | 27 | 25 | 35 |
| Somewhat high | 34 | 36 | 28 |
| About right | 35 | 36 | 28 |
| Don't know | 4 | 3 | 9 |
| Doctors' fees generally are | 100% | 100% | 100% |
| Much too high | 16 | 14 | 23 |
| Somewhat high | 33 | 33 | 28 |
| About right | 48 | 50 | 42 |
| Don't know | 3 | 3 | 7 |
| Hospital charges are | 100% | 100% | 100% |
| Much too high | 39 | 39 | 43 |
| Somewhat high | 31 | 31 | 25 |
| About right | 21 | 22 | 15 |
| Don't know | 9 | 8 | 17 |
| Dentists' fees are | 100% | 100% | 100% |
| Much too high | 24 | 24 | 24 |
| Somewhat high | 30 | 31 | 25 |
| About right | 37 | 38 | 26 |
| Don't know | 9 | 7 | 25 |

TABLE 5.9—*Continued*

| Attitude Question | Age | | |
|---|---|---|---|
| | 21 and Over | 21 to 64 | 65 and Over |
| Cost of prescriptions at drugstores is..........100% | 100% | 100% | |
| Much too high........................... 38 | 38 | 39 | |
| Somewhat high........................... 28 | 28 | 24 | |
| About right............................. 26 | 27 | 23 | |
| Don't know............................. 8 | 7 | 14 | |
| Reasons for not seeing doctor when perhaps should................................100% | 100% | 100% | |
| Didn't want to spend money unless had to... 38 | 38 | 43 | |
| Might prescribe expensive drug or treatment.. 10 | 10 | 13 | |
| Being sick in bed for a week would make things, for self and family......................100% | 100% | 100% | |
| Very difficult............................. 17 | 17 | 22 | |
| Somewhat difficult........................ 21 | 21 | 15 | |
| Get along fairly well...................... 62 | 62 | 63 | |
| If sick in bed for a week, for care..............100% | 100% | 100% | |
| Somebody is here........................ 49 | 49 | 46 | |
| Could get someone easily................... 30 | 30 | 29 | |
| Hard to get somebody..................... 20 | 20 | 23 | |
| Don't know............................. 1 | 1 | 2 | |
| If a housewife and sick in bed for a week, managing the household for rest of family would be. 100% | 100% | 100% | |
| Great deal of trouble...................... 21 | 20 | 22 | |
| Some trouble............................ 29 | 31 | 18 | |
| Not much trouble........................ 50 | 49 | 60 | |
| If the family suddenly had to pay out a $500 medical bill, to pay it would be................100% | 100% | 100% | |
| Not too much trouble...................... 43 | 43 | 44 | |
| Very difficult............................. 40 | 41 | 29 | |
| Just couldn't pay........................ 17 | 16 | 27 | |
| Does the family............................100% | 100% | 100% | |
| Save regularly........................... 31 | 32 | 21 | |
| Save occasionally......................... 31 | 32 | 27 | |
| Not able to save......................... 38 | 36 | 52 | |
| Have had to borrow money to pay doctor, dentist or hospital bills*........................100% | 100% | 100% | |
| No.................................... 80 | 79 | 87 | |
| Yes, total.............................. 20 | 21 | 13 | |

TABLE 5.9—*Continued*

| Attitude Question | Age | | |
|---|---|---|---|
| | 21 and Over | 21 to 64 | 65 and Over |
| Yes, doctor | 14 | 15 | 10 |
| Yes, dentist | 2 | 3 | 1 |
| Yes, hospital | 11 | 11 | 6 |
| When was last time had to borrow money for medical or dental bills | 100% | 100% | 100% |
| Within last 2 years | 30 | 30 | 13 |
| 2–5 years ago | 24 | 24 | 21 |
| Over 5 years ago | 46 | 46 | 66 |
| How much was borrowed on last occasion for medical or dental bills | 100% | 100% | 100% |
| Under $100 | 21 | 20 | 26 |
| $100–$199 | 26 | 26 | 19 |
| $200–$299 | 19 | 20 | 16 |
| $300–$499 | 15 | 15 | 13 |
| $500 and over | 15 | 14 | 21 |
| Don't know | 4 | 5 | 5 |
| Attitude toward medical, surgical or hospital insurance by those who do not have it | 100% | 100% | 100% |
| Good idea | 60 | 61 | 58 |
| As well without it | 37 | 36 | 37 |
| Don't know | 3 | 3 | 5 |
| Use of insurance to pay all or part of doctor or hospital bills | 100% | 100% | 100% |
| Yes, have now | 65 | 69 | 39 |
| No, used to have | 11 | 10 | 13 |
| No, never had | 24 | 21 | 48 |
| Members of family covered by any medical, surgical or hospital insurance held† | 100% | 100% | 100% |
| Respondent | 97 | 97 | 96 |
| Spouse | 81 | 83 | 59 |
| Child | 54 | 59 | 2 |
| Other | 2 | 2 | 4 |
| In general, having health insurance makes difference in manner of treatment when sick† | 100% | 100% | 100% |
| Agree | 15 | 16 | 7 |
| Don't agree | 78 | 78 | 81 |
| Don't know | 7 | 6 | 12 |

TABLE 5.9—*Continued*

| Attitude Question | Age | | |
|---|---|---|---|
| | 21 and Over | 21 to 64 | 65 and Over |
| How long has health insurance been held† | 100% | 100% | 100% |
| Less than 2 years | 16 | 16 | 8 |
| 2–4 years | 21 | 21 | 18 |
| 5–9 years | 30 | 31 | 24 |
| 10 or more years | 33 | 32 | 50 |
| How was first health insurance acquired† | 100% | 100% | 100% |
| Through place of work | 65 | 69 | 28 |
| Pay directly | 29 | 25 | 68 |
| Both | 6 | 6 | 4 |
| Attitude toward health insurance held† | 100% | 100% | 100% |
| Don't like some things | 25 | 25 | 25 |
| Completely satisfied | 69 | 69 | 66 |
| Don't know | 6 | 6 | 9 |
| Have any family members ever received any benefits from health insurance held† | 100% | 100% | 100% |
| Yes | 69 | 70 | 61 |
| No | 31 | 30 | 39 |
| Attitude toward health insurance which would cover all of medical expenses of family | 100% | 100% | 100% |
| Good idea | 65 | 66 | 53 |
| As well without it | 27 | 26 | 38 |
| Qualified | 6 | 6 | 6 |
| Don't know | 2 | 2 | 3 |
| For those believing health insurance to cover all of medical expenses a good idea or qualified, amount willing to pay each month for family | 100% | 100% | 100% |
| Nothing | 5 | 4 | 14 |
| $5 or less | 27 | 25 | 40 |
| $5.01–$10 | 38 | 40 | 25 |
| $10.01–$15 | 13 | 14 | 5 |
| Over $15 | 9 | 9 | 5 |
| Don't know | 8 | 8 | 11 |

\* Since each respondent may give more than one reason, the percentages shown are not additive. All respondents, whether or not stating a reason, are taken as 100%.
† Asked only if any medical, surgical, or hospital insurance is held.
Source: Unpublished data from the 1955 survey by the National Opinion Research Center sponsored by the Health Information Foundation; the figures for ages 21 to 64 were computed from source data by the author.

place was at least as good as that received from a private doctor. The greater medical care needs of the aged and their reduced circumstances very likely influenced the large proportion who considered medical care costs much too high, 35
per cent; for persons at the main productive ages, the same
opinion was held by 25 per cent. A larger proportion of the
aged regarded hospital charges as high (43 per cent much too
high, 25 per cent somewhat high) than they did of doctors'
fees (23 per cent much too high, 28 per cent somewhat
high). The aged also considered dentists' fees and the cost of
prescriptions at drugstores rather high (49 per cent and 63
per cent, respectively, either much too high or somewhat
high). In view of opinions on the cost of living in general, the
survey also inquired into attitudes on other expenditure
items. In the case of food, for example, 81 per cent of all
adults considered prices as high, compared with only 61 per
cent in the case of medical care. Since this question was asked
of all persons in the survey, the day-to-day impact of food
prices may have left a greater impression than the occasional
medical care expenditures. Perhaps different attitudes
would have been expressed by those who recently incurred
more than ordinary medical care costs.

Although the impact of a large medical bill usually creates
problems, 44 per cent of the aged thought that there would
not be too much trouble if the family suddenly had to pay a
bill of $500.[19] On the other hand, for 29 per cent of the aged
such a bill would be very difficult to pay and 27 per cent could
not pay it. However, most of the aged (87 per cent) never
had to borrow to pay a medical care bill; most borrowing,
when done, was to pay the doctor. Also, most of the borrowing by the aged was five or more years prior to interview (66
per cent), and relatively little within the two prior years (13
per cent). Whenever the borrowing was done, for one fourth
of the aged it was less than $100 and for one fifth $500 or
more.

---

[19] In this connection, see pp. 30–33 of Chapter 2.

Many other aspects in the 1955 survey of the National Opinion Research Center were confirmed in its later survey of the aged alone in 1957 (summarized in Table 5.10), when account is taken of the chance fluctuations due to the small numbers involved in the samples. Thus in the earlier survey, 39 per cent of the aged reported that they have insurance to

TABLE 5.10

ATTITUDES OF PERSONS AT AGES 65 AND OVER TOWARD THE FINANCING OF HEALTH SERVICES, UNITED STATES, 1957

| Attitude Question | Both Sexes | Males | Females |
|---|---|---|---|
| Use of insurance to pay all or part of medical, surgical or hospital bills | 100% | 100% | 100% |
| Have now | 39 | 42 | 35 |
| Used to have | 16 | 18 | 14 |
| Never had | 45 | 40 | 51 |
| Feeling toward insurance that helps pay hospital and medical costs[a] | 100% | — | — |
| Would like but | | | |
| Can't afford | 34 | — | — |
| Can't obtain | 16 | — | — |
| Don't want it | 23 | — | — |
| Never thought of it | 26 | — | — |
| Other | 1 | — | — |
| Reason for terminating insurance[b] | 100% | 100% | 100% |
| Retired | 26 | 32 | 19 |
| Could not afford it | 31 | — | — |
| Dissatisfied with it | 24 | 19 | 29 |
| All other | 19 | — | — |
| How long ago was insurance given up[b] | 100% | — | — |
| Within five years | 47 | — | — |
| All other | 53 | — | — |
| Insurance in relation to bills[c] | 100% | — | — |
| Hospital | 93 | — | — |
| Doctor, while in hospital | 67 | — | — |
| Doctor, home or office visits | 21 | — | — |
| How long has insurance been held[c] | 100% | — | — |
| Less than five years | 24 | — | — |
| 5–9 years | 22 | — | — |
| 10–14 years | 20 | — | — |
| 15 or more years | 28 | — | — |
| Don't know, no answer | 6 | — | — |

TABLE 5.10—*Continued*

| Attitude Question | Both Sexes | Males | Females |
|---|---|---|---|
| Where health insurance was heard of[d] | 100% | — | — |
| Advertising, direct mail, or mass media | 18 | — | — |
| Salesman called | 42 | — | — |
| Friend or relative | 25 | — | — |
| Fraternal order | 3 | — | — |
| No answer | 12 | — | — |
| How much does this insurance cost per month[c] | 100% | — | — |
| Less than $2.00 | 13 | — | — |
| $2–$2.90 | 11 | — | — |
| $3–$3.90 | 20 | — | — |
| $4–$4.90 | 14 | — | — |
| $5–$5.90 | 12 | — | — |
| $6–$7.90 | 11 | — | — |
| $8–$9.90 | 6 | — | — |
| $10 or more | 5 | — | — |
| Don't know, no answer | 8 | — | — |
| How insurance paid for[c] | 100% | | |
| All costs paid by the insured | 76 | — | — |
| Others paying all or part | 24 | — | — |
| Would like insurance to cover all of medical expenses | 100% | — | — |
| Yes | 65 | — | — |
| Why not interested in health insurance for all medical expenses[e] | 100% | — | — |
| Has enough insurance now | 7 | — | — |
| Now insured; this type costs too much | 4 | — | — |
| Cannot afford it | 19 | — | — |
| Has enough money to take care of costs | 12 | — | — |
| Can have costs met another way | 7 | — | — |
| Does not consider self insurable | 14 | — | — |
| Does not have costs so not interested | 12 | — | — |
| Objects to idea of insurance | 10 | — | — |
| No answer | 15 | — | — |
| How much willing to pay per month for insurance covering all medical expenses | 100% | — | — |
| Reported an amount | 62 | — | — |
| Total | 100% | — | — |
| Nothing | 17 | — | — |
| Under $4 | 17 | — | — |
| $4–$6 | 27 | — | — |
| $7–$12 | 29 | — | — |
| $13 and over | 10 | — | — |
| Median | $5.00 | — | — |
| Mean | $6.84 | — | — |

TABLE 5.10—*Continued*

| Attitude Question | Both Sexes |
|---|---|
| Government insurance | 100% |
| Don't know, no answer | 4 |
| Against it | 43 |
| Favors it for all | 29 |
| Favors it for certain people | 24 |
| All people who cannot afford insurance | 14 |
| Older people who cannot afford insurance | 4 |
| All others | 6 |
| Favors it, not further specified | 1 |

ᵃ Asked only of those who did not hold such insurance at interview.
ᵇ Asked only of those who used to have insurance.
ᶜ Asked only of those now insured.
ᵈ Asked only of those who acquired insurance through other than place of work (or of husband or wife).
ᵉ Asked only of those who would not like insurance to cover all of medical expenses.

Source: "Voluntary Health Insurance Among the Aged," *Progress in Health Services*, Vol. 8 (January, 1959), Health Information Foundation, New York. The detailed data corresponding to those in the charts of this report were supplied by the Health Information Foundation. The bases used in the report for "Favors it for certain people" under "Government insurance" were revised by the author to relate to all respondents.

pay all or part of doctor or hospital bills, another 13 per cent stated that they once held such insurance, but not presently, and 48 per cent were never protected in this way. For the later survey, the corresponding proportions were 39, 16, and 45 per cent respectively.[20] Among the aged in the 1955 survey who did not have insurance to cover medical, surgical, or hospital expenses, 58 per cent regarded such insurance as a good idea and 37 per cent thought they would be as well off without it; the percentages for the younger ages were similar.

Pertinent, in connection with the situation of the uninsured, are the findings from the 1957 NORC survey. This showed that, among the uninsured, 34 per cent could not afford it although they would like to be covered, over 25 per cent had not thought about it, 16 per cent could not obtain it although they desired it, and somewhat under 25 per cent did not want it. Not far different are the observations from the national survey of aged beneficiaries on the rolls of the Old-

---

[20] *Progress in Health Services,* Vol. 8 (January, 1959), Health Information Foundation, New York.

Age and Survivors Insurance program in December, 1956. Among those without health insurance,

. . . 39 percent said they could not afford it, and 37 percent said they had never had the opportunity to purchase it, had not thought much about it, or the like. The remaining 23 percent were not insured because the policy had been canceled, could not be continued after retirement, and so forth. The first two reasons were cited by a larger proportion of the beneficiaries who came on the rolls in the 1940's than of those who had retired more recently.[21]

Apparently the aged currently entering the ranks of the retired are in a better position than their predecessors to afford health insurance, in their opportunities to purchase it, and in their awareness of it.

The NORC survey of 1957 indicated a number of reasons for the termination of the insurance among the aged who had been formerly insured. Thus, 31 per cent stated that they could not afford it, 26 per cent had their insurance terminated because they retired or stopped working, and 24 per cent terminated because of dissatisfaction with the insurance. A variety of other reasons for the termination was also cited. Nearly half of the aged who had been insured terminated their protection within five years before the interview.

In the 1955 NORC survey, most of the insured aged (81 per cent) did not believe that the ownership of health insurance made any difference in the way they would be treated when they were sick. The same survey also showed that two thirds of the insured aged were completely satisfied with the insurance and one fourth stated there were some things about it they did not like; the proportions were practically the same for younger persons.

In both NORC surveys, about one half of the insured aged

[21] National Survey of Old-Age and Survivors Insurance Beneficiaries, 1957, *Highlights from Preliminary Tabulations—Health Insurance and Hospital Utilization,* Bureau of Old-Age and Survivors Insurance and Office of the Commissioner, Social Security Administration, Washington, D.C., November, 1958.

held their health insurance for ten or more years and almost one fourth for 5–9 years. According to the 1957 survey, 56 per cent of the insured aged acquired their health insurance through a place of work (64 per cent for males and 49 per cent for females). The rest, who obtained their insurance by other means, had their attention drawn to it by salesmen in about two fifths of the cases, by friends or relatives in one fourth, or by some advertising approach in one sixth of the cases. Among the insured aged, 76 per cent bore the cost of their insurance alone, and the rest had all or part paid by children or relatives, employers (past or present), unions, or fraternal orders. The average monthly payment for the insurance by all insured persons was $4.62; somewhat over two fifths paid less than $4.00.

According to the 1957 NORC survey, 65 per cent of the aged had a preference for health insurance that would cover all medical care expenses. Many (about 40 per cent) among those without such a preference did not need it because they had means of their own, had no medical costs, could meet their costs in other ways, or felt they had enough insurance. About one fourth of those without a preference for complete coverage were worried about its costs, one seventh considered themselves uninsurable, and one tenth were against the concept of health insurance.

The 1955 NORC survey showed that younger people had a more favorable attitude toward complete coverage of medical care expenses by insurance than did older people, perhaps because of their greater family responsibilities. However, the lower proportion with this attitude at the older ages may reflect also a belief that they would not be eligible for such insurance or that it would be too costly. The younger people in favor of such insurance were willing to pay more than the older people. Thus, 40 per cent of the younger persons were willing to pay between $5 and $10 a month for health insurance covering all members of the family; among the aged, 40 per cent would pay $5 or less each month. It is an anomaly that as much as 14 per cent of the aged believing in such

complete insurance protection were not willing to pay for it.[22]
Similar findings were reported from the 1957 NORC survey;
44 per cent of the aged were willing to pay $6 or less and 17
per cent would not pay anything.

An inquiry into the matter of government health insurance
in the 1957 NORC survey showed that 43 per cent of all aged
were against it, 29 per cent favored it for all persons, 18 per
cent favored it for those with an economic need (this included 4 per cent for old people in need), 6 per cent for other
categories of people, and 4 per cent did not take a stand or
did not answer.

[22] E. Freidson and J. J. Feldman, *Public Attitudes Toward Health Insurance,* Research Series 5 (New York: Health Information Foundation,
1958). This source has limited data with regard to age; however, it is
valuable for its findings on the evaluation that physicians make of the
significance of insurance to medical care.

# Mechanisms for Financing Medical Care of the Aged

6

DURING THE working lifetime of most of today's aged, medical care was paid for principally out of pocket as incurred, either from immediate resources or by borrowing. Although this is still the approach for many of the aged, increasing use is being made of the risk-sharing or prepayment mechanism for the accumulation of funds to pay for their medical care. The agencies developing these mechanisms are insurance companies, Blue Cross and Blue Shield associations, medical societies, and a variety of others acting independently, such as some employers, unions, community groups, and consumer associations. For certain categories of the population, principally veterans of the armed forces, the federal government provides medical care services as a right under specific conditions. The aged without means of their own are aided in their medical care problems through programs of public or general assistance supported by federal, state, and local government. Also contributing to the medical care of the needy aged are many voluntary agencies operating under private auspices.

## THE DEVELOPMENT OF VOLUNTARY HEALTH INSURANCE

*Some Insurance Principles.* The primary purpose of an insurance, or risk-sharing mechanism, is to spread the individual loss arising upon the occurrence of an unpredictable

162

event among the members of a large group formed to share the risk. There is no generally accepted convention on the underlying principles of an insurance. However, it should be evident that for a sound insurance:

(1) The event insured must be clearly defined and its occurrence clearly recognized. Obviously, the event occasioning a benefit should be reasonably described in advance in such terms that both the insured and the insurer have a mutual understanding of what it encompasses. Such an understanding would leave no ambiguities upon the occurrence of the event.

(2) The benefit to be provided upon the occurrence of the event must be stated. The insured expects to know in advance the benefits to which he will be entitled and the insurer wants an understanding of the limit to his liability.

(3) The loss involved upon the occurrence of the event must not be trivial. The use of the administrative procedures of insurance to spread the risk of casual losses that can easily be borne out of pocket seems an economic waste. The costs of such insurance might be applied advantageously toward the more significant risks. No borderline can distinguish the trivial from the significant; the rule of reason applies.

(4) For the insured group as a whole, the chances for the occurrence of the event must be predictable within reasonable limits. Basic to the risk-sharing mechanism is the assumption that the insurer can estimate in advance the probable loss to which he is liable. Since the insurer cannot expect precision in the estimate he is satisfied with an estimate that may vary, within reasonable limits, from the loss eventually experienced. Unless sizable numbers are insured, the random fluctuations of actual experience may fall far from the estimate.

(5) For the insured group as a whole, the chances for the occurrence of the event within a short period must be relatively small; for insurance extending over a long period, the chances of the occurrence may be **large** but the time **of its**

occurrence must be uncertain. To incur the administrative costs of an insurance for an event that can be practically foretold within the near future is hardly economic. Expenditures for such events can be budgeted. However, the insurer may add such a budgeting program to the insurance program.

(6) Neither the chances for the occurrence of the event nor the size of the loss should be enlarged because of the insurance. For the individual covered by the insurance, the occurrence of the insured event must be unpredictable and very largely beyond his control. Although a vendor of goods or services required upon the occurrence of the event is free to fix his charge, the insurer expects that the usual and customary charge will be made for the occasion. To introduce an overcharge because of the presence of the insurance necessarily defeats its purpose.[1] In other words, pooling the costs of medical services should not lessen individual responsibility for their use, either by the consumer or by the provider of the services.

*The Background.* The history of voluntary risk-sharing and prepayment mechanisms to anticipate the costs of medical care is one of continual experiment, with the focus first on the problems of the working population and later on its dependents and others of the population. The most obvious need for the wage earner was a mechanism to make up for loss of income during a period of illness or disability.[2] In due

---

[1] For a further discussion of insurance principles, see J. B. Maclean, *Life Insurance* (8th ed.; New York: McGraw-Hill Book Co., Inc.), chap. i; "Report of the Commission on Medical Care Plans, Findings, Conclusions, and Recommendations," *Journal of the American Medical Association,* January 17, 1959, Special Edition, p. 59; H. H. Wolfenden, *The Problems of Medical Economics* (Toronto: Canadian Medical Association, 1941), pp. 13–14; F. Goldmann, *Voluntary Medical Care Insurance in the United States* (New York: Columbia University Press, 1948), chap. i; *Health Insurance Plans in the United States,* Report of the Committee on Labor and Public Welfare (U.S. Senate, 82d Cong., 1st sess., Report No. 359, Part 2, May 28, 1951), pp. 116–20; *A Look at Modern Health Insurance* (Washington, D.C.: Chamber of Commerce of the United States, 1954), chap. v.

[2] Since the present concern is with the aged, the history of voluntary insurance in general will not be traced here. Convenient references are:

course, experimentation with the risk-sharing and prepayment mechanisms was extended to the costs of medical care for the wage earner and his dependents. The developments in this area were cautious, but rapid. They began with plans to cover limited costs of the hospital stay and routine services, and then grew to include lengthier stays and more services. In short order there followed, in sequence, plans to cover the costs of surgery, regular medical expense, and then major medical expense. Most recent is the comprehensive plan which encompasses, in one program, hospital costs, surgical costs, and both regular and major medical expense. Although caution at first dictated restrictions in the benefits paid under these plans, accumulating experience soon pointed the way to broad liberalizations which were at the same time adapted to advances in medical care practice.[3] For example, plans have been developed which provide benefits for nursing home care, nursing and home care, dental care, drugs, and vision care.[4] It was also possible to adapt the details of the

---

P. Williams, *The Purchase of Medical Care Through Fixed Periodic Payment* (New York: National Bureau of Economic Research, Inc., 1932); E. J. Faulkner, *Health Insurance* (New York: McGraw-Hill Book Co., Inc., to be published July, 1960); L. S. Reed, *Blue Cross and Medical Service Plans,* Division of Public Health Methods, Public Health Service, Federal Security Agency, Washington, D.C., 1947, chaps. ii and xiv; F. Goldmann, *Voluntary Medical Care Insurance in the United States* (New York: Columbia University Press, 1948), chap. ii; *A Look at Modern Health Insurance* (Washington, D.C.: Chamber of Commerce of the United States, 1954), chaps. ix, x, and xi; H. Becker (ed.), *Financing Hospital Care in the United States* (New York: McGraw-Hill Book Co., Inc., 1955) Vol. 2, chap. i; J. H. Miller, *et al., Accident and Sickness Insurance Provided Through Individual Policies* (Chicago: Society of Actuaries, 1956), pp. 1–5.

[3] For details, see J. F. Follmann, Jr., *Voluntary Health Insurance and Medical Care, Five Years of Progress, 1952–1957,* Health Insurance Association of America, Chicago, New York, Washington, February, 1958.

[4] J. F. Follmann, Jr., *Health Insurance and Nursing Home Care,* March 5, 1958: *Health Insurance and Nursing and Home Care,* May, 1959: *Health Insurance and Vision Care,* August, 1958, Health Insurance Association of America, Chicago, New York, Washington. See also J. F. Follmann, Jr., "Insuring Dental Care Costs," *Journal of the American Dental Association,* Vol. 56, p. 194 (February, 1958). References to the insurance of the cost of drugs are made in *Medical Economics Briefs* of the Health Insurance Association of America, September 27, 1957 and August 28, 1959, and T. P. Weil and U. F. Caruso, "Health Insurance," *Journal of the American Pharmaceutical Association,* Vol. 18, p. 661 (November, 1957).

plans to suit local circumstances. A stimulus to the liberalizations was produced by the competitive efforts of the various voluntary insurers. By this approach, which is unique to the United States and Canada, voluntary health insurance has won wide public acceptance, as reflected in the record of growth described later. Under the same impetus, further developments are in prospect.

*Types of Coverage.*   The concern here is only with those types of coverage that are applicable to the aged and the retired, as well as to younger persons.[5] Thus, this account excludes benefit features distinct for dependent children and for childbirth and also insurance against loss of income because of sickness or injury. Because there is great variety in the plans issued by insurers for each type of coverage, the description is necessarily in general terms.

(1) *Hospital Expense.*   The usual hospital expense benefit has two elements: one, a provision for the daily charge for room and board, including routine nursing care, for a stated maximum period; the other, a miscellaneous expense benefit which reimburses for such other hospital expenses as the use of the operating room, anesthetics, laboratory tests and services, X rays, drugs, dressings, and other medical supplies.

The maximum duration of hospital stay may vary, according to plan, from 30 days to one year; a maximum of 90 or 120 days is common. Any succession of hospital stays for the same cause that are separated by less than some stipulated period may be regarded as a continuous stay. The amount of the daily benefit provided varies from one plan to another according to the type of hospital accommodation desired and the local level of hospital charges; a plan can therefore be selected to suit the needs of the insured. It is usual for insurance companies to pay a cash benefit, or indemnity, applicable toward the daily hospital charge up to a maximum,

---

[5] This section is restricted to the coverages of insurance companies and Blue Cross and Blue Shield plans; the coverages of independent plans are noted later.

either to the beneficiary or directly to the hospital, irrespective of the type of accommodation used. Blue Cross plans commonly pay the hospital directly for semiprivate accommodations and grant an allowance toward private accommodations, but generally restrict the miscellaneous benefits to a number of specified services.[6] Insurance companies pay the miscellaneous expense benefit for charges up to some specified limit with each hospital stay, or, more usual, up to a maximum specified in terms of a certain number of times the daily room and board benefit; other variations are sometimes made.

A usual requirement for hospital benefits is that the patient stay in the hospital overnight, except for cases of emergency or surgery, in which event only the miscellaneous expense benefit is paid.

(2) *Surgical Expense.*  Generally, the surgical expense benefit provides an indemnity for the charges of a surgeon according to a schedule in the insurance contract which shows the maximum payable for a list of the more frequent operations. For any surgical procedures not stated on the list, the maximum indemnity is on a basis consistent with those specified. Multiples of the basic indemnity schedule may be used, with corresponding changes in the insurance premium. If more than one operation is performed at any time, the total indemnity is sometimes limited to the maximum benefit allowed for the costliest procedure shown on the schedule, or to some other arrangement totaling less than the sum of the individual benefits. The same restrictions may

---

[6] The cash benefit, or indemnity, and service benefit approaches are discussed by G. W. Fitzhugh in *Accident and Sickness Insurance* (D. McCahan, ed.) (Homewood, Ill.: Richard D. Irwin, Inc., 1954), pp. 51–69; L. S. Reed, *Blue Cross and Medical Service Plans,* Division of Public Health Methods, Public Health Service, Federal Security Agency, Washington, D.C., 1947, chap. xxi; F. Goldmann, *Voluntary Medical Care Insurance in the United States* (New York: Columbia University Press, 1948), chap. i; and *Health Insurance Plans in the United States,* Report of the Committee on Labor and Public Welfare (U.S. Senate, 82d Cong., 1st sess., Report No. 359, Part 2, May 28, 1951), pp. 121–24.

also apply if two operations for the same cause are performed within some stipulated period.

Insurance companies commonly make surgical expense benefits available together with hospital expense benefits, both room and board and miscellaneous expenses. Blue Shield plans, which pay the charge for surgical care including that for anesthetics, are frequently co-ordinated with the local Blue Cross plans in their activities.

(3) *Regular Medical Expense.* The most usual form of regular medical expense benefit is a cash payment applicable to the fees charged by a physician, other than the surgeon, for his calls while the beneficiary is confined to a hospital. Limits on the total cash benefit during a hospital stay may be placed in various ways: for example, by excluding the first few calls or days of call and by specifying the cash benefit for each call or day of stay, the total number of calls or days of stay, and the total amount of benefit allowed. Some plans also indemnify for the physicians' fees on office visits or home calls. The benefit is usually fixed below the general level of physicians' fees in the locality; it may also be smaller for office visits than for house calls. Insurance companies sometimes make regular medical expense benefits available in one contract together with surgical and hospital expense benefits; in such instances, the regular medical expense benefit may be restricted to hospital calls. Blue Shield plans offer surgical and regular medical expense benefits in one contract; other features of Blue Shield plans are described later in this chapter.

(4) *Major Medical Expense.* In most instances of illness or injury requiring medical care, the charges involved can be met in large measure by means of hospital, surgical, or regular medical expense benefits. For the infrequent cases involving very large charges inside or outside the hospital, the risk-sharing mechanism developed is known as "major medical expense insurance." Under this plan, the medical charges within some stated period must exceed some stipu-

lated amount varying from about $200 to $500, according to plan, which is deducted in computing the insurance benefit. This deductible feature assumes that the insured either has the basic forms of hospital, surgical, and regular medical expense protection, or will bear the risk of these charges himself. The use of the deductible feature also makes it possible to offer this form of insurance at an economically feasible premium to the public. A large maximum amount of benefit is generally stated for each spell of illness or for a lifetime, or both.[7] In most plans, provision is made for reinstatement of the maximum benefit after a certain lesser amount of benefit has been received, provided satisfactory evidence of insurability is presented. Besides the elements of a deductible charge and a maximum benefit, major medical expense contracts usually have a coinsurance feature which limits the benefits paid to a high percentage (75 per cent or 80 per cent) of the medical care charges in excess of the deductible amount. With coinsurance, it is expected that the beneficiary will seek to minimize the use of unneeded expensive care.

Because of the inclusive character of the major medical expense contract, the charges covered are not itemized in great detail. The more commonly mentioned charges are those for hospital room and board and general nursing, the miscellaneous hospital expenses cited previously, physician's services inside and outside the hospital for medical and surgical treatment, prescribed drugs, private registered nurses in the hospital and at home, oxygen, blood, physiotherapy, radiological treatments, ambulance service, appliances, and rental of wheel chairs. In fact, the major medical expense contract provides benefits for almost all forms of customary medical expense considered necessary by the physician. Benefits are not usual for periodic checkups, for the fitting and

---

[7] The imposition of a limit may influence some to pay directly from their own resources for a moderate amount of medical expenses covered by this insurance in order to conserve their protection against possible large expenses.

purchase of eyeglasses and hearing aids, or for cosmetic surgery and dental treatment unless it is a consequence of an accidental injury.[8]

(5) *Comprehensive Medical Expense.* A natural subsequent development of voluntary health insurance is a plan for comprehensive medical expense coverage which, in essence, combines features of the basic hospital and surgical expense plans with those of the major medical expense plan. It is characterized by a low deductible amount from medical expenses covered by insurance (ranging from about $25 to $50), after which coinsurance applies. In some plans, there is an area of full reimbursement before coinsurance applies. In this sense, "comprehensive" medical expense protection does not imply 100 per cent coverage of the total of medical expenses. The comprehensive medical expense plan is a recent significant development in the progress of voluntary health insurance.

*The Record for Growth.* Although some forms of health insurance were attempted in this country about 1850 and further activity was in evidence around the turn of the century, the modern era dates only from about 1930. The growth in the number of people covered under various types of health insurance since 1940 is shown in Table 6.1. By the end of 1958, each type of coverage ranked, in number of people protected, according to its chronological development. Over 123 million persons had protection for hospital expense, 111.4 million for surgical expense, 75.4 million for regular medical expense, and 17.4 million for major medical expense. On the other hand, the more recently developed plans have the greater rate of growth. Thus, the number protected against

---

[8] For further discussions, see *Major Medical Expense Insurance* (Washington, D.C.: Chamber of Commerce of the United States, February, 1956); E. Hess, "Comprehensive or Single Plan Major Medical Insurance," *Journal of the American Medical Association,* Vol. 166, p. 472 (February 1, 1958); and C. A. Siegfried, "Major Medical Expense Insurance," *American Journal of Public Health,* Vol. 48, p. 1636 (December, 1958). For a critique, see J. Pollack, "Major Medical Expense Insurance: An Evaluation," *ibid.,* Vol. 47, p. 322 (March, 1957).

hospital expense in 1958 was 1.4 times that in 1951; for surgical expense it was 1.7; for regular medical expense, 2.7; and for major medical expense, over 160 times.

The growth in voluntary insurance since 1940 was stimu-

TABLE 6.1

NUMBER OF PERSONS WITH VOLUNTARY HEALTH INSURANCE PROTECTION ACCORDING TO TYPE OF COVERAGE; UNITED STATES FROM 1940 TO 1958*

| Year (as of December 31) | Number (in Thousands)† | | | |
|---|---|---|---|---|
| | Hospital Expense | Surgical Expense | Regular Medical Expense | Major Medical Expense |
| 1940 | 12,312 | 5,350 | 3,000 | — |
| 1941 | 16,349 | 6,775 | 3,100 | — |
| 1942 | 19,695 | 8,140 | 3,200 | — |
| 1943 | 24,160 | 10,069 | 3,411 | — |
| 1944 | 29,232 | 11,713 | 3,840 | — |
| 1945 | 32,068 | 12,890 | 4,713 | — |
| 1946 | 42,112 | 18,609 | 6,421 | — |
| 1947 | 52,584 | 26,247 | 8,898 | — |
| 1948 | 60,995 | 34,060 | 12,895 | — |
| 1949 | 66,044 | 41,143 | 16,862 | — |
| 1950 | 76,639 | 54,156 | 21,589 | — |
| 1951 | 85,348 | 64,892 | 27,723 | 108 |
| 1952 | 90,965 | 72,459 | 35,670 | 689 |
| 1953 | 97,303 | 80,982 | 42,684 | 1,220 |
| 1954 | 101,493 | 85,890 | 47,248 | 2,198 |
| 1955 | 107,662 | 91,927 | 55,506 | 5,241 |
| 1956 | 115,949 | 101,325 | 64,891 | 8,876 |
| 1957 | 121,432 | 108,931 | 71,813 | 13,262 |
| 1958 | 123,038 | 111,435 | 75,395 | 17,375 |

* Data relate to all persons protected, including dependents.
† Data relate to coverage provided by insurance companies; Blue Cross–Blue Shield and plans approved by Medical Societies; and independent plans. However, data for major medical expense relate to coverage by insurance companies only.

Source: Health Insurance Council.

lated by a number of factors. The wage stabilization regulations of World War II permitted employers to grant certain health and welfare benefits which included insurance payments for such purposes. In the period since World War II, such "fringe benefits" have been extended widely among workers by employers seeking better relations with their employees and also as a result of collective bargaining between employers and unions. Favoring this extension has been not only the increasing productivity of the economy, but also a liberal income tax treatment to employers contributing toward such benefits. Furthermore, such benefits for workers were, in effect, additional wages free of tax.

In some forms, voluntary insurance against the costs of medical care was available to the aged before World War II, but it was generally incidental to plans designed primarily for workers and their dependents. In the postwar period, the health insurance needs of the aged and retired received increasing attention only after considerable headway had been made with the programs for workers during their productive years. At first, these plans were concerned only with the workers during their retirement, but extensions were soon made to include dependents of the retired, and the beginnings of health insurance for surviving dependent spouses of the retired are in evidence.

### INSURANCE COMPANIES

The categories of insurance companies that issue health insurance policies or contracts are life companies, casualty companies, and companies that write only accident and health insurance. These companies may write individual policies, group policies covering many lives, or both.

Table 6.2 shows that at the end of 1958, insurance companies provided protection for hospital expense to 71.8 million persons, for surgical expense to 69.1 million, for regular medical expense to nearly 35.1 million, and for major medical expense to 17.4 million. Thus, in relation to total coverage by all types of insuring organizations, insurance companies accounted for 58 per cent of those with hospital expense protection, 62 per cent in the case of surgical expense protection, 47 per cent in the case of regular medical expense protection, and for practically all with major medical expense protec-

## TABLE 6.2

NUMBER OF PERSONS WITH VOLUNTARY HEALTH INSURANCE PROTECTION IN INSURANCE COMPANIES ACCORDING TO TYPE OF COVERAGE; UNITED STATES FROM 1940 TO 1958*

| Year (as of December 31) | Number (in Thousands) | | | | | |
|---|---|---|---|---|---|---|
| | Hospital Expense | | | Surgical Expense | | |
| | Total† | Group | Individual | Total† | Group | Individual |
| 1940 | 3,700 | 2,500 | 1,200 | 2,280 | 1,430 | 850 |
| 1941 | 5,350 | 3,850 | 1,500 | 3,300 | 2,300 | 1,000 |
| 1942 | 6,880 | 5,080 | 1,800 | 4,475 | 3,275 | 1,200 |
| 1943 | 8,900 | 6,800 | 2,100 | 6,100 | 4,700 | 1,400 |
| 1944 | 10,800 | 8,400 | 2,400 | 7,225 | 5,625 | 1,600 |
| 1945 | 10,504 | 7,804 | 2,700 | 7,337 | 5,537 | 1,800 |
| 1946 | 14,315 | 11,315 | 3,000 | 10,661 | 8,661 | 2,000 |
| 1947 | 21,127 | 14,190 | 7,584 | 15,558 | 11,103 | 4,875 |
| 1948 | 26,786 | 16,741 | 11,286 | 20,379 | 14,199 | 6,944 |
| 1949 | 30,216 | 17,697 | 14,729 | 23,881 | 15,590 | 9,315 |
| 1950 | 36,955 | 22,305 | 17,296 | 33,428 | 21,219 | 13,718 |
| 1951 | 44,288 | 26,663 | 20,802 | 40,280 | 26,376 | 15,623 |
| 1952 | 46,842 | 29,455 | 21,412 | 44,919 | 29,621 | 18,354 |
| 1953 | 52,218 | 33,575 | 23,475 | 50,464 | 34,039 | 20,212 |
| 1954 | 55,282 | 35,090 | 25,338 | 52,806 | 35,723 | 21,442 |
| 1955 | 59,654 | 39,029 | 26,706 | 56,645 | 39,725 | 22,445 |
| 1956 | 66,259 | 45,211 | 27,629 | 62,996 | 45,906 | 23,074 |
| 1957 | 70,192 | 48,439 | 28,673 | 67,456 | 48,955 | 24,928 |
| 1958 | 71,798 | 49,508 | 29,372 | 69,125 | 49,917 | 25,819 |
| | Regular Medical Expense | | | Major Medical Expense | | |
| | Total† | Group | Individual | Total | Group | Individual |
| 1944 | 200 | 100 | 100 | — | — | — |
| 1945 | 535 | 335 | 200 | — | — | — |
| 1946 | 867 | 567 | 300 | — | — | — |
| 1947 | 2,116 | 1,098 | 1,111 | — | — | — |
| 1948 | 3,538 | 1,927 | 1,810 | — | — | — |
| 1949 | 4,827 | 2,736 | 2,350 | — | — | — |
| 1950 | 8,001 | 5,587 | 2,714 | — | — | — |
| 1951 | 11,711 | 7,946 | 4,230 | 108 | 96 | 12 |
| 1952 | 14,220 | 10,157 | 4,965 | 689 | 533 | 156 |
| 1953 | 18,361 | 13,787 | 5,824 | 1,220 | 1,044 | 176 |
| 1954 | 20,721 | 15,778 | 6,513 | 2,198 | 1,892 | 306 |
| 1955 | 25,031 | 20,678 | 6,264 | 5,241 | 4,759 | 482 |
| 1956 | 29,756 | 25,177 | 6,789 | 8,876 | 8,294 | 582 |
| 1957 | 33,240 | 28,317 | 7,371 | 13,262 | 12,428 | 834 |
| 1958 | 35,142 | 29,868 | 7,869 | 17,375 | 16,229 | 1,146 |

* Data relate to all persons protected, including dependents.
† Net total, after deduction for duplication in persons with both group insurance and individual insurance.

Source: Health Insurance Council.

tion. However, some persons with these types of coverage in insurance companies also have the same type of coverage with other kinds of insurers.

*Group Health Insurance in General.* A characteristic of group insurance is that the lives covered are banded together for some purpose other than the insurance. Group health insurance followed the development of group life insurance, which was originally issued to cover the employees, or specified classes of employees, of an employer.[9] In group insurance, the contract is made between the insurer and the employer, who pays all or part of the premium and receives a master contract; employees are given certificates that describe the benefits to which they are entitled. The concept of group insurance has been extended to include labor unions, associations, and trustees acting for more than one union or for more than one employer, all of whom are in the same industry. The minimum number of lives covered by the group plan, which varies according to state regulation, may be as small as 25; a few states permit insurance for groups as small as three. By dealing with groups instead of individuals as units of administration, the insurer can effect a number of economies in operation which lower appreciably the cost of the group insurance as compared with individual insurance.

The importance of group insurance in the business of companies offering health insurance is evident in Table 6.2. For example, in 1958 the proportions covered by group health insurance were 69 per cent in the case of hospital expense, 72 per cent for surgical expense, 85 per cent for regular medical expense, and 93 per cent for major medical expense.[10] The actual significance of the group insurance mechanism in voluntary health insurance becomes even more evident when it is considered that it encompasses much larger proportions

---

[9] D. W. Gregg, *Group Life Insurance* (rev. ed.; Homewood, Ill.: Richard D. Irwin, Inc., 1957).

[10] The proportions of persons with group insurance who are also protected by individual insurance for the same types of coverage are relatively small.

of the coverage provided by Blue Cross, Blue Shield, medical society plans, and the independent plans.[11]

***Group Health Insurance for the Aged.*** The mechanism of group insurance has been adapted in several ways to provide health insurance for the aged and the retired.[12]

(1) The coverage provided under group contracts to active employees may be continued into the older ages as long as they remain at work. In 1954, the Bureau of Accident and Health Underwriters (later merged into the Health Insurance Association of America) collected data from its member insurance companies regarding group coverage available to older active employees.[13] Their summary report is based upon the returns of 43 companies then writing 72 per cent of all group health insurance. Of these, 37 continued their usual program of health insurance coverage for older active employees. At that time, the other six companies also continued coverage on older active employees, but with various limitations on benefits; only one then terminated all coverage at age 70. Although there is no more recent survey to indicate the trend of group coverage for older active employees, such coverage has become generally available in group contracts. By continuing older active employees in group coverage, the cost of the insurance to the employer will increase as the average age of his work force rises. However, this usually will not affect the contribution rate of the active employees, where such is made.

(2) Because of its characteristics, the insured group is a convenient means for making health insurance available to the aged as they retire by continuing them in the group. Usu-

---

[11] Details for New York State at the end of 1956 are described in *Voluntary Health Insurance and the Senior Citizen: A Report on the Problem of Continuation of Medical Care Benefits for the Aged in New York State*, Insurance Department, State of New York, February 26, 1958, pp. 3–7.

[12] J. F. Follmann, Jr., *Voluntary Health Insurance and Medical Care, Five Years of Progress, 1952–1957, op. cit.,* pp. 30–36.

[13] Bureau of Accident and Health Underwriters, Group Disability Insurance Bulletins Nos. 137 and 138, Health Insurance Association of America, Chicago, New York, and Washington, March, 1955.

ally, a period of several years of membership in the group before retirement is required to establish eligibility for benefits. Many employers introducing such a group plan will also include in the coverage those already retired. The 1954 survey of 43 companies just cited also showed that 36 companies then had plans providing insurance to retired employees and their dependents. Among these companies, 19 had the same benefits for the retired as for active lives, and the remaining had plans with reduced or limited benefits for the retired. Some new features of this development were reported by the Insurance Department of the State of New York on the basis of a survey conducted among insurers writing hospital, surgical, and medical care coverage in the state.[14] Although the findings relate only to one state they are indicative of the developing situation.

According to Table 6.3, provision for continuing health in-

TABLE 6.3

YEAR IN WHICH MEDICAL CARE BENEFITS FOR RETIRING EMPLOYEES WERE INTRODUCED IN GROUP CONTRACTS OF LIFE AND CASUALTY COMPANIES, FOR CONTRACTS IN FORCE AS OF DECEMBER 31, 1956, NEW YORK STATE*

| Year Introduced | Number of Group Contracts | Number of Persons with Medical Care Benefits Available on Retirement (Thousands) |
|---|---|---|
| Total | 424 | 1,340 |
| 1956 | 73 | 188 |
| 1955 | 79 | 264 |
| 1954 | 64 | 215 |
| 1953 | 58 | 130 |
| 1952 | 40 | 68 |
| 1951 and prior† | 110 | 475 |

* Data relate only to companies writing group medical care insurance in New York State.
† Reporting incomplete due to lack of company records.

Source: *Voluntary Health Insurance and the Senior Citizen: A Report on the Problem of Continuation of Medical Care Benefits for the Aged in New York State*, Insurance Department, State of New York, February 26, 1958, p. 24.

[14] *Voluntary Health Insurance and the Senior Citizen, op. cit.*

surance protection at retirement was available to 1,340,000 employees in New York State covered under group plans by life and casualty companies at the end of 1956; almost two thirds received this continuance benefit within the preceding five years. Considering this recent development, Table 6.4 is

TABLE 6.4

PROPORTION OF ACTIVE PERSONS WITH MEDICAL CARE BENEFITS IN GROUP CONTRACTS WHO HAVE THESE GROUP BENEFITS AVAILABLE UPON RETIRE-MENT; CONTRACTS WITH LIFE AND CASUALTY COMPANIES IN FORCE AS OF DECEMBER 31, 1956; UNITED STATES AND NEW YORK STATE*

| Type of Coverage | Number of Persons with Specified Type of Coverage (Thousands) | | Per Cent of Persons with Specified Type of Coverage Available on Retirement | |
|---|---|---|---|---|
| | United States | New York State | United States | New York State |
| Hospital expense......35,081 | 4,424 | | 30.0 | 32.4 |
| Surgical expense......35,458 | 4,614 | | 29.2 | 32.5 |
| Regular medical expense...........22,142 | 2,738 | | 32.8 | 42.2 |
| Major medical expense  7,773 | 1,391 | | 41.4 | 53.6 |

* Data relate only to companies writing group medical care insurance in New York State.

Source: *Voluntary Health Insurance and the Senior Citizen: A Report on the Problem of Continuation of Medical Care Benefits for the Aged in New York State*, Insurance Department, State of New York, February 26, 1958, p. 25.

pertinent since it shows the proportions of active employees protected by health insurance who may continue the same type of coverage into retirement; the data relate only to life and casualty insurance companies. At the end of 1956, in the country as a whole, hospital expense coverage during retirement was available to 30.0 per cent of those who had it during their active years; the corresponding percentages are 29.2 for surgical expense, 32.8 for regular medical expense, and 41.4 per cent for major medical expense. On the basis of these returns and those from Blue Cross, Blue Shield, and other medical plans writing group contracts, the report of the Insurance Department estimated that, at the end of 1956, one third of the covered employees in the state of New York were eligible to continue their hospital and surgical coverage at retirement.

Since the number of companies which include provision for continued protection during retirement in group contracts has been increasing, by reason of this growth alone the proportion of aged covered by health insurance will mount in time. The trend toward continuation of retired employees in the group was also observed in a survey conducted by the Health Insurance Association of America among eight companies writing approximately 60 per cent of the group health insurance business in the United States.[15]

The Insurance Department study also concerned itself with the contribution required of the employee for continuing his health insurance into retirement, since this is a period of reduced income. According to its survey, for 54 per cent of the employees, contributions would not be required during retirement. For those expected to contribute during their retirement years, 68 per cent would pay the same as active employees, 27 per cent would pay more, and 5 per cent would pay less. A convenient mechanism for collecting the contribution of the retired employee is by a deduction from his pension income. Where the retired employee is not expected to contribute, some insurers permit the employer to purchase a paid-up policy for the employee.

As the proportion of retired lives included under an employer's group health insurance plan rises, his costs will also rise. In most instances, for the purpose of reducing cost, the life and casualty insurance companies reduce the scale of benefits for retired employees with continued health insurance coverage. In the survey by the Insurance Department of the State of New York this was found to be the case for 80 per cent of those with hospital expense coverage and 70 per cent of those with surgical expense coverage. However,

---

[15] *Trend in Medical Care Benefits Provided to Active Employees and at Retirement Through Group Insurance Plans, January 1953 and December 1956,* Health Insurance Association of America, Chicago, New York and Washington, December 28, 1956.

the rise in employer's costs with the rise in the proportion of retired lives included in the group insurance can be avoided by a program whereby a fund is created during the active years to pay for the retirement years.

(3) In those instances where a death benefit is provided after retirement, it is possible to integrate this with hospital and surgical benefits.[16] The arrangement is that any hospital and surgical benefits paid on behalf of the retiree or his dependent are deducted from the death benefit. In effect, the extra cost of this plan, beyond that of the death benefit, is the interest on the amount of the hospital or surgical benefit from the time of its payment to the death of the retired employee. Since the amount of the death benefit is stipulated, the employer can have an estimate of the limit of his liability to retired employees. Under the plan, the retired employee has access to funds that would not be available until his death. It conforms closely, therefore, to the concept that part of the death benefit from life insurance is intended to pay for terminal expenses.

(4) There are cases where group health insurance was issued to groups of retired persons associated for some purpose other than the insurance, such as Golden Age Clubs. An active program in this direction is being pursued by the National Retired Teachers Association, which had an enrollment of about 100,000 of the 170,000 retired teachers in the United States in 1959.[17] In order to extend the benefits of its experience to other retired persons, this association founded the American Association of Retired Persons in late 1958; the latter had a membership of 50,000 by mid-1959. Another step in the same direction is found in several states whereby, under permissive legislation, an appropriate state or local agency is authorized to obtain group health insurance

---

[16] J. H. Braddock, "Post Retirement Death-Hospital-Surgical Plan Packages," *Journal of Commerce*, New York, June 17, 1958, second section, p. 10.

[17] Statement of E. P. Andrus, U.S. House Committee on Ways and Means, *Hospital, Nursing Home and Surgical Benefits for OASI Beneficiaries* (Hearings, 86th Cong., 1st sess., July, 1959), p. 509.

coverage with an insurer for retired public employees, teachers, and school employees; the premiums would be deducted from pensions paid by the agency.[18] In at least one instance, the premiums would be shared by the local government.[19] Where the costs are not shared by an employer, they will tend to be higher for the participants than otherwise; however, the costs are less than on individually purchased coverage.

(5) Another development in group health insurance contracts is the inclusion of a right to convert to an individual policy, without evidence of insurability or physical examination, upon leaving the group. Where this right is available, it relates to termination of employment for any reason, including retirement. In this regard, the survey by the Insurance Department of the State of New York yielded the data in Table 6.5. The last column of this table shows that about 80 per cent of the persons in New York State with this right at the end of 1956 received it within the two preceding years. Of the 64 life and casualty companies writing group health insurance in New York State, the survey by the Insurance Department found that 31 made the right to convert to an individual policy available to the group policyholder. At the end of 1956, this right was available to more than one fifth of all persons covered by group health insurance benefits; there are indications that this proportion is growing.

The right to convert to an individual policy is usually not restricted to any maximum age, although some companies may specify some limit between ages 65 and 75. The conversion right generally applies also to dependents and sometimes to the surviving spouse. Frequently, the maximum benefits available after conversion may not be as liberal as under the previous group contract. Most insurance companies which permit conversion to an individual policy in their group contract retain the right to cancel the converted policy at a sub-

---

[18] Recent (1959) examples of such legislation are Chapter 319, laws of Oregon (House Bill No. 392) and laws of Ohio (Senate Bill No. 256).

[19] Chapter 595, laws of Massachusetts, 1959 (House Bill No. 3106).

sequent anniversary. The right to cancel, which is seldom exercised, is of some importance to the insurance company when it finds evidence of duplication of health insurance coverage on the part of the individual. However, the survey by the Insurance Department showed that only a little over

TABLE 6.5

Year in Which Right to Convert to an Individual Health Insurance Contract upon Leaving a Group Was Introduced in Group Contracts of Life and Casualty Companies, for Contracts in Force as of December 31, 1956; New York State*

| Year Introduced | Number of Group Contracts | Number of Persons with Right to Convert to Individual Contracts upon Leaving a Group (Thousands) |
|---|---|---|
| Total...................655 | | 737 |
| 1956.....................393 | | 232 |
| 1955.....................119 | | 361 |
| 1954..................... 58 | | 88 |
| 1953..................... 10 | | 12 |
| 1952..................... 13 | | 6 |
| 1951 and prior†........... 62 | | 38 |

* Data relate only to companies writing group medical care insurance in New York State.
† Reporting incomplete due to lack of company records.
Source: *Voluntary Health Insurance and the Senior Citizen: A Report on the Problem of Continuation of Medical Care Benefits for the Aged in New York State*, Insurance Department, State of New York, February 26, 1958, p. 28.

1 per cent of the converted policies in force in New York State during 1956 were canceled or refused renewal.

It has been found, in hospital expense coverage, that the subsequent experience of persons who had converted to individual policies from a group contract is not as favorable as that of persons of the same ages who held individual policies originally. Thus, a study by the Metropolitan Life Insurance Company showed that persons covered by individual hospital and surgical expense policies after physical examination had a hospital admission rate of 125 per 1,000 at ages 65 and over in 1957. For persons who had converted from group to individual policies without physical examination at any time, the corresponding rate at ages 65 and over was 184 per 1,000.[20] Although those who formerly held group coverage had the benefit of that protection for a number of years, their higher rate after conversion is indicative of some self-selection on the part of those entitled to the conversion right. In other words, those who sensed a need for hospital care took advantage of their option to continue protection on an individual basis, while many of the others failed to exercise the option. Since the persons in the Metropolitan experience with converted policies are largely in the same social strata as those who had individual policies originally, social factors are a minor influence in the difference noted between the two categories.

*Individual Health Insurance in General.* Those in the population who do not fall within the scope of group insurance coverage for their costs of medical care may secure this protection for themselves and their dependents (wife and children) through individual health insurance. Most individual health insurance is held with insurance companies. Because each policy requires the services of an agent and also separate underwriting and administrative attention in the insurance office, individual health insurance is more costly than group insurance. Table 6.2 shows the growth of individual health insurance issued by insurance companies for the several types of coverage. Not only are the numbers covered by individual insurance smaller than those for group insurance, but since about 1950 they have been growing at a lesser rate. Nevertheless, at the end of 1958 nearly 30 million persons had hospital expense coverage with insurance companies, almost 26 million had surgical expense coverage, close to eight million had regular medical expense protection, and over one million had major medical expense protection.

---

[20] J. C. Horan, "Complaints of the Senior Citizen," presented before the Annual Individual Insurance Forum, Health Insurance Association of America, Chicago, October 27–29, 1958.

Much individual health insurance has been sold on a one-year term basis, renewable at the option of the insured and the insurer, in a fashion similar to that of some lines of casualty insurance. Thus, both parties have annually an opportunity to reconsider the desirability of renewing the contract.[21] By exercising its right when necessary on such occasions in order to maintain a satisfactory level of claim experience, the insurer is in a position to offer its coverage at a low cost; this does not interfere with the payment of benefits on claims that have already been incurred. Although exercise of the cancellation option might vary from one company to another, a study covering a six-month period in 1957 showed that cancellations and nonrenewals averaged only 0.26 per 100 policies in force and 2.0 per 100 policies with claims paid.[22] About half of these cancellations and nonrenewals were because of deterioration of health.[23] Among other reasons for termination are false claims, a high frequency of claims, the presence of pre-existing conditions, overinsurance, fraud in the application, and the expiration of the age limit where that age is not stated in the policy.

Insurance companies are continually studying their nonrenewal practices and experience in order to liberalize their procedures, since it is their desire to increase the persistence of insurance in force. To meet the need for individual health insurance that continues irrespective of the extent of physical deterioration or of frequency of claims, companies have introduced policies that are noncancellable and guaranteed renewable for the term of the contract. These are issued at a cost somewhat above that of the corresponding cancellable

---

[21] J. F. Follmann, Jr., *Voluntary Health Insurance and Medical Care, Five Years of Progress, 1952–1957, op. cit.,* pp. 52–56.

[22] *Individual Accident and Health Insurance: A Report of Practices With Respect to Cancellation and Non-Renewability of Insurance Companies in the United States,* Based upon a Survey Conducted by the Health Insurance Association of America on Behalf of the National Association of Insurance Commissioners, New York, June, 1958.

[23] For a further discussion of the termination of individual health insurance, see *Voluntary Health Insurance and the Senior Citizen, op. cit.,* pp. 33–43.

policy.[24] Also, because of the trend in the costs of medical care, the company reserves the right to change the premium scale for all policies of any one class or form of contract. Since about 1950, the issue of guaranteed renewable insurance has grown more rapidly than that of cancellable insurance.

***Individual Health Insurance for the Aged.*** Individual insurance to protect against the costs of medical care during the later years is available not only to those already in old age but also to those who plan ahead during their working life. This individual protection may be secured in several ways:

(1) Those who have the right to convert to an individual policy upon leaving an insured group, a method previously mentioned, are required to pay the premium applicable to their attained age. For the retired, this may be high in relation to income.

(2) Several companies are issuing health insurance to individuals at ages after 65 up to some maximum which, in a few instances, may run up to 85 years. The practice to 1956 in this regard, derived from the previously cited report by the Insurance Department of the State of New York, is summarized in Table 6.6. Among the reporting life and casualty companies that had individual health insurance available, 20 per cent stated that their principal forms of policies had maximum ages at issue greater than 65 years, and almost 12 per cent issued at ages 71 and over. For individual insurance at these advanced ages, the premiums are naturally high, and there is also the need to pass a health examination. To meet these situations, a few companies have adapted group insurance principles for selecting applicants, although individual policies are issued. The premiums are not varied with age and pre-existing conditions are covered after a waiting period of a few months. Sales are effected by intensive advertising campaigns within a limited time period, using various mass me-

---

[24] For a comparison of these costs, see *Voluntary Health Insurance and the Senior Citizen, op. cit.,* pp. 92–97.

dia, such as newspapers and radio. The benefits provided by the policies issued after age 65 are usually of the same scope as those for the older ages in contracts continued from the younger ages. The policies are not subject to individual consideration at renewal; however, premiums may be adjusted on the basis of the experience of classes of policyholders.

TABLE 6.6

DISTRIBUTION OF MAXIMUM AGES AT ISSUE ON CONTRACT FORMS OF INDIVIDUAL HEALTH INSURANCE AND OF AGES AT EXPIRATION OF COVERAGE FOR LIFE AND CASUALTY COMPANIES WRITING IN NEW YORK STATE, 1956

| Age | Maximum Age at Issue | | Age at Expiration of Coverage | |
|---|---|---|---|---|
| | Number of Contract Forms* | Per Cent | Number of Contract Forms* | Per Cent |
| Total................196 | | 100.0 | 196 | 100.0 |
| Up to 55.............. | 48 | 24.5 | 0 | — |
| 56–60................ | 85 | 43.4 | 14 | 7.2 |
| 61–65................ | 23 | 11.7 | 88 | 44.9 |
| 66–70................ | 17 | 8.7 | 23 | 11.7 |
| 71 and over........... | 23 | 11.7 | 71 | 36.2 |

* Number of contract forms represents the number of forms which produced the largest volume of premiums during 1956 for each of the following types of coverage for each insurer: loss of income with hospital, surgical or medical benefits; hospital only; surgical-medical only; hospital and surgical-medical; and major medical. The figures present the combined results for these contract forms.

Source: *Voluntary Health Insurance and the Senior Citizen: A Report on the Problem of Continuation of Medical Care Benefits for the Aged in New York State*, Insurance Department, State of New York, February 26, 1958, p. 32.

(3)  The survey summarized in Table 6.6 also shows that nearly half of the policy forms available continued health insurance coverage beyond age 65 and that over one third continued to ages 71 and over; some may be continued for life. Several companies follow the practice of increasing the premiums at the older ages to meet the higher claim costs, while some reduce the benefit in order to avoid increasing the premium.

(4)  For those still at the main working ages, a few companies have available individual health insurance policies with premiums payable up to age 65, after which they are paid-up

for life. In such policies, the scale of benefits payable during the productive years may be reduced after attaining age 65. Since there is a fixed scale of benefit, the proportion of medical expenses that would be met depends upon the trend in costs of medical care.

## BLUE CROSS, BLUE SHIELD AND OTHER MEDICAL SOCIETY APPROVED PLANS

It is characteristic of the Blue Cross, Blue Shield, and other medical society plans for the prepayment of medical care that they operate in local areas generally not larger than a state, are nonprofit, and for the most part base their premiums on the experience of the area or community they serve.[25] At the end of 1958, these plans provided 55.2 million persons with protection against hospital expense, over 46.4 million against surgical expense, and 38.9 million against regular medical expense, as shown in Table 6.7.[26]

*Blue Cross Plans in General.* Blue Cross plans must meet the requirements of the American Hospital Association; in most states, there are also legislative requirements.[27] Each plan arranges with hospitals in its area to provide specified services to its subscribers on hospitalization; the subscriber pays for any services beyond those specified that may be needed. The contracting hospitals in the area served are

---

[25] For a description of community rating in relation to insurance of the aged, see *Hospitalization Insurance for OASDI Beneficiaries,* Report submitted to the Committee on Ways and Means by the Secretary of Health, Education, and Welfare, Washington, D.C., April 3, 1959, p. 48.

[26] For the development and problems of these plans, see L. S. Reed, *Blue Cross and Medical Service Plans, op. cit.;* D. L. MacDonald, "Blue Cross Troubles: A Price of Delusion," *The Weekly Underwriter,* November 17, 1956; and O. D. Dickerson, *Health Insurance* (Homewood, Ill.: Richard D. Irwin, Inc., 1959).

[27] For a survey of these legislative requirements, see *Blue Cross and Blue Shield in Wisconsin,* a special report by the Insurance Department of the State of Wisconsin, January, 1959, p. 99; also pertinent is a report by T. L. Wenck, *Comparative Analysis of Costs of the Blue Cross and Blue Shield Plans in Wisconsin with the Private Insurance Industry,* Insurance Department of the State of Wisconsin, August, 1959.

TABLE 6.7

Number of Persons with Voluntary Health Insurance
Protection in Blue Cross, Blue Shield, and
Medical Society Plans According to Type of Coverage;
United States from 1940 to 1958*

| Year (as of December 31) | Number (in Thousands) | | |
|---|---|---|---|
| | Hospital Expense | Surgical Expense | Regular Medical Expense |
| 1940 | 6,012 | 370 | 200 |
| 1941 | 8,399 | 775 | 300 |
| 1942 | 10,215 | 965 | 400 |
| 1943 | 12,600 | 1,235 | 600 |
| 1944 | 15,772 | 1,768 | 800 |
| 1945 | 18,899 | 2,845 | 1,300 |
| 1946 | 24,707 | 5,000 | 2,350 |
| 1947 | 27,986 | 7,380 | 2,985 |
| 1948 | 31,246 | 10,608 | 5,712 |
| 1949 | 34,315 | 14,628 | 8,508 |
| 1950 | 38,822 | 19,690 | 11,428 |
| 1951 | 40,933 | 24,095 | 14,347 |
| 1952 | 41,475 | 27,773 | 18,321 |
| 1953 | 45,829 | 31,511 | 21,674 |
| 1954 | 47,484 | 34,899 | 24,668 |
| 1955 | 50,726 | 39,165 | 29,451 |
| 1956 | 53,162 | 42,570 | 33,907 |
| 1957 | 54,923 | 45,383 | 36,926 |
| 1958 | 55,205 | 46,424 | 38,860 |

* Data relate to all persons protected, including dependents.
Source: Health Insurance Council.

reimbursed by the plan on a per diem basis agreed upon in
advance. This per diem payment, with an addition for administration and reserves, is the basis for the premium rate.[28]
The Blue Cross plans thus sell their subscribers hospital services rather than cash benefits applicable to hospital expense;
there are a few Blue Cross plans that also offer insurance
against surgical expense. Exchange of information among

---

[28] The problems involved in arriving at the per diem charge and premium
rates are discussed by E. A. van Steenwyk, *op. cit.*; see also *Blue Cross and
Blue Shield in Wisconsin, op. cit.*, p. 23.

the plans is effected through the Blue Cross Commission of the American Hospital Association.

Although Blue Cross plans obtain their subscribers principally by group enrollment, most will also accept subscribers on a nongroup basis either by direct enrollment during stated periods or by community campaigns with or without a minimum participation requirement.[29] In many plans, enrollment is accepted at any time from individuals or families upon meeting stated qualifications, such as a health statement, and also with some restriction, usually exclusion from coverage because of pre-existing conditions or coverage after a waiting period.

In order to sell and service large employee groups extending over more than one Blue Cross area, the plans developed a number of mechanisms. Since 1956, the Blue Cross Association has acted as consultant and assisted plans in enrolling large group accounts. The plans which are members of the Association have agreed, among other things, "to offer to all national accounts all of the hospital benefit contracts which may be approved by the Board of Governors of the Association," according to the Blue Cross Guide. Health Service, Incorporated, will provide a portion of the coverage which exceeds the benefits that a local plan is able to underwrite for a given account. A Blue Cross subscriber who happens to be hospitalized in an area outside that served by his plan will receive benefits accorded by the plan of the area in which the hospital is located. To effect the financial interchange on a national basis, the Blue Cross plans have established an Inter-Plan Service Benefit Bank. For those who move from one area to another, coverage is transferred immediately through the Inter-Plan Transfer Program.

*Blue Cross Plans for the Aged.* It has been estimated by the Blue Cross Commission that 24 per cent of the population at ages 65 and over was covered by its plans toward the

---

[29] S. Levine, O. W. Anderson, and G. Gordon, *Non-Group Enrollment For Health Insurance* (Cambridge, Mass.: Harvard University Press, 1957).

end of 1958; the number of aged so covered then totaled about 3½ million.[30] About half of these aged obtained their coverage through group plans by continuing in employment after age 65 or by being retained in the group after retirement. In the latter case, the retired employee may pay the same premium as an active employee through his former employer and receive the same benefits. The extra cost of the benefits of these older people is borne by all covered by Blue Cross since the contributions are not graded by age in a group plan. Some of the other half of the aged covered by Blue Cross obtained their protection by direct enrollment at an earlier age, but most by conversion from a group to an individual contract upon retirement, a privilege available in all plans. This privilege is subject to restriction of benefits after some stated age in a few plans. Several plans have developed special contract certificates for aged subscribers.

Among the 79 Blue Cross plans in the United States in 1958, no age limits were placed on group enrollments in 41 plans; an additional four without age limits placed restrictions on benefits after a stated age (Table 6.8). An age limit on group enrollment was placed in 26 plans; in 22 it was age 65. There were eight plans with an age limit for certain types of contract or size of group.

All but three of the 79 Blue Cross plans accept nongroup enrollment either through application at any time or by periodic campaigns. Age limits on nongroup enrollment were stated in 67 plans; 12 were at age 60 and 51 at age 65. Only six plans had no age limits and no restrictions of benefits, and an additional three without age limits had either a special contract or reduced benefits.

In view of the high and continually rising costs of hospital care, a few Blue Cross plans have introduced nursing home

---

[30] Cited by A. W. Brewster and R. Bloodgood, "Blue Cross Provisions for Persons Aged 65 and Over, Late 1958," *Research and Statistics Note No. 5,* Division of Program Research, Social Security Administration, March 12, 1959; see also *Social Security Bulletin,* May, 1959. Further data in this and the next two paragraphs were derived from a report of the Blue Cross Commission.

TABLE 6.8

Distribution of Blue Cross Plans According to Maximum Ages at Issue, Separately for Group and Nongroup Enrollment, United States, 1958

| Age Limitation | Number of Plans |
|---|---|
| Group enrollment, total | 79 |
| With an age limit | 26 |
| Age limit at 65 years | 22 |
| With age limit for certain types of contract or size of group | 8 |
| With no age limit, but restricted benefits over a stated age | 4 |
| With no age restrictions | 41 |
| Nongroup enrollment, total | 79 |
| With an age limit | 67 |
| Age limit at 55 years | 1 |
| Age limit at 60 years | 12 |
| Age limit at 65 years | 51 |
| Age limit at 66 years | 1 |
| Age limit at 70 years | 2 |
| With no age limit, but special contract or reduced benefit | 3 |
| With no age limit and no restrictions of benefit | 6 |
| No nongroup enrollment, total | 3 |

Source: Blue Cross Commission of the American Hospital Association, "Extent and Availability of Blue Cross Coverage for Those 65 and Over," *Research & Technical Assistance Service Bulletin*, January 8, 1959.

benefits under certain limitations.[31] These limitations are classified by Brewster as:

(1) sale only to groups—a provision which excludes most retired persons and elderly persons; (2) discharge from a hospital directly to a nursing home as a prerequisite, which tends to confine the cases to certain diagnoses and excludes the chronically ill except following an acute episode; (3) a lifetime limit on the

[31] J. F. Follmann, Jr., *Health Insurance and Nursing Home Care*, Health Insurance Association of America, New York, March 5, 1958, and A. W. Brewster, "Care in Nursing Homes Through Prepayment Hospital Plans," *Research and Statistics Note No. 41*, Division of Program Research, Social Security Administration, November 25, 1958. According to J. F. Follmann, Jr., reporting in *Best's Insurance News, Life Edition*, July, 1958, there may be no insurance companies providing for nursing home care in their policy plans, although they may pay for such benefits in special circumstances under their hospital, major medical, and comprehensive policies by administrative arrangements. However, since this article was written, at least one large insurance company has introduced nursing home care as part of its coverage for those over age 65.

benefit; (4) coinsurance, so that the insured pays 20% of the nursing home charges.

The use of a coinsurance feature in this instance is reasonable, not only as a means of reducing the insurance prepayment charge and as a deterrent to unneeded use of this service, but also because the insured is relieved of many usual living costs while maintained in a nursing home. Without coinsurance, a person maintained in a nursing home would be better off financially than living at home.

The concern with medical care costs also led to a study by Associated Hospital Service of New York, the local Blue Cross plan, on the problems arising with the early discharge of hospital patients who are provided with visiting nurse services.[32] The study reports on 500 patients selected for early discharge and subsequent visiting nurse service at home. The study showed that patient care was improved, in addition to the benefit of the home environment, by the requirement of an evaluation of nursing needs before discharge and the individual attention each patient was given in continuing his care from hospital to home. This program also showed a reduction in the costs of illness "for older patients who suffered from long-term diseases." By extending the resources of the aged in need of prolonged medical care in this way, the community saves by decreasing its burden of medically indigent. Early discharge, and therefore shortened hospital stay, also gives more of the population access to the hospital beds in the community. The success of this approach obviously requires close cooperation between the hospital, the nursing service, and the insurer.[33]

---

[32] *Report of a Study Concerning the Feasibility of Providing Visiting Nurse Service Following Hospitalization for Blue Cross Subscribers,* Associated Hospital Service of New York, New York City, May 1, 1957. For a general review, see J. F. Follmann, Jr., "Visiting Nurse Service," *Best's Insurance News, Life Edition,* Vol. 60, p. 75 (May, 1959), and *Health Insurance and Nursing and Home Care,* Health Insurance Association of America, Chicago, New York, Washington, May, 1959.

[33] M. Phaneuf, Associated Hospital Service of New York, "Visiting Nurse Service Following Hospitalization for Blue Cross Subscribers," presented at the Annual Meeting of the American Public Health Association at St. Louis, October, 1958.

*Blue Shield and Other Medical Society Approved Plans in General.* As is the case with Blue Cross plans, in most states Blue Shield plans must meet legislative requirements.[34] Any physician who is a member of the local medical society is eligible to participate in its Blue Shield plan. Blue Shield Medical Care Plans, Inc., provides the medium for exchange of information among the individual Blue Shield plans.

Whereas most Blue Shield plans and other plans approved by medical societies provide both surgical and in-hospital medical benefits (a few include also home and office visits), several provide surgical benefits only, and a few will also cover hospitalization. A small number of Blue Shield plans are experimenting with major medical expense benefits by adding them in the form of endorsements or riders to their basic contract. Although some plans provide their benefits in the form of services, without the necessity of an additional fee to the physician, these cover only a small fraction of the total enrollment of Blue Shield and other plans having the approval of medical societies.[35] Many plans pay benefits only in the form of a cash indemnity toward the physicians' fee. These benefits are made according to a schedule of allowances that varies on the basis of the service rendered. Most plans, and over two thirds of the enrollment, operate under a combination of service and cash indemnity benefits. By this arrangement, subscribers with incomes below a specified level are given service benefits while those over that level are provided cash indemnities according to a schedule of allowances.[36] The arrangements for Blue Shield subscribers requiring medical care services outside the area of their plan are very much like those for Blue Cross. The conditions for enrollment in Blue Shield plans also correspond closely to

---

[34] *Blue Cross and Blue Shield Plans in Wisconsin, op. cit.,* p. 99.

[35] *Voluntary Prepayment Medical Benefit Plans,* American Medical Association, Chicago, published annually.

[36] A. W. Brewster, "Income Ceilings for Service Benefits in Blue Shield Plans, End of 1958," *Research and Statistics Note No. 7,* Division of Program Research, Social Security Administration, March 17, 1959.

those for Blue Cross plans. In many areas, the administration of Blue Shield and Blue Cross is co-ordinated, although the two are legally independent.

**Blue Shield Plans for the Aged.**  According to Blue Shield Medical Care Plans, Inc., about 2½ million persons at ages 65 and over were covered by their plans at the end of 1957; these represented one sixth of the total population at those ages. Of the 66 more common group contracts issued by Blue Shield that are described in Table 6.9, all permit conversion to an individual plan upon retirement. In somewhat over one fifth of these contracts, no additional premium is required after conversion. The retired, under some Blue Shield contracts, may also be continued in the group by their past employers, as in the case of some Blue Cross contracts. About three fifths of the plans have no age limit on group enrollment; most others set the limit at age 65, but this is generally waived for the larger groups.

All but two of the 66 Blue Shield plans accepted nongroup enrollment about the end of 1956. Although only five plans had no age limit on nongroup enrollment at that time, the number has since increased.[37] Table 6.9 shows that three fourths of the nongroup contracts limited enrollment to age 65, most others having a lower limit. In nearly one fifth of the nongroup contracts the premiums were the same as for group contracts; for all others there was an additional charge.

In order to assist the individual plans in the development of programs to provide protection against medical care expenses for the aged, the Blue Shield Medical Care Plans, Inc. established a study committee in 1958.[38] For the attention

---

[37] Statement of Blue Shield Medical Care Plans to the Council on Medical Service of the American Medical Association, October 17, 1958.

[38] Late in 1958, the American Medical Association recommended that: ". . . physicians everywhere expedite the development of an effective voluntary health insurance or prepayment program for the group over 65 with modest resources or low family income; that physicians agree to accept a level of compensation as full payment for medical service rendered to this group, which will permit the development of such insurance and prepayment plans at a reduced premium rate . . ." *Journal of the American Medical Association,* Vol. 168, p. 2148 (December 20, 1958).

## TABLE 6.9

| Age Limit for Enrollment; Premium Level | Type of Benefit | | | |
|---|---|---|---|---|
| | All Types | Surgical Only | Surgical and in-Hospital Medical[b] | Hospital and Physician[c] |
| **Group Contracts** | | | | |
| Number of plans............. | 66 | 11 | 51 | 4 |
| Plans with group conversion.. | 66 | 12 | 50 | 4 |
| Additional premium after conversion | | | | |
| One person contracts | | | | |
| None required........... | 16 | 3 | 10 | 3 |
| Addition required........ | 50 | 9 | 40 | 1 |
| Family contracts | | | | |
| None required........... | 13 | 3 | 9 | 1 |
| Addition required........ | 53 | 9 | 41 | 3 |
| Age limit for enrollment[d] | | | | |
| None.................... | 38 | 8 | 27 | 3 |
| 60 years................. | 1 | — | 1 | — |
| 65 years................. | 23 | 5 | 17 | 1 |
| 66 years................. | 2 | — | 2 | — |
| **Nongroup Contracts** | | | | |
| Number of plans............. | 64 | 13 | 47 | 4 |
| Additional premium over group premium | | | | |
| One person contracts | | | | |
| No addition............. | 12 | 4 | 5 | 3 |
| Some addition........... | 52 | 9 | 42 | 1 |
| Family contracts | | | | |
| No addition............. | 10 | 4 | 5 | 1 |
| Some addition........... | 54 | 9 | 42 | 3 |
| Age limit for enrollment | | | | |
| None.................... | 5 | 1 | 4 | — |
| 56 years................. | 1 | — | 1 | — |
| 60 years................. | 7 | — | 5 | 2 |
| 61 years................. | 1 | — | 1 | — |
| 65 years................. | 48 | 11 | 35 | 2 |
| 66 years................. | 2 | 1 | 1 | — |

[a] Prepared from plan summaries in the *Blue Shield Manual*, revised June 1, 1957. Group contracts selected for analysis were those offered in the most widely held contracts in each plan; group conversion and nongroup contracts were those most nearly resembling the group contracts in benefits.

[b] Includes one plan which also provides limited indemnity payments for physicians' home and office visits; another plan limits such benefits to employed subscribers (not dependents) under group contracts, provided they are unable to work. All other plans restrict benefits to in-hospital medical care.

[c] Physicians' benefits consist of surgery in all cases; of in-hospital medical care in all group contracts and in three group conversion and two nongroup contracts; and of limited home and office medical care in three group contracts and in the group conversion and nongroup contracts of one plan.

[d] Data relate to 64 plans offering both group and nongroup enrollment.

Source: C. E. Ortmeyer, "Blue Shield Provisions for Retired Persons," *Research and Statistics Note No. 25*, Division of Program Research, Social Security Administration, July 30, 1957.

of the individual plans, there was developed a special, or model, program suited to the medical care needs of those over age 65.[39] The benefits would consist of surgery wherever performed; anesthesia; in-hospital medical care for 120 days; diagnostic X ray as a hospital inpatient or outpatient, or in a doctor's office if followed by hospitalization; and radiation therapy. The income level for entitlement to service benefits in an area generally depends upon its economic situation. In order to produce a premium rate for this insurance that would conform with the low income of the aged, an appropriate scale had to be set to reimburse physicians for their services. For this purpose, use was made of a relative value schedule, with a proposal that the dollar charge per unit value be fixed by taking into account the medical practices in the locality. In effect, the medical profession would be subsidizing the care of a low-income group, as in the past, but on a uniform program.[40] One Blue Shield plan announced, early in 1959, that it would accept, on an experimental basis, individual enrollment of persons over 65 at the same premiums and with the same benefits as younger persons; there is a requirement of apparent good health at time of application.

## INDEPENDENT PLANS

The "independent" plans comprise those miscellaneous plans that provide health insurance and operate outside the sphere of private insurance companies and Blue Cross and Blue Shield plans as previously described.[41] A survey con-

---

[39] *The AMA News,* published by the American Medical Association, February 9, 1959, p. 1.

[40] An interesting allied development by the National Retired Teachers Association and its affiliate, the American Association of Retired Persons, is the establishment of a service whereby its members may purchase pharmaceuticals at reduced prices (Health Insurance Association of America, *Medical Economics Briefs,* August 28, 1959).

[41] For a comprehensive review, see A. W. Brewster, "Independent Plans Providing Medical Care and Hospital Insurance: 1957 Survey," *Social Security Bulletin,* April, 1958.

ducted during the summer of 1958 jointly by the Health Information Foundation and the National Opinion Research Center showed that 6 per cent of the population then had group hospital insurance with independent plans and 1 per cent had such individual insurance.[42]

*Independent Plans in General.* Independent industrial plans are those operated for the benefit of employees in specific industries. These may operate under the sponsorship of employers alone, employers and employees acting jointly, employee benefit associations, or unions, the last covering the largest number of enrollees. Largest among the independent nonindustrial plans are those with community sponsorship; also included in this category are private group clinics, medical society plans without Blue Shield affiliation, and consumer and fraternal organizations. Except for the last two, the independent nonindustrial plans are open to the general public under various group or individual enrollment bases.

The scope of benefits provided by the independent plans varies widely with regard to provisions for hospitalization, surgery, and medical care. The benefits range from a full complement of benefits provided on a service basis to cash indemnity for a few days of hospital stay. A feature of a great many independent plans, not common in plans of private insurance companies or of Blue Cross or Blue Shield plans, is the availability of diagnostic services. Dental services are also provided in several independent plans; there may be other benefits, such as nursing care, vision care, and the provision of drugs.

The independent plans account for a relatively small proportion of the total number in the country protected by voluntary health insurance. At the end of 1958, out of a total of over 123 million persons covered against the costs of hospital expense, almost 5 million, or about 4 per cent, were in independent plans. These plans covered over 5½ million out

---

[42] Unpublished data from the Health Information Foundation; see also *Progress in Health Services,* Vol. 8 (May, 1959).

of a total of more than 111 million protected against surgical expense, and 6 million out of a total of over 75 million protected against regular medical expense. These estimates of numbers covered by independent plans, which are published by the Health Insurance Council, exclude those protected by medical society plans not affiliated with Blue Cross or Blue Shield.[43] Also, some persons covered by one type of health insurance under an independent plan may be protected for other types by another form of insurer. The trend in the numbers with health insurance protection in independent plans is shown in Table 6.10.

*Independent Industrial Plans for the Aged.* Analysis of the returns of a survey of independent health insurance plans made by the Division of Program Research of the Social Security Administration yielded the results in Tables 6.11 and 6.12 for industrial plans as of the end of 1956. The data relate, for the most part, to plans with programs for retired workers.[44]

Returns were received from 97 plans covering about $2\frac{1}{2}$ million active and retired workers. Of this total, 79 plans with over $2\frac{1}{3}$ million members provided for health insurance benefits to retired workers and their dependents. For about one fifth of the members in these plans the benefits are reduced upon retirement. Although only half of these plans also provided benefits for dependents of the retirees, three fourths of the active and retired workers covered had this coverage available. At the end of 1956, the 72 plans reporting on the number of retirees and dependents then covered claimed a total of 182,100 persons entitled to benefits.

Over three fifths of the members of independent industrial plans with health insurance benefits for retirees were in plans

---

[43] Such plans are included in Table 6.7 along with Blue Cross and Blue Shield; Health Insurance Council, *The Extent of Voluntary Health Insurance Coverage in the United States,* issued annually.

[44] In this connection, see also *Older Workers Under Collective Bargaining: Part II—Health and Insurance Plans, Pension Plans,* Bulletin No. 1199–2, Bureau of Labor Statistics, Washington, D.C., October, 1956.

TABLE 6.10

NUMBER OF PERSONS WITH VOLUNTARY HEALTH INSURANCE
PROTECTION IN INDEPENDENT PLANS ACCORDING TO TYPE OF
COVERAGE; UNITED STATES FROM 1940 TO 1958*

| Year (as of December 31) | Number (in Thousands) | | |
|---|---|---|---|
| | Hospital Expense | Surgical Expense | Regular Medical Expense |
| 1940 | 2,600 | 2,700 | 2,800 |
| 1941 | 2,600 | 2,700 | 2,800 |
| 1942 | 2,600 | 2,700 | 2,800 |
| 1943 | 2,660 | 2,734 | 2,811 |
| 1944 | 2,660 | 2,720 | 2,840 |
| 1945 | 2,665 | 2,708 | 2,878 |
| 1946 | 3,090 | 2,948 | 3,204 |
| 1947 | 3,775 | 3,829 | 3,844 |
| 1948 | 3,765 | 3,824 | 3,839 |
| 1949 | 3,760 | 3,820 | 3,835 |
| 1950 | 3,619 | 2,919 | 2,873 |
| 1951 | 3,531 | 2,790 | 2,791 |
| 1952 | 5,364 | 4,794 | 5,150 |
| 1953 | 4,834 | 4,995 | 5,260 |
| 1954 | 5,196 | 4,801 | 4,908 |
| 1955 | 4,530 | 4,340 | 4,639 |
| 1956 | 4,654 | 4,909 | 5,276 |
| 1957 | 4,947 | 5,597 | 6,019 |
| 1958 | 4,865 | 5,572 | 6,015 |

* Data relate to all persons protected, including dependents. These data
exclude medical society plans not affiliated with Blue Cross or Blue Shield;
such plans are included in Table 6.7.

Source: Health Insurance Council.

sponsored by 25 unions.[45] The 24 plans whose source of financing is the sponsor alone account for over half the total
membership in the industrial plans with health insurance

---

[45] Many unions have established health centers to provide diagnostic
and other services to ambulatory patients among their membership. Some
of these centers also make their services available to retired workers from
their union. For a description of their operation see Committee on Medical
Care for Industrial Workers, *A Survey of Union Health Centers* (Chicago:
American Medical Association, 1954). For a more general discussion, see
*The Physician and Labor Health Plans* (New York: American Labor
Health Association, 1959).

benefits. There were also 24 plans where the retiree was expected to finance his benefits alone and 21 where the sponsor of the plan and the retiree contributed jointly. In eight plans the cost of the retiree benefits were borne by the plan spon-

TABLE 6.11

DISTRIBUTION OF INDEPENDENT INDUSTRIAL PLANS AND OF THEIR ACTIVE
AND RETIRED WORKERS AND DEPENDENTS ACCORDING TO SPONSOR, SOURCE
OF FINANCING, AND PROVISION AT RETIREMENT, DECEMBER, 1956*

| Sponsor; Source of Financing; Provision at Retirement | Number of Plans | | Number of Persons (Thousands) | | | |
|---|---|---|---|---|---|---|
| | | | Active and Retired | | Retirees and Dependents | |
| | Total | With Reduced Benefits† | Total | With Reduced Benefits† | Total | With Reduced Benefits† |
| All plans.......... | 79‡ | 27‡ | 2354.6 | 486.5 | 182.1 | 35.7 |
| Sponsor | | | | | | |
| Union........... | 25 | 10 | 1509.5 | 194.5 | 113.7 | 2.4 |
| Employer-employee...... | 27 | 13 | 391.0 | 272.0 | 43.2 | 31.4 |
| Employer........ | 7 | — | 113.5 | — | 3.4 | — |
| Employee....... | 20 | 4 | 340.6 | 20.0 | 21.8 | 1.9 |
| Source of financing | | | | | | |
| Sponsor only..... | 24 | 8 | 1248.9 | 73.8 | 119.6 | 1.5 |
| Retiree only..... | 24 | 11 | 463.3 | 121.7 | 16.0 | 6.0 |
| Sponsor and retiree jointly.... | 21 | 4 | 401.6 | 165.0 | 23.0 | 10.5 |
| Sponsor and active employees..... | 8 | 4 | 193.2 | 126.0 | 18.4 | 17.7 |
| Active employees only.......... | 1 | — | 41.0 | — | 5.1 | — |
| Not reported.... | 1 | — | 6.5 | — | — | — |
| Provision at retirement | | | | | | |
| Retiree only..... | 39 | 17 | 612.5 | 389.5 | 52.9 | 32.5 |
| Retiree and dependents...... | 39 | 10 | 1735.5 | 97.0 | 129.2 | 3.2 |
| Not reported..... | 1 | — | 6.5 | — | — | — |

* Data relate to plans with benefits to retired workers.
† With reduced benefits to retirees and dependents.
‡ Includes plans not reporting on number of retirees and dependents, as indicated in Table 6.12.

Source: Compiled by the author from returns used by A. W. Brewster, "Independent Plans Providing Medical Care and Hospital Insurance: 1957 Survey," *Social Security Bulletin*, April, 1958, p. 3. The current compilation includes returns received since this article appeared.

## TABLE 6.12

DISTRIBUTION OF INDEPENDENT INDUSTRIAL PLANS AND OF RETIRED WORKERS AND DEPENDENTS IN THESE PLANS ACCORDING TO SPONSOR AND TYPE OF BENEFIT, DECEMBER, 1956*

| Benefit for Retiree and Dependents | Sponsor | | | | |
|---|---|---|---|---|---|
| | Total | Union | Employer-Employee | Employer | Employee |
| | Number of Plans | | | | |
| Total plans............. | 79 | 25 | 27 | 7 | 20 |
| With reduced benefits† | 27 | 10 | 13 | — | 4 |
| Hospital benefits........ | 64 | 19 | 22 | 7 | 16 |
| Surgical benefits........ | 64 | 19 | 20 | 7 | 18 |
| Medical benefits......... | 67 | 17 | 25 | 6 | 19 |
| Diagnostic benefits...... | 63 | 17 | 24 | 7 | 15 |
| Dental benefits.......... | 17 | 5 | 6 | 3 | 3 |
| Benefits not reported.... | 1 | — | 1 | — | — |
| Not reporting number of retirees and dependents | 7 | 5 | 1 | 1 | — |
| | Number of Retirees and Dependents in Reporting Plans (Thousands) | | | | |
| Total plans............. | 182.1 | 113.7 | 43.2 | 3.4 | 21.8 |
| Hospital benefits........ | 169.7 | 111.3 | 33.7 | 3.4 | 21.3 |
| Surgical benefits........ | 159.1 | 111.3 | 22.7 | 3.4 | 21.7 |
| Medical benefits......... | 180.7 | 112.6 | 43.0 | 3.4 | 21.7 |
| Diagnostic benefits...... | 174.9 | 113.0 | 42.9 | 3.4 | 15.5 |
| Dental benefits.......... | 15.6 | .9 | 8.5 | .7 | 5.4 |
| | Number of Active and Retired Members in Plans (Thousands) | | | | |
| All reporting plans (97).. | 2551.7 | 1648.6 | 418.4 | 124.5 | 360.1 |
| Plans with benefits for retirees and dependents (79)................ | 2354.6 | 1509.5 | 391.0 | 113.5 | 340.6 |
| Plans stating number of retirees and dependents (72)................ | 2173.2 | 1336.9 | 384.5 | 111.2 | 340.6 |
| With reduced benefits (25).............. | 471.2 | 179.2 | 272.0 | — | 20.0 |
| Plans not stating number of retirees and dependents (7)............. | 181.4 | 172.6 | 6.5 | 2.3 | — |
| With reduced benefits (2)............... | 15.3 | 15.3 | — | — | — |
| Not reporting (1)...... | 6.5 | — | 6.5 | — | — |

* Data relate to plans with benefits to retired workers.
† With reduced benefits to retirees and dependents.

Source: Compiled by the author from returns used by A. W. Brewster, "Independent Plans Providing Medical Care and Hospital Insurance: 1957 Survey," *Social Security Bulletin*, April, 1958, p. 3. The current compilation includes returns received since this article appeared.

sor and the active employees jointly, and one plan by the active employees alone.

The extent of variation in the scope of benefits to retirees in independent industrial plans is evident in Table 6.12. Only 64 out of the total of 79 provide hospital benefits, a like number have surgical benefits, and 67 have medical benefits. However, 63 of these plans offer diagnostic benefits and 17 dental benefits. On the whole, this distribution does not vary much with the sponsorship of the plan. Most retirees and dependents entitled to benefits under these plans at the end of 1956 had coverage for hospital, surgical, medical, and diagnostic care, but less than one tenth had coverage for dental care.

*Independent Nonindustrial Plans for the Aged.*    There has been no systematic survey of the practices of the independent nonindustrial plans with regard to health insurance of the aged. The private group clinics and medical society plans not affiliated with either Blue Shield or Blue Cross may vary in their policies regarding the aged very much like these major organizations. Several co-operative health insurance plans operating in rural areas have indicated that they provide protection to the aged.[46] Among the community-sponsored independent plans, the largest ones (the Kaiser Foundation Health Plan and the Health Insurance Plan of Greater New York) will include aged persons in their group enrollment and permit conversion to individual contracts upon retirement.

*Medical Care Utilization after Conversion from Group to Individual Insurance.*    Although the right may be exercised to convert from group insurance to an individual health insurance contract upon retiring from employment, many fail to use the privilege. According to the experience of the

---

[46] R. E. Van Goor, "Meeting the Medical Costs of Older People With Cooperative Plans," *Studies of the Aged and Aging: Volume II, Health and Health Services,* Committee on Labor and Public Welfare, U.S. Senate, Washington, D.C., 1957, p. 30; H. L. Johnston, *Rural Health Cooperatives,* Farm Credit Administration and Public Health Service, Washington, D.C., June, 1950.

Health Insurance Plan of Greater New York during 1952–54, only 37 per cent of those aged 65 and over who had this right actually converted.[47] This low proportion converting at a period of life when health needs begin to rise rapidly may result from a changed economic situation upon retirement. At a time when income is reduced, in most instances the retiree finds he must pay the entire insurance cost; during employment at least part of it was borne by his employer.

Even among those who do convert after retirement, many drop their insurance within a short time. Thus, the same study showed that of those who converted to individual contracts at ages 65 and over, 11 per cent dropped their insurance within one year, 18 per cent within two years, and 23 per cent within three years; these figures do not include deaths.[48]

In view of the low conversion rate and the drop-out rates just cited, it might be expected that those who use the right to take an individual contract would contain a large proportion of lives in need of immediate medical attention. This is borne out by the experience summarized in Table 6.13, which compares the utilization of physicians' services by persons at ages 65 and over who obtained an individual contract by conversion with those of the same ages still under a group contract. Most of the latter are still at work. Among the males who converted, 81 per cent were seen by a doctor of the Plan during the year and physicians' services averaged

---

[47] S. Shapiro and M. Einhorn, "Experience with Older Members in a Prepaid Medical Care Plan," *Public Health Reports*, Vol. 73, p. 687 (August, 1958).

[48] Another study of the Health Insurance Plan of Greater New York showed lower retention rates for new entrants at ages 65 and over than for all other ages except 15–24 years. Possibilities offered in explanation are retirement from employment and consequent drop in income, desire to maintain established medical contacts on the part of older new entrants, and greater likelihood of incapacity to continue working because of chronic disease. P. M. Densen, N. R. Deardorff, and E. Balamuth, "Longitudinal Analyses of Four Years of Experience of a Prepaid Comprehensive Medical Care Plan," *Milbank Memorial Fund Quarterly*, Vol. 36, p. 5 (January, 1958).

10.75 per enrollee per year. On the other hand, for the aged males still protected by a group contract, only 66 per cent saw a physician, and physicians' services averaged 7.0 per enrollee.

Although both categories of aged males received most of

TABLE 6.13

INCIDENCE OF PHYSICIANS' SERVICES AT AGES 65 AND OVER, BY SEX, SEPARATELY UNDER GROUP CONTRACTS AND UNDER INDIVIDUAL CONTRACTS BY CONVERSION FROM GROUP CONTRACTS, HEALTH INSURANCE PLAN OF GREATER NEW YORK, 1955–56

| Service | Individual Contract by Conversion | | Group Contract | |
|---|---|---|---|---|
| | Males | Females | Males | Females |
| Per cent of enrollees seen by HIP doctor during the year | 81.3 | 85.9 | 65.9 | 65.0 |
| Physician services per enrollee per year, total | 10.75 | 7.66 | 7.03 | 6.50 |
| Place of service: | | | | |
| Office | 6.98 | 5.81 | 5.06 | 4.99 |
| Home | .53 | .88 | .42 | .48 |
| Hospital | 3.24 | .96 | 1.55 | 1.03 |
| Physician specialty: | | | | |
| Family physician | 5.94 | 4.56 | 3.76 | 3.78 |
| Internist | .88 | .72 | .63 | .52 |
| Ophthalmology, otolaryngology | .59 | .62 | .55 | .54 |
| Radiology | .68 | .60 | .55 | .50 |
| Surgery | .87 | .28 | .48 | .35 |
| Urology | .96 | .05 | .63 | .06 |
| Orthopedy | .23 | .31 | .15 | .40 |
| Other | .60 | .52 | .28 | .35 |

Source: S. Shapiro and M. Einhorn, "Experience With Older Members in a Prepaid Medical Care Plan," *Public Health Reports*, Vol. 73, p. 687 (August, 1958).

their services in the office of the physician, the difference between the two was greatest for hospital visits, those on individual contracts obtaining twice the attention of those on group contracts. Also, males on individual contracts received more attention from physicians in each of the specialties. Among aged females, the differentials in physicans' services between those who converted to individual contracts and those remaining in a group are not as marked as for males.

In fact, there are only small differences in the case of services in the hospital and for many of the specialties. This evidence of self-selection with regard to the use of physicians' service by those entitled to the conversion right confirms the experience previously cited from insurance experience with hospitalization.[49]

---

[49] See p. 181 of this chapter.

# Mechanisms for Financing
# Medical Care
## of the Aged (Continued)

### THE EXTENT OF VOLUNTARY HEALTH INSURANCE
### AMONG THE AGED

AT THE END of 1958, somewhat over 70 per cent of the total population of the United States had some form of voluntary health insurance. The proportions insured vary with age and sex, and are highest for married men at the main productive ages, where family responsibility is greatest.[1] At no period of life is the proportion insured as low as among the aged. Health insurance, in some form, was held by about 6 million persons at ages 65 and over, of whom over 2 million were covered by insurance companies, 3.5 by Blue Cross, and 400,000 by independent plans.[2]

*Age, Sex, and Race.* According to a survey of the noninstitutional population of the United States conducted September, 1956, the proportion then with health insurance at ages 65 and over was 36.5 per cent, compared with 63.6 per cent for all ages.[3] Among aged males, the proportion covered

---

[1] A. W. Brewster, "Characteristics of the Population with Hospitalization Insurance, September 1956," *Research and Statistics Note No. 14,* Division of Program Research, Social Security Administration, Washington, D.C., May 27, 1958.

[2] *Hospitalization Insurance for OASDI Beneficiaries,* Report submitted to the Committee on Ways and Means by the Secretary of Health, Education, and Welfare, Washington, D.C., April 3, 1959, p. 43.

[3] The institutional population includes those in mental and tuberculosis hospitals, residents of homes for the aged, and persons in penal institutions.

by health insurance ranged from practically 50 per cent at ages 65–69 years to somewhat over 25 per cent at ages 75 and over (Table 7.1). The respective figures for females were somewhat lower, namely 45.5 per cent and 22.5 per cent. Over two thirds of the insured aged were covered against both hos-

TABLE 7.1

PER CENT OF NONINSTITUTIONAL POPULATION WITH HEALTH INSURANCE AT AGES 65 AND OVER, BY SEX, ACCORDING TO TYPE OF COVERAGE, RACE, MARITAL STATUS, AND LABOR FORCE STATUS, UNITED STATES, SEPTEMBER, 1956

| Characteristic | Males | | | | Females | | | |
|---|---|---|---|---|---|---|---|---|
| | 65 and Over | 65–69 | 70–74 | 75 and Over | 65 and Over | 65–69 | 70–74 | 75 and Over |
| Type of coverage, total | 39.2 | 49.8 | 39.5 | 25.3 | 34.2 | 45.5 | 33.6 | 22.5 |
| Hospital only...... | 8.8 | 10.6 | 8.6 | 6.8 | 8.2 | 10.3 | 7.1 | 6.8 |
| Hospital and surgical......... | 27.1 | 34.7 | 27.4 | 17.1 | 23.4 | 31.6 | 24.5 | 13.7 |
| Other*............ | 3.3 | 4.5 | 3.5 | 1.4 | 2.6 | 3.6 | 2.0 | 2.0 |
| Not insured......... | 60.8 | 50.2 | 60.5 | 74.7 | 65.8 | 54.5 | 66.4 | 77.5 |
| | | | | | | | | |
| Race | | | | | | | | |
| White............. | 40.8 | 52.1 | 41.5 | 25.9 | 35.5 | 46.8 | 35.1 | 23.5 |
| Nonwhite......... | 18.1 | 19.2† | 17.5† | 17.3† | 16.6 | 26.2† | 14.2† | 8.3† |
| | | | | | | | | |
| Marital status | | | | | | | | |
| Married........... | 44.2 | 54.5 | 44.7 | 26.4 | 40.9 | 50.6 | 36.1 | 23.3 |
| Not married....... | 27.7 | 33.7 | 26.5 | 24.3 | 30.5 | 40.8 | 32.0 | 22.2 |
| | | | | | | | | |
| Labor force status | | | | | | | | |
| In labor force...... | 50.8 | 58.3 | 46.9 | 33.0 | 48.3 | 54.1 | 41.7† | 33.3† |
| Not in labor force.. | 31.1 | 38.6 | 34.8 | 23.2 | 32.4 | 43.5 | 32.7 | 22.1 |

* Hospitalization and surgical expense insurance plus other benefits.
† Per cent based on small sample.

Source: A. W. Brewster, "Health Insurance Coverage by Age and Sex, September 1956" and "Health Insurance in the Population 65 and Over," *Research and Statistics Notes Nos. 13 and 17*, Division of Program Research, Social Security Administration, May 21 and June 11, 1958; A. W. Brewster and L. M. Kramer, "Health Insurance and Hospital Use Related to Marital Status," *Public Health Reports*, Vol. 74, p. 721 (August, 1959).

pital and surgical expenses, only one fourth against hospital expenses only, and the rest against a variety of other medical care expenses including both hospitalization and surgery.

The proportions covered among nonwhite lives were substantially lower than among white lives. Thus, at ages 65 and over, more than 40 per cent of the white males had some health insurance, compared with 18 per cent for nonwhite males. Similarly among aged females, 35.5 per cent of the whites were insured, but only 16.6 per cent of the nonwhites. These racial differences may reflect variations in health insurance coverage according to geographic region and income status. For example, a survey conducted for the Health Insurance Institute during October and November, 1957, showed that, for the noninstitutional population of all ages, only 58 per cent were insured in the South, where the proportion of nonwhite population is highest.[4] On the other hand, the proportion was 78 per cent for the Northeast and 69 per cent for the North Central and Western states. Also pertinent are the findings of an earlier survey made of the aged in the general population in March, 1952.[5] At that time, among all persons 65 and over, hospitalization insurance was held by only 15.2 per cent of those in farm areas and 22.0 per cent in rural-nonfarm areas, where large proportions of nonwhites live, compared with 30.4 per cent in urban centers. Reference will be made later to the variation in coverage with income status.

**Marital Status and Labor Force Status.**  Throughout the higher ages, larger proportions of the married than of the unmarried are insured. However, for each sex the differential practically disappears by ages 75 and over. It is interesting to note in Table 7.1 that, among the unmarried at ages 65–74, the females have larger proportions insured than males, a result possibly produced by a better recognition of need for this protection.

The aged who remain in the labor force are much more likely to continue their health insurance than those outside of it. Thus, about half of the aged at work or seeking work were insured, compared with less than one third for those

---

[4] *A Profile of the Health Insurance Public* (New York: Health Insurance Institute, 1959), p. 8.

[5] I. S. Falk and A. W. Brewster, *Hospitalization and Insurance Among Aged Persons, A Study Based on a Census Survey in March 1952,* Bureau Report No. 18, Division of Research and Statistics, Social Security Administration, Washington, D.C., April, 1953.

who left work. Again, it is found that among those at ages 65–69 not in the labor force, the females have the larger proportion insured.

*Income.* The proportion covered by health insurance among the aged rises with the income of the families with which they live or with their own income if living without relatives in the household; this income picture very likely reflects, in some degree, the effect of labor force participation. Table 7.2, also from the September, 1956 survey, shows

TABLE 7.2

PER CENT OF NONINSTITUTIONAL POPULATION WITH HEALTH INSURANCE AT AGES 65 AND OVER, BY SEX, ACCORDING TO FAMILY STATUS AND ANNUAL MONEY INCOME, UNITED STATES, SEPTEMBER, 1956

| Annual Money Income | Aged Persons in Primary Families* | | | Aged Primary Individuals | | |
|---|---|---|---|---|---|---|
| | Both Sexes | Males | Females | Both Sexes | Males | Females |
| Total................. | 38.6 | 41.5 | 35.7 | 30.7 | 30.9 | 30.6 |
| Under $1,000............ | 17.4 | 19.3 | 15.4 | 19.5 | 17.1 | 20.3 |
| $1,000–$1,999............ | 32.3 | 34.5 | 29.7 | 37.9 | 33.7 | 40.1 |
| $2,000–$2,999............ | 43.2 | 46.8 | 39.4 | 46.8 | 43.4 | 48.1 |
| $3,000 and over.......... | 46.8 | 50.9 | 42.5 | 54.8 | 55.7 | 54.3 |
| $3,000–$3,999.......... | 46.1 | 49.1 | 43.0 | — | — | — |
| $4,000–$4,999.......... | 46.2 | 47.8 | 45.0 | — | — | — |
| $5,000 and over........ | 47.7 | 53.4 | 42.6 | — | — | — |

* The income shown for the family unit in which the aged person lives is not necessarily that of the aged person but would include his income.

Source: A. W. Brewster, "Health Insurance in the Population 65 and Over," *Research and Statistics Note No. 17*, Division of Program Research, Social Security Administration, June 11, 1958.

that only a little over one sixth of the aged in families with an annual income of less than $1,000 had some health insurance, compared with almost half where the income was $3,000 or more.[6] A like situation is found for the aged living without relatives present. For each income bracket up to

[6] A study of the expenditures of farm-operator families showed, among families headed by persons aged 65 and over, an increase in the proportion of families purchasing health insurance with rise in family income; see *Farmers' Expenditures in 1955, by Regions*, U.S. Department of Agriculture Statistical Bulletin No. 224, Washington, D.C., April, 1958, p. 99.

$3,000, females living alone have larger proportions insured than all other categories of the aged. For higher incomes, their proportion is exceeded, by a small margin, only by males living alone.

A corresponding variation of insurance coverage with income was noted in the 1957 survey of aged OASDI beneficiaries.[7] Thus, among aged couples with an annual money income of less than $1,200, only 20.5 per cent had hospitalization insurance and 15.7 per cent had surgical or medical insurance. On the other hand, where the annual income was $5,000 or more, the respective proportions were 65.0 per cent and 54.0 per cent.

**Type of Insurance.**  The importance of group insurance in the health insurance picture has already been indicated. According to the survey made for the Health Insurance Institute late in 1957, over three fourths of the population at ages 30–49 years, when family responsibility is greatest, had some health insurance (Table 7.3). Group insurance, either alone or with individual insurance, protected almost three fifths of these people. These proportions drop with advance in age. At ages 60–64, somewhat over 63 per cent were still insured, and 40 per cent had group insurance; the proportions are about the same at age 65, when a great many begin their retirement. Largely as a result of this withdrawal from the labor force, the proportion with health insurance dropped to 32 per cent at ages 66 and over, and only 10 per cent had group insurance. On the other hand, Table 7.3 shows that the proportion with individual insurance only is at a level near or above 20 per cent from age 20 onward.

This survey of late 1957, showing a sharp drop in health insurance coverage from age 65 to ages 66 and over, does not reflect the full impact of the recently introduced medical care benefits for retiring employees in group contracts and for individuals at ages 65 and over. It will be recalled, in this connection, that almost two thirds of the employees in New

---

[7] *Hospitalization Insurance for OASDI Beneficiaries, op. cit.,* p. 46.

York State insured under group plans by life and casualty companies at the end of 1956 had such benefits added only within the five years preceding. The low proportion insured at the higher ages may also reflect an unwillingness, for one reason or another, to continue coverage held during the

TABLE 7.3

PER CENT OF NONINSTITUTIONAL POPULATION WITH HEALTH INSURANCE, BY AGE, ACCORDING TO TYPE OF INSURANCE, UNITED STATES, OCTOBER AND NOVEMBER, 1957

| Age | Per Cent (Total Population for Age = 100%) | | | | | |
|---|---|---|---|---|---|---|
| | Insured | | | | | Not Insured |
| | All Types | Group Only | Individual Only | Group and Individual | Type Not Stated | |
| All ages........... | 67.3 | 44.8 | 18.4 | 3.8 | .3 | 32.7 |
| Under 18.......... | 66.1 | 49.1 | 14.7 | 2.1 | .2 | 33.9 |
| 18–19............. | 61.3 | 42.2 | 13.9 | 3.5 | 1.7 | 38.7 |
| 20–29............. | 71.2 | 47.5 | 19.5 | 4.1 | .1 | 28.8 |
| 30–39............. | 77.5 | 53.8 | 18.2 | 5.5 | — | 22.5 |
| 40–49............. | 76.9 | 48.5 | 21.5 | 6.5 | .4 | 23.1 |
| 50–59............. | 69.4 | 36.6 | 25.9 | 6.1 | .8 | 30.6 |
| 60–64............. | 63.3 | 35.5 | 21.9 | 5.1 | .8 | 36.7 |
| 65 and over....... | 34.7 | 10.8 | 22.0 | 1.3 | .6 | 65.3 |
| 65*............. | 63.6 | 31.8 | 25.0 | 6.8 | — | 36.4 |
| 66 and over...... | 32.1 | 8.9 | 21.7 | .9 | .6 | 67.9 |

* Per cent based on small sample.

Source: Unpublished data from the Health Insurance Institute Survey conducted in October and November, 1957 on a sample of 2,000 families including over 6,600 persons.

working years into later life. Pertinent to this is the finding of the Health Insurance Plan of Greater New York that a relatively small fraction of the aged with the right to convert from a group to an individual contract used this privilege, and that many of those who converted dropped their protection within a few years.[8]

*Trends.* Data regarding the trend of health insurance coverage among the aged are available from several surveys

---

[8] See p. 201 of Chapter 6.

of the general population. Since these were conducted on relatively small samples of the population, their results are subject to sampling fluctuations. Moreover, the comparability of the data is affected by differences in the form of the questions asked regarding health insurance coverage and also in the interviewing practices. Table 7.4 compares the coverage of the aged observed in these surveys with that of the total population of all ages.

The first survey of the extent of voluntary health insurance among the noninstitutional population at ages 65 and over was conducted by the Bureau of the Census in March, 1952; at that time 26.3 per cent had some insurance against hospital expenses. Another survey, conducted by the National Opinion Research Center for the Health Information Foundation in July, 1953, showed that 31 per cent then held hospitalization insurance. On the basis of a survey only two years later, in 1955, the National Opinion Research Center reported that 39 per cent of the aged had insurance to pay all or part of doctor or hospital bills. However, the figure for hospitalization insurance, whether or not any other health insurance was held, was only 36.5 per cent in a later survey made by the Bureau of the Census in September, 1956. When account is taken of the sampling fluctuations in these surveys, not much different is the finding that 34.7 per cent of the aged were covered by health insurance in the survey made during October–November, 1957 by National Analysts, Inc., for the Health Insurance Institute. A different survey in 1957, by the National Opinion Research Center, yielded an estimate that 38.6 per cent of the aged had health insurance. One year later, in the summer of 1958, a joint survey by the NORC and the Health Information Foundation reported that 43 per cent of the aged had insurance against hospital expense. These comparisons relate only to the proportions of the population covered by health insurance. They do not take into account the interim extensions in the scale and scope of benefits.

It will be noted in Table 7.4 that the rate of growth of

## TABLE 7.4

PER CENT OF POPULATION AT AGES 65 AND OVER* AND AT ALL AGES WITH
HEALTH INSURANCE ACCORDING TO VARIOUS SURVEYS AND ESTIMATES FROM
1951 TO 1958

| Ages 65 and Over | | | All Ages | |
|---|---|---|---|---|
| Date of Survey | Per Cent Insured | Survey Agency and Sponsor | Date of Estimate (Dec. 31) | Per Cent Insured for Hospitalization |
| March, 1952[a] | 26.3 | Bureau of the Census for Social Security Administration | 1951 | 56.9 |
| July, 1953[b] | 31.0 | National Opinion Research Center and Health Information Foundation | 1953 | 62.4 |
| 1955[c] | 39.0 | National Opinion Research Center and Health Information Foundation | 1955 | 66.3 |
| September, 1956[d] | 36.5 | Bureau of the Census for Social Security Administration | 1956 | 70.1 |
| October–November, 1957[e] | 34.7 | National Analysts, Inc. for Health Insurance Institute | 1957 | 72.1 |
| 1957[e] | 38.6 | National Opinion Research Center and Health Information Foundation | | |
| Summer, 1958[f] | 43.0 | National Opinion Research Center and Health Information Foundation | | |

* These percentages are derived from relatively small samples of the population and are therefore subject to sampling fluctuations.

Source for ages 65 and over:

[a] I. S. Falk and A. W. Brewster, *Hospitalization and Insurance Among Aged Persons, A Study Based on a Census Survey in March 1952*, Bureau Report No. 18, Division of Research and Statistics, Social Security Administration, April, 1953.

[b] O. W. Anderson and J. J. Feldman, *Family Medical Costs and Voluntary Health Insurance; A Nationwide Survey* (New York: McGraw-Hill Book Co., Inc., 1956), p. 107.

[c] Unpublished data.

[d] A. W. Brewster, "Health Insurance Coverage by Age and Sex, September 1956," *Research and Statistics Note No. 13*, Division of Program Research, Social Security Administration, May 21, 1958.

[e] "Voluntary Health Insurance Among the Aged," *Progress in Health Services*, Vol. 8 (January, 1959), Health Information Foundation, New York.

[f] "Voluntary Health Insurance: 1953 and 1958," *Progress in Health Services*, Vol. 8 (May, 1959), Health Information Foundation, New York.

Source for all ages: A. W. Brewster, "Voluntary Health Insurance—Estimated Enrollment and Rates per 1,000 Population, 1939–57," *Research and Statistics Note No. 26*, Division of Program Research, Social Security Administration, July 24, 1958.

voluntary health insurance among the aged during a comparable period was more rapid than that for the general population. For several reasons, the proportions of aged protected by health insurance will undoubtedly continue to rise at a rapid rate in the near future. Thus, it has been noted that over one fifth of the aged have individual health insurance, practically the same proportion as at the earlier ages; accordingly, individual health insurance for the aged may be expected to grow with its expansion at the earlier ages. Then, within a relatively short period there should be evident the effects of recently introduced rights for the retired to continue their group health insurance or to convert to individual contracts. Further stimulating this trend is the growing recognition of the health needs of retired workers on the part of employers and unions. Also, larger proportions of aged are entering the ranks of the retired with an appreciation of the benefits of health insurance from their earlier experience. As a result, there should be apparent, in coming years, an increasing willingness on the part of the aged to carry this protection into later years.

Some results of the two surveys by the Bureau of the Census are compared in Table 7.5, since they present detail with regard to age, sex, race, and labor-force status. It should be recognized that the differences noted may be subject to large sampling fluctuations. In the 4½ year period from March, 1952 to September, 1956, the proportion of aged covered by health insurance rose by two fifths—from 26.3 per cent to 36.5 per cent. Although aged females have the smaller proportion insured, the extent of their coverage in 1956 was just 1½ times that of 1952, compared with 1⅓ for males. Likewise, the coverage of the nonwhite population in 1956 was over 1⅔ times that of 1952; the ratio was over 1⅓ for the white population.

Of special significance is the relatively large gain in health insurance coverage among the aged not in the labor force. The proportion covered among them in September, 1956— namely 32.0 per cent—was over 1½ times that only 4½ years earlier;[9] each sex shared equally in both the extent and rise in coverage. Although the rise in coverage among the aged still in the labor force was slow in comparison—the ratio between the two surveys being 1¼ in this instance—one half

TABLE 7.5

PER CENT OF NONINSTITUTIONAL POPULATION WITH HEALTH INSURANCE AT AGES 65 AND OVER, BY SEX, ACCORDING TO AGE, RACE, AND LABOR FORCE STATUS, SEPTEMBER, 1956 AND MARCH, 1952 COMPARED

| Characteristic | Both Sexes | | | Males | | | Females | | |
|---|---|---|---|---|---|---|---|---|---|
| | September, 1956 | March, 1952 | Increase | September, 1956 | March, 1952 | Increase | September, 1956 | March, 1952 | Increase |
| Ages 65 and over....... | 36.5 | 26.3 | 10.2 | 39.2 | 30.2 | 9.0 | 34.2 | 22.8 | 11.4 |
| 65–69..... | 47.6 | 36.4 | 11.2 | 49.8 | 42.3 | 7.5 | 45.5 | 30.9 | 14.6 |
| 70–74..... | 36.3 | 24.8 | 11.5 | 39.5 | 28.2 | 11.3 | 33.6 | 21.7 | 11.9 |
| 75 and over. | 23.7 | 15.0 | 8.7 | 25.3 | 15.8 | 9.5 | 22.5 | 14.4 | 8.1 |
| White....... | 37.9 | 27.5 | 10.4 | 40.8 | 31.4 | 9.4 | 35.5 | 24.2 | 11.3 |
| Nonwhite.... | 17.3 | 10.5 | 6.8 | 18.1 | 15.7 | 2.4 | 16.6 | 6.3 | 10.3 |
| In labor force. | 50.2 | 43.9 | 6.3 | 50.8 | 44.5 | 6.3 | 48.3 | 41.2 | 7.1 |
| Not in labor force..... | 32.0 | 21.0 | 11.0 | 31.1 | 20.4 | 10.7 | 32.4 | 21.3 | 11.1 |

Source: A. W. Brewster, "Health Insurance Coverage by Age and Sex, September 1956" and "Health Insurance in the Population 65 and Over," *Research and Statistics Notes Nos. 13 and 17*, Division of Program Research, Social Security Administration, May 21 and June 11, 1958; I. S. Falk and A. W. Brewster, *Hospitalization and Insurance Among Aged Persons, A Study Based on a Census Survey in March 1952*, Bureau Report No. 18, Division of Research and Statistics, Social Security Administration, April, 1953, Tables 26 and 30.

of them had some protection against their medical care expenses.

This picture of the extent of voluntary health insurance coverage among all aged in the general population does not take into account those segments that have access to medical care by other means. Thus, very few among those on Old-Age Assistance would have such insurance since their medical care is provided by governmental programs;[10] in 1957 and 1958, about one sixth of the population at ages 65 and over

---

[9] It is worth noting that the figure for coverage among those at ages 65 and over not in the labor force in September, 1956 is practically identical with that observed for all persons 66 and over in the survey of October–November, 1957. A large proportion of the latter population is presumably out of the labor force.

[10] See p. 220 of this chapter.

were such recipients. A further category of aged not likely to purchase health insurance is the institutional population, that is, persons in mental and tuberculosis hospitals, residents of homes for the aged, and those in penal institutions. There may also be many among the growing population of aged veterans who do not feel a need for voluntary health insurance because of a reliance upon the program of the Veterans Administration. Then there are those who feel that they would be as well off without health insurance; 37 per cent of the aged without such insurance reported so in the 1955 survey of the National Opinion Research Center.[11] Another segment, though relatively small, may be those who regard their means to be ample enough for their possible medical care problems. Thus, the extent of voluntary health insurance among the aged taken in relation to those who have or feel a need for such protection, instead of the entire population of aged, is greater than indicated by the surveys just cited.[12]

*Aged Beneficiaries of Old-Age and Survivors Insurance.* A closer picture of the extent of voluntary health insurance coverage among the retired is available from the results of a survey conducted on a sample of aged beneficiaries in receipt of benefits of Old-Age and Survivors Insurance in December, 1956. The data, shown in Table 7.6, relate to the insurance status at the time of the survey in the fall of 1957. Altogether, 43 per cent of these aged beneficiaries were then covered by health insurance—41 per cent of the males and 45.1 per cent of the females. Just one half of the beneficiaries at ages 65–69 had some coverage, and even at ages 70–74 years it amounted to 44.7 per cent. However, the proportion then covered fell to 37.2 per cent at ages 75–79 and further to 26.5 per cent at ages 80 and over. This variation in coverage

---

[11] See p. 158 of Chapter 5.

[12] W. Polner, "Critique of Some Statistics on Health Insurance Among the Aged," *Journal of the American Medical Association,* Vol. 169, p. 507 (January 31, 1959), and U.S. House, Committee on Ways and Means, *Hospital, Nursing Home, and Surgical Benefits for OASI Beneficiaries* (Hearings, 86th Cong., 1st sess., July, 1959), Statement of E. J. Faulkner, p. 434.

with advance in age reflects the course of the recent development of health insurance. When those now at the advanced
ages were in their later productive years, health insurance
was still in its formative period. As those now entering re-

TABLE 7.6

PER CENT OF AGED BENEFICIARIES UNDER OLD-AGE AND SURVIVORS
INSURANCE WHO CARRY HEALTH INSURANCE, BY SEX, ACCORDING TO
MARITAL STATUS, AGE, AND TYPE OF COVERAGE; FALL OF 1957*

| Age; Type of Coverage | Both Sexes | Males† | | | Females† | | | |
|---|---|---|---|---|---|---|---|---|
| | | Total | Single | Married | Total | Single | Married | Widowed |
| 65 and over, total..... | 43.0 | 41.0 | 30.3 | 46.0 | 45.1 | 49.8 | 45.4 | 38.5 |
| Hospital and surgical | 28.5 | 28.4 | 19.2 | 32.7 | 28.6 | 30.0 | 31.3 | 21.3 |
| Hospital only...... | 14.5 | 12.6 | 11.1 | 13.3 | 16.5 | 19.8 | 14.1 | 17.2 |
| 65–69, total......... | 49.5 | 48.3 | 32.8 | 53.6 | 50.4 | 57.9 | 49.3 | 43.1 |
| Hospital and surgical | 33.8 | 35.0 | 20.7 | 39.9 | 32.8 | 37.8 | 33.1 | 24.7 |
| Hospital only...... | 15.7 | 13.3 | 12.1 | 13.7 | 17.6 | 20.1 | 16.3 | 18.4 |
| 70–74, total......... | 44.7 | 41.2 | 33.2 | 44.5 | 48.1 | 53.7 | 46.0 | 44.5 |
| Hospital and surgical | 29.3 | 28.1 | 20.6 | 31.2 | 30.6 | 31.7 | 32.6 | 24.8 |
| Hospital only...... | 15.3 | 13.1 | 12.6 | 13.4 | 17.6 | 21.9 | 13.3 | 19.7 |
| 75–79, total......... | 37.2 | 39.2 | 33.2 | 42.4 | 34.8 | 36.3 | 36.3 | 31.3 |
| Hospital and surgical | 24.3 | 26.6 | 23.0 | 28.5 | 21.4 | 21.0 | 25.7 | 16.7 |
| Hospital only...... | 12.9 | 12.6 | 10.1 | 13.9 | 13.4 | 15.3 | 10.6 | 14.7 |
| 80 and over, total..... | 26.5 | 24.7 | 17.4 | 32.6 | 29.0 | 31.7 | 29.8 | 26.4 |
| Hospital and surgical | 15.6 | 15.7 | 9.0 | 22.9 | 15.5 | 12.7 | 21.1 | 13.8 |
| Hospital only...... | 10.9 | 9.0 | 8.4 | 9.7 | 13.5 | 19.0 | 8.8 | 12.6 |

* Data on age and marital status of beneficiary, as well as ownership of health insurance,
are as of the end of the survey year.

† Divorced, separated, or widowed beneficiaries are classified as single persons, except that
women entitled to widow's benefits are shown separately. Widows entitled to benefits on their
own employment record are included with other "single" women.

Source: "Aged Beneficiaries of Old-Age and Survivors Insurance: Highlights on Health
Insurance and Hospitalization Utilization, 1957 Survey," *Social Security Bulletin*, December,
1958, p. 3.

tirement move forward in life, the proportions covered at
the very high ages will continue to mount.

Contrary to the situation of the aged in the general population (see Table 7.5), the proportions with health insurance
coverage among female aged beneficiaries are generally
higher than for male aged beneficiaries. Also, the "single"

among the female aged beneficiaries, which includes also the divorced, separated, and widowed who are entitled to benefits through their own employment record, have higher proportions insured than married women and those with widow's benefits. The situation of aged male beneficiaries with

TABLE 7.7

PER CENT OF AGED BENEFICIARIES UNDER OLD-AGE AND SURVIVORS INSURANCE WHO CARRY HEALTH INSURANCE, ACCORDING TO MONEY INCOME AND TYPE OF COVERAGE; FALL OF 1957[a]

| Money Income;[b] Type of Coverage | Beneficiary Couples[c] | | Nonmarried Beneficiaries[d] |
|---|---|---|---|
| | Husbands | Wives | |
| All incomes, total................... | 46.1 | 48.9 | 39.3 |
| Hospital and surgical.............. | 32.9 | 34.5 | 23.5 |
| Hospital only................... | 13.2 | 14.4 | 15.8 |
| Less than $600, total............... | | | 26.3 |
| Hospital and surgical............. | | | 14.3 |
| Hospital only................... | 20.5 | 20.8 | 12.0 |
| $600–$1,199, total................. | 15.3 | 15.2 | 31.6 |
| Hospital and surgical............. | 5.2 | 5.6 | 16.7 |
| Hospital only................... | | | 14.9 |
| $1,200–$1,799, total................ | 33.2 | 36.9 | 40.8 |
| Hospital and surgical.............. | 22.4 | 24.6 | 23.9 |
| Hospital only................... | 10.8 | 12.3 | 16.9 |
| $1,800–$2,399, total................ | 43.1 | 49.1 | 60.3 |
| Hospital and surgical............. | 27.2 | 32.7 | 42.2 |
| Hospital only................... | 15.9 | 16.4 | 18.1 |
| $2,400–$2,999, total................ | 55.8 | 55.4 | 65.2 |
| Hospital and surgical............. | 40.5 | 38.2 | 46.7 |
| Hospital only................... | 15.3 | 17.2 | 18.5 |
| $3,000–$4,999, total................ | 62.6 | 67.4 | |
| Hospital and surgical............. | 45.0 | 47.7 | |
| Hospital only................... | 17.6 | 19.7 | 66.9 |
| $5,000 or more, total............... | 66.5 | 70.1 | 45.8 |
| Hospital and surgical............. | 55.3 | 58.9 | 21.1 |
| Hospital only................... | 11.2 | 11.2 | |

[a] Data on ownership of health insurance are as of the end of the survey year.

[b] Represents cash receipts from all sources except sale of property, tax refunds, large cash gifts, lump-sum inheritances and insurance payments, and cash contributions by relatives within the household. Includes, if known, the value of bills, except medical, paid by relatives outside the household.

[c] A couple consists of a beneficiary drawing a retired worker's benefit and a spouse, whether or not entitled to benefits.

[d] Includes those never married, widowed, divorced, or separated as of the end of the survey year.

Source: *Highlights from Preliminary Tabulations—Medical Care Costs of Aged Beneficiaries,* National Survey of Old-Age and Survivors Insurance Beneficiaries, 1957, Social Security Administration, 1959.

regard to marital status resembles that of males in the general population. On the whole, two thirds of the insured aged beneficiaries had both hospital and surgical coverage and one third had hospital coverage only.

As is the case for the aged in the general population, the proportion of aged beneficiaries covered by health insurance rises with their income level. This may reflect, to some extent, an effect of age since those with the lower incomes may be concentrated at the higher ages. Table 7.7 shows that among couples where one spouse or both were beneficiaries, only one fifth of those with annual incomes of less than $1,200 had some health insurance. This rose to at least two thirds where the income was $5,000 or more. For beneficiaries who were not married, even higher proportions were covered at each income level, ranging from more than one fourth for incomes less than $600 to two thirds for incomes of $3,000 and over.

## GOVERNMENT PROGRAMS

It was mentioned at the outset of Chapter 6 that government has programs for the public financing or direct provision of medical services for the indigent and for certain categories of veterans. The general population of aged also has some relief from heavy medical expenses through the income tax program. In addition, a wide variety of activities are carried on by federal, state and local government which, although not designed with regard to age, provide a measure of medical care to the aged.[13] These include, among other ac-

---

[13] A. W. Brewster, *Health Insurance and Related Proposals for Financing Personal Health Services,* Division of Program Research, Social Security Administration, Department of Health, Education, and Welfare, Washington, D.C., 1958, p. 46, and *Studies of the Aged and Aging:* Vol. I, "Federal and State Activities," pp. 122–37, and Vol. X, "Surveys of State and Local Projects," pp. 107–19, Committee on Labor and Public Welfare, U.S. Senate, Washington, D.C., 1956 and 1957; see also *Programs of the Department of Health, Education, and Welfare Affecting Older Persons,* Special Staff on Aging, Washington, D.C., January, 1958; *Programs and Resources for Older People,* Federal Council on Aging, Washington, D.C.,

tivities, a state-federal program of rehabilitation and special state and local programs in the areas of mental disease, tuberculosis, heart disease, cancer, diabetes, and other chronic diseases. The concern here will be principally with programs for aged indigents and veterans.

*The Indigent—Background and Definition.* It has been traditional in the United States, following the pattern of the Poor Laws of England, to have local government take on the responsibilities for the relief of the indigent; this includes their medical care.[14] In this situation, the programs that developed were necessarily suited to local circumstances, with the result that they varied greatly in dimension. However, in most instances, voluntary charitable assistance and free services from physicians were important elements of the program, and informal arrangements with relatives, friends, and neighbors were common.[15]

The difficulties which these varied local arrangements for the care of the indigent ran into during the severe economic depression of the early 1930's were a significant influence in the inclusion of provisions for public assistance in the Federal Social Security Act of 1935. Meanwhile, the organization of medical care programs was being improved generally and, under the impetus of the Social Security Act, agencies at all levels of government were increasing their roles in providing medical care for the indigent.

The indigent include those who receive aid for basic living needs as public assistance cases under the terms of the Social

September 30, 1959; and *Federal Programs for the Aged and Aging* (Hearings Before the Subcommittee on the Problems of the Aged of the Committee on Labor and Public Welfare, U.S. Senate, 86th Cong., 1st sess., July 23, 24, 28–30, 1959).

[14] H. E. Raynes, *Social Security in Britain, A History* (London: Sir Isaac Pitman & Sons, Ltd., 1957).

[15] The responsibility of relatives for the needy is a matter of state legislation; see, for example, M. Windhauser and G. J. Blaetus, "State Public Assistance Legislation, 1957," *Social Security Bulletin,* January, 1958, and S. Kaplan, "Old-Age Assistance: Children's Contributions to Aged Parents," *Social Security Bulletin,* June, 1957. Also, *A Report of the Advisory Council on Public Assistance,* made to Congress and the Secretary of Health, Education, and Welfare, January 1, 1960, Appendix H.

Security Act and also those who have been accepted by local government either as relief cases or as medically indigent. Whereas relief cases must be provided all their basic living needs, including medical care, the medically indigent require aid only for their medical care. However, those claiming medical indigency are required to establish their right to public medical care through a means test of some kind, which may inquire into family income, property ownership, insurance held, and size of family. Furthermore, medical indigency will depend upon the kind of medical care that is needed and its extent. Being a local matter, there are wide variations among communities in the practices of ascertaining medical need; these arise from financial considerations of the community, traditions, and public attitudes.[16]

From a community viewpoint, it would be desirable to provide needed public medical care for the medically indigent early enough to minimize the likelihood of public assistance or relief. However, individual attitudes also enter the picture. One aged person requiring medical care may exhaust his resources before seeking public aid, while another with a like condition may appeal as soon as he begins to feel a strain on his funds. The latter falls back upon his own means for his daily living after his medical care needs are met, while the former remains a public charge.

*Medical Care within Old-Age Assistance under the Social Security Act.* Under the Social Security Act of 1935 and its amendments, the federal government matches, by formula, the financial aid given by the individual states to certain categories of their indigent.[17] The program for the indigent aged

---

[16] The difficulty in defining medical indigency is described in a letter from the Medical Care Committee of the American Public Welfare Association in U.S. Senate, 82d Cong., 1st sess., Committee on Labor and Public Welfare, *Health Insurance Plans in the United States,* Part 3, p. 33, Washington, D.C., 1951.

[17] The categories, according to the Act of 1935, include needy persons at ages 65 and over, the needy blind, and dependent children. An amendment of 1950 added the needy permanently and totally disabled. See, *A Report of the Advisory Council on Public Assistance,* made to Congress and the Secretary of Health, Education, and Welfare, January 1, 1960, Appendix F.

is known as Old-Age Assistance. The changes in the federal matching proportions for Old-Age Assistance since 1935 are set forth in Table 7.8.

Prior to the 1950 amendments, the federal government shared only in funds granted by the states directly to Old-

TABLE 7.8

MAXIMUM MATCHABLE AMOUNTS AND FEDERAL MATCHING PROPORTIONS
FOR OLD-AGE ASSISTANCE UNDER VARIOUS LAWS*

| Law | Maximum Matchable Individual Payment per Month | Federal Matching Proportion† |
|---|---|---|
| 1935 Act | $30 | ½ |
| 1939 Act | 40 | ½ |
| 1946 Act | 45 | ⅔ of first $15 + ½ of remainder |
| 1948 and 1950 Acts | 50 | ¾ of first $20 + ½ of remainder |
| 1952 and 1954 Acts | 55 | ⅘ of first $25 + ½ of remainder |
| 1956 Act | 60 | ⅘ of first $30 + ½ of remainder |
| 1958 Act | None | ⅘ of first $30 + variable grant ranging between 50% and 65% on next $35‡ |

* Certain exceptions to these matching provisions are applicable to Puerto Rico, the Virgin Islands, Hawaii, and Alaska.

† Dollar figures relate to average matchable payment.

‡ The Federal matching basis under the variable grant procedure is formulated as

$$P = 100 - 50 \cdot \frac{S^2}{N^2}, \text{ except that } 50 \leq P \leq 65,$$

where $P$ is the Federal grant percentage applicable to the upper portion of the state-wide average payment, and $N$ and $S$ are the national and state per capita income figures.

Source: Adapted from R. J. Myers, "1958 Amendments to the Social Security Act," *Transactions of the Society of Actuaries*, Vol. 11, p. 1 (1959).

Age Assistance recipients who were expected, in turn, to pay for their own medical care. In effect, since the recipients were free to use as they pleased the limited funds given by the state, they could barely budget for irregular medical care needs. The federal government did not match then any funds that the states paid hospitals or physicians on behalf of Old-Age Assistance recipients. This was changed with the 1950 amendments which extended federal matching for any portion of a recipient's grant paid by the state directly to a hospital or physician; however, the total matchable limit was not changed. Another change affecting the financing of medical care for Old-Age Assistance recipients came with the

1956 amendments. Under this arrangement, the federal government reimbursed the states for one half of their payments made directly to hospitals, physicians and certain other vendors of medical care because of services to Old-Age Assistance recipients. However, the total amount subject to sharing each month was limited to $6 times the number of OAA recipients on the rolls; again, the matchable amount was subject to a maximum. This change worked to the disadvantage of some states with high vendor payments for medical care, and a further modification was introduced in 1957 which permitted each state to base its computation according to the provisions of either the 1950 or 1956 amendments.[18] However, this alternative procedure was eliminated with the extension of the maximum matchable payments allowed under the 1958 amendments. In other words, matching for medical care financing is no longer apart from that for money payments to OAA recipients. Also, in place of matching on the basis of payments to individuals, the federal share would be computed according to the average amount of expenditure per recipient. The effect of the 1958 amendments is not only to increase the funds available for public assistance in all states, particularly those with low income, but also to give the states greater freedom in arranging their programs for vendor payments.[19]

***The Population of Aged Indigents.*** The numbers of aged who may be regarded as currently eligible for tax-supported medical care are available only for Old-Age Assistance recipients. Data regarding the medical indigents among the aged are lacking because of variations in the systems of record-keeping among communities.

As a result of the extension of the OASI program by way of increased benefits and greater numbers in receipt of bene-

---

[18] Council on Medical Service, "Medical Care for the Indigent in 1957," *Journal of the American Medical Association,* Vol. 164, p. 772 (June 15, 1957), and Vol. 167, p. 350 (May 17, 1958).

[19] Council on Medical Service, "Medical Care for the Indigent in 1958," *ibid.,* Vol. 168, p. 2151 (December 20, 1958).

fit, the proportion of OAA recipients among the aged has declined rapidly in recent years. Thus, the proportion of aged receiving OASI benefits rose from 17 per cent in 1950 to nearly 63 per cent in 1959; meanwhile, the proportion who were OAA recipients fell from 22.6 per cent to 15.6 per cent, and their number from 2,779,000 to 2,420,000.[20] According to the projections in Table 7.9, it is expected that in com-

TABLE 7.9

Old-Age, Survivors, Insurance Beneficiaries (OASI), Old-Age Assistance Recipients (OAA), and Those Receiving Both Payments, United States, 1955–59, and Projections for 1965 and 1970*

| Year (June) | Number Aged 65 and Over (Thousands) | | | Percentage of Population Aged 65 and Over Receiving | | | Concurrent Recipients of Both OASI and OAA as Per Cent of | |
|---|---|---|---|---|---|---|---|---|
| | OASI Beneficiaries | OAA Recipients | Concurrent Recipients of OASI and OAA | OASI | OAA | Both OASI and OAA Concurrently | OASI Beneficiaries | OAA Recipients |
| 1955..... | 5,923 | 2,544 | 505 | 41.7 | 18.0 | 3.6 | 8.5 | 19.9 |
| 1956..... | 6,646 | 2,519 | 526 | 45.7 | 17.3 | 3.6 | 7.9 | 20.9 |
| 1957..... | 7,866 | 2,500 | 571 | 52.8 | 16.8 | 3.8 | 7.3 | 22.8 |
| 1958..... | 8,903 | 2,456 | 612 | 58.6 | 16.2 | 4.0 | 6.9 | 24.9 |
| 1959..... | 9,726 | 2,420 | 646 | 62.7 | 15.6 | 4.2 | 6.6 | 26.7 |
| 1965..... | 12,520 | 2,230 | 830 | 70.3 | 12.6 | 4.7 | 6.6 | 37.2 |
| 1970..... | 14,650 | 2,230 | 960 | 74.4 | 11.3 | 4.9 | 6.6 | 43.0 |

* The data include Alaska and Hawaii before statehood, Puerto Rico, and the Virgin Islands.

Source: "Projections to 1970 of the Number of Aged Persons Receiving OAA and OASDI," *Research and Statistics Note No. 24*, August 19, 1959, and "Persons Receiving OASDI, OAA, or Both, June 30, 1959, *Rearch and Statistics Note No. 4*, January 25, 1960, Division of Program Research, Social Security Administration.

ing years the number of OAA recipients relative to the aged population will continue to decline so that, "Old-age assistance will increasingly be a program primarily for aged persons who do not qualify for insurance benefits and for beneficiaries who have special needs that cannot be met from their insurance benefits and whatever other resources they may have."[21]

---

[20] R. J. Myers, "1958 Amendments to the Social Security Act," *Transactions of the Society of Actuaries*, Vol. 11, p. 1 (1959).

[21] S. Ossman, "Concurrent Receipt of Public Assistance and Old-Age and Survivors Insurance," *Social Security Bulletin*, September, 1958; see also *Social Security Bulletin*, November, 1959.

As a result of the declining role of OAA, there has been a reduction in the relative numbers of aged entitled to tax-supported medical care without a further means test. However, the number of aged receiving concurrent OASI and OAA benefits has been rising, and these form an increasing proportion of the total OAA recipients. This situation results from the addition of many to the OASI rolls, following recent extensions of coverage, who receive small benefits and therefore need some OAA aid to supplement their resources. Although unusual medical care requirements may be a significant factor in these needs among persons receiving OASI and OAA concurrently, they may be no greater than among those who are only OAA recipients. Thus, according to a study of Public Assistance recipients in New York State, among those receiving only OAA income, 58 per cent were chronically ill or disabled but not hospitalized and 5 per cent were hospitalized or acutely ill; among those with both OAA and OASI income, the percentages were not much different, being 55 and 7 respectively.[22]

***State and Local Government Medical Care Programs for the Indigent.***    At the level of state and local government, there is wide diversity in the approach to financing and administering medical care for the indigent.[23] The financial responsibility for this care is shared variously by state and local government. Some states, functioning through a state public assistance agency, support programs of medical care

---

[22] E. M. Snyder, *Public Assistance Recipients in New York State, January–February, 1957,* Interdepartmental Committee on Low Incomes, State of New York, October, 1958, pp. 63 and 98. For this study, "Persons who have been continuously ill for a period of 30 days or longer are to be classified as chronically ill. Include here also persons who are diagnosed as having a recurrent chronic disabling condition," p. 93.

[23] P. Bierman, *Role of the State Public Assistance Agency in Medical Care,* a series of eight reports, American Public Welfare Association, Chicago, 1953 to 1955; "Tax-Supported Medical Care for the Needy," a statement of the Joint Committee on Medical Care of the American Public Health Association and the American Public Welfare Association, *Public Welfare,* Vol. 10, p. 87 (October, 1952), and "Tax-Supported Personal Health Services for the Needy," *American Journal of Public Health,* Vol. 45, p. 1593 (December, 1955).

for indigents according to defined standards and without total monthly expenditure limits, while others operate within limits. Several states participate financially only in small degree in providing medical care, while a number do not provide state public assistance funds specifically for this purpose. However, in some of the latter states, medical care for indigents is provided by local funds. Outside their public assistance program, most states operate tuberculosis and mental hospitals and institutions for their population generally, and thus their indigents, and many provide a variety of outpatient services. Tax funds, at the local level, may come from the community, county, or two or more neighboring communities or counties acting jointly.

A state may arrange to give any of its public assistance funds set aside for medical care directly to the recipient, who will then pay for his medical care costs, or it may make the payment to the vendor of medical services. Also, according to local or individual circumstances, a state may use both of these methods of disbursing for medical care. Several states operate pooled funds for the medical care of public assistance recipients. The pooled fund has paid into it monthly a specified amount for each person on the public assistance rolls. Disbursements are made as needed, thus permitting payment of large medical care bills.

Great diversity is also evident in the responsibility for administration of medical care for indigents. A number of states administer all of their public assistance program, in others it is all administered locally, and several divide the responsibility between the state for some phases and the locality for other phases. The responsibilities for medical care usually lie in the public assistance agency. Sometimes they may be shared with the health department, but rarely do the health departments bear the major responsibility.

The arrangements with the providers of medical care services vary greatly among the states and localities, and may be made by the public assistance agency, the health department, or both, according to agreement. Thus, the agency or department arranges with individual physicians, hospitals, medical societies, and other professional bodies to have the indigent provided with authorized services; payment is made on the basis of agreed schedules. In a few instances, physicians and allied professional personnel are employed on either a full-time or part-time basis by the public assistance agency or health department to provide medical care directly to indigents. In Colorado, use is made of an existing insurance mechanism in providing medical care for its aged indigents.

Marked diversity also characterizes the services available in the provision of medical care to the indigent. In setting standards for the various phases of their public assistance policy, most states also specify the medical services included and many go further to set standards for quality, quantity, and cost; these vary widely. Local variations in services within the state may also be wide. Since local services may be available from both voluntary and public agencies, a local health council is often created to co-ordinate their activities;[24] in some areas, the voluntary agencies may provide more services than the public agencies. The services at the state or local level may include any combination of those of the physician in the home, office, or clinic, hospital care, nursing home care, ambulance, nursing services, laboratory services, drugs, dental services, and rehabilitation.[25]

*Voluntary Health Insurance for the Indigent.* Voluntary health insurance held by the aged has the effect of reducing the potential number of medical indigents among them.[26]

---

[24] J. C. Haldeman, "Local Health Organization—A Progress Report," *Public Health Reports,* Vol. 69, p. 1047 (November, 1954); J. C. Haldeman and E. Flook, "The Development of Community Health Services," *American Journal of Public Health,* Vol. 49, p. 10 (January, 1959).

[25] *Special Types of Public Assistance: Types of Medical Care Covered by State Public Assistance Plan Provisions and Method(s) of Payment, Early 1957 and January 1958,* Table 10, Division of Program Statistics and Analysis, Bureau of Public Assistance, Social Security Administration, Washington, D.C., March 17, 1958.

[26] L. S. Reed, *Blue Cross and Medical Service Plans,* Division of Public Health Methods, Public Health Service, Federal Security Agency, Washington, D.C., 1947, p. 230.

For those whose insurance benefits are exhausted, the claim of medical indigency is made at a later date than would have been the case without such insurance. Some public assistance agencies arrange that those aged who are covered by health insurance purchased before they became public assistance recipients have their premium payments included in their allowances. The advantage of such insurance was recognized at a Conference on Financing Health Costs for the Aged held in Albany, New York, on December 6–7, 1956, where it was recommended that:[27]

1. Local welfare departments should continue to pay insurance premiums for those people who have had coverage at the time they commenced receiving assistance.
2. Welfare departments should consider purchasing voluntary health insurance for public assistance recipients who are undergoing rehabilitation, with the assumption that the coverage will be continued by the recipient after he becomes self-supporting.
3. Pending provisions of adequate voluntary health insurance for older people, the State and local governments should increase their participation and direct payments for medical care of the ordinarily self-supporting medically indigent persons.

These recommendations also imply an expectation of growth of voluntary health insurance among the aged and a consequent mitigation of medical indigency. There are very few instances where an insurance or prepayment plan was made available for those who come on the public assistance roles without coverage.[28] However, an insurer may perform the necessary administrative functions for a public assistance agency in carrying out medical care programs for its recipients, as in the case of Colorado.

Colorado Blue Cross acts as the agent of the Department of Public Welfare in making payments to hospitals and for

---

[27] *Financing Health Costs for the Aged,* Office of the Special Assistant, Problems of the Aging, State Capitol, Albany, N.Y., 1957, p. 142.

[28] P. Bierman, *Role of the State Public Assistance Agency in Medical Care: VI, Physicians' Services* (Chicago, Ill.: American Public Welfare Association, September, 1954).

this service receives a fixed fee for each hospital admission. The aged welfare recipient entitled to benefits is given an identification card. The Colorado Blue Cross Comprehensive coverage plan is operative with regard to regulations and rates, except that the waiting period for pre-existing conditions is waived; also the maximum period of hospitalization is reduced, but extension is possible when need is certified by a physician. Similarly, Colorado Blue Shield acts as the agent of the Department of Public Welfare in making payments for the services of the physician in the hospital. Again, pre-existing conditions are waived. The Colorado Blue Shield Standard coverage plan is followed with regard to regulations and fee schedules, except that services are paid for from the first day of hospitalization through the authorized period of stay. The Department of Public Welfare is charged a fee by Blue Shield for each billing. Both Blue Cross and Blue Shield are reimbursed not less often than monthly for amounts paid out on behalf of eligible participants.

*Veterans.*  Under current federal legislation, the Veterans Administration is providing eligible veterans of the armed forces with inpatient and outpatient medical services and with domiciliary care. The services are made available through an integrated system of hospitals, clinics, and homes. Veterans with service-connected disabilities requiring treatment are eligible, without condition, for medical and hospital care at government expense.[29] Another class of veteran, eligible for care in a hospital of the Veterans Administration only if a bed is available, includes those requiring treatment for a nonservice-connected condition who were discharged for a disability incurred or aggravated in the course of their duties or who have a compensable service-connected disability. A third category comprises wartime veterans requiring treatment for a nonservice-connected disability; these are eligible for care in a Veterans Administration hospital only if a bed is available and they are unable to

---

[29] See latest Annual Report of the Administrator of Veterans Affairs.

pay. Only veterans with service-connected disabilities are eligible for outpatient treatment and for home nursing care where it can be arranged through a public health nursing service. In some areas, the local medical society or Blue Shield is used as an agent to pay for medical care on the basis of fee schedules plus administrative costs.

Within the Veterans Administration, the aging of the veteran population is increasing the demand for inpatient care. Using recent experience, a projection was made of veterans in hospitals for every fifth year to 1986; the results are summarized in Table 7.10. Data regarding age are available only for war service veterans with nonservice-connected disabilities; these constitute a very large and increasing proportion of all veterans using hospital facilities. Considering only war service veterans over age 65, their numbers in hospitals are expected to rise from 30,500 in 1957 to 183,700 in 1986, when they will constitute well over half of all hospitalized war service veterans. With the increase of veterans in proportion to the total aged population, in time the Veterans Administration will carry a significant share of the nation's burden of medical care for the aged.

*Income Tax Relief.*   The lowering of income status in the later ages is recognized, in federal tax policy, by doubling the amount of personal income tax exemption at ages 65 and over. Further recognition is given to the special needs of the aged by increasing the amount allowed as a deduction for medical expenses.[30] This is effected by eliminating, for persons 65 and over, the provision that medical expenses are deductible only to the extent that they exceed 3 per cent of adjusted gross income, but the maximum deduction allowed is not changed. Moreover, for those who are 65 and over and also disabled, there is an appreciable increase in the maximum deduction. For this purpose, ". . . an individual shall be considered to be disabled if he is unable to engage in any substantial gainful activity by reason of any medically de-

---

[30] 1954 Internal Revenue Code Section 213 and amendments.

TABLE 7.10

VETERANS IN HOSPITALS OF ALL KINDS, ACCORDING TO ELIGIBILITY STATUS
AND TYPE OF PATIENT, ESTIMATED FOR 1957 AND PROJECTED TO 1971 AND 1986

| Type of Patient | Number (Thousands) in Hospital as of June 30 | | |
|---|---|---|---|
| | 1957 | 1971 | 1986 |
| | All Classes of Disability | | |
| All patients, all ages...................... | 187.8 | 258.0 | 328.1 |
| | Service-Connected Disability | | |
| All patients, all ages...................... | 39.0 | 29.7 | 23.6 |
| Tuberculosis............................ | 3.1 | .8 | .3 |
| Psychiatric............................. | 31.3 | 26.6 | 22.0 |
| General medical, surgical, and neurological.. | 4.6 | 2.3 | 1.3 |
| | Non-Service-Connected Disability | | |
| All patients, all ages...................... | 148.8 | 228.3 | 304.5 |
| Tuberculosis............................ | 15.1 | 13.1 | 14.4 |
| Psychiatric............................. | 53.6 | 78.5 | 100.5 |
| General medical, surgical, and neurological.. | 80.1 | 136.7 | 189.6 |
| War service veterans, all ages.............. | 148.0 | 226.6 | 302.2 |
| Tuberculosis............................ | 15.0 | 13.0 | 14.4 |
| Psychiatric............................. | 53.1 | 77.7 | 99.5 |
| General medical, surgical, and neurological.. | 79.9 | 135.9 | 188.3 |
| War service veterans, ages 65 and over....... | 30.5 | 94.4 | 183.7 |
| Tuberculosis............................ | 2.2 | 3.4 | 7.6 |
| Psychiatric............................. | 10.8 | 31.3 | 60.8 |
| General medical, surgical, and neurological.. | 17.5 | 59.7 | 115.3 |

Source: Veterans Administration, Department of Medicine and Surgery, and Bureau of the Budget, Hospital Programs, Labor and Welfare Division, *Current and Projected Veteran Patient Load Through 1986*, Washington, D.C., June 4, 1958.

terminable physical or mental impairment which can be expected to result in death or to be of long-continued and indefinite duration."[31]

Premiums paid for health insurance may be included among medical expenses, both for current benefits during active years and for benefits payable during retirement. How-

---

[31] Compare with definitions in footnote 16, p. 50 of Chapter 3.

ever, benefits received must be used as an offset against medical expenses. The contributions made by employers to an insurance plan or fund providing medical care benefits for retired employees are deductible as a business expense.[32]

A number of proposals for federal legislation would have provided special exemptions as credits on income taxes for health insurance premiums that have been paid.[33] Some of these proposals would have allowed them as a deduction apart from medical expenses, while others would have established them as deductions against income tax payments, sometimes varying inversely with income. *Stop*

## VOLUNTARY HEALTH AGENCIES

To define voluntary health agencies categorically is no easy task. One study defined a voluntary health agency as:

> . . . an organization that is administered by an autonomous board which holds meetings, collects funds for its support chiefly from private sources, and expends money, whether with or without paid workers, in conducting a program directed primarily to furthering the public health by providing health services or health education, or by advancing research or legislation related to health, or by a combination of these activities.[34]

This definition, according to the source, is intended to exclude voluntary hospitals, nursing homes, homes for the aged, nonprofit insurers of medical services, and professional organizations. Voluntary health agencies may be local, statewide, or national in scope. Co-operation with official health agencies at these levels of government is effected through health councils, or similarly termed bodies. Included among the voluntary health agencies are visiting nurse associations,

---

[32] Regulations issued on Subsection 1.162–10 of 1954 Internal Revenue Code.

[33] A. W. Brewster, *Health Insurance and Related Proposals for Financing Personal Health Services . . . A Digest of Major Legislation and Proposals for Federal Action, 1935–1957, op. cit.,* p. 16.

[34] S. M. Gunn and P. S. Platt, *Voluntary Health Agencies* (New York: Ronald Press Co., 1945), p. 15.

Red Cross chapters, and many thousands of groups whose attention is given to specialized health problems. Among these are heart disease, cancer, mental health, arthritis, tuberculosis, diseases of the central nervous system, and many other specific conditions. It has been estimated that the United States had about 20,000 voluntary agencies in 1957, but their distribution within the country is uneven, with a concentration in urban areas. Voluntary agencies may be organized along sectarian or nonsectarian lines, and by civic, fraternal, and other groups of citizenry.

Among the voluntary health agencies, there are some that provide medical care services directly to the public. Those concerned primarily with the chronic conditions have facilities or services available to the aged, as well as to the general population of the community, the more outstanding examples being bedside nursing care for cancer patients, and cardiovascular and diabetes clinics.[35] The aged in a community may also receive services, where such exist, from the local visiting nurse associations, homemaker service organizations, and Red Cross volunteers which provide a wide variety of services either in the home or the hospital.[36] Some activities related to health are also carried on by many social and recreational centers organized for the aged.

On the whole, very little is known regarding the scope, quantity, and quality of health services available to the aged through voluntary agencies. In some communities they may be fairly well organized, though not adequate to meet all the needs; in others, they may be very meager, if not completely lacking. As an institution, the voluntary agency has a vital role in the health and welfare program of the nation. However, there is much room for a further development

---

[35] C. H. Greve, J. R. Campbell and K. J. Cannon, *Report of Local Public Health Resources, 1952,* Public Health Service, Department of Health, Education, and Welfare, Washington, D.C., 1954.

[36] *Studies of the Aged and Aging:* Vol. I, "Federal and State Activities," Committee on Labor and Public Welfare, United States Senate, Washington, D.C., 1956, p. 123.

which should give a fair share of attention to the health needs of the aged.[37]

## MEDICAL CARE PROGRAMS FOR THE AGED IN FOREIGN COUNTRIES[38]

The approaches used in countries other than the United States for insuring the costs of medical care for their aged are widely varied. Some rely wholly on voluntary insurance, several use voluntary insurance as part of their social security program, and others integrate health insurance fully with their social security program. Although there is no consistent pattern of benefits under the social security programs, they commonly provide for hospitalization, surgery, general practitioner care, essential drugs and medicines, and occasionally specialist care, laboratory services, and dental care. Likewise, variations are found in the methods of providing the benefits, and combinations of methods in one country are not unusual. One method (A) is to have the social insurance system reimburse the insured for the services he purchases, either according to a fee schedule or on a percentage basis, or a combination of both. Another approach (B) has the social insurance system pay the providers of medical care directly for the services they give, either on a fee-for-service basis or on a per capita basis which takes into account the number of insured entitled to service. Under a third approach (C) the social security program maintains a medical care system which renders services directly to those covered by it.

Gerig and Farman have adopted the classification noted

[37] G. Mathiasen, "Assessment of Services in the Voluntary Agency Field As Seen by A National Committee," *Journal of Gerontology Supplement No. 2*, Vol. 13, p. 58 (July, 1958).

[38] This section is based upon *Social Security Programs Throughout the World, 1958*, Division of Program Research, Social Security Administration, Washington, D.C., 1958, and D. S. Gerig and C. H. Farman, "Provision of Medical Benefits to Old-Age Pensioners Under Foreign Social Security Programs," *Research and Statistics Note No. 10*, Division of Program Research, Social Security Administration, April 17, 1959.

below with regard to the provision of medical benefits for the aged by countries with social security programs. The letter following a country refers to the chief method of providing the benefit, as indicated in the preceding paragraph.[39]

(1) Countries covering old-age insurance beneficiaries under sickness insurance, without payment of contribution after retirement; coverage is generally incidental to employment:

| Western Europe | Eastern Europe |
|---|---|
| Belgium (A) | Albania (C) |
| France (A) | Czechoslovakia (C) |
| Federal Republic of Germany (B) | East Germany (C) |
| many (B) | Hungary (C) |
| Greece (C) | Poland (C) |
| Italy (B) | Rumania (C) |
| | Yugoslavia (C) |

(2) Countries covering old-age insurance beneficiaries under sickness insurance, but requiring them to contribute after retirement:

| | |
|---|---|
| Austria (B) | Panama (C; A for hospital and surgery) |
| Chile (C) | |
| Luxembourg (B; A in part) | Spain (B; C for hospital in part) |
| Mexico (C; B in part) | |

(3) Countries permitting old-age pensioners to insure voluntarily under the public sickness insurance program by paying a contribution:

| | |
|---|---|
| Denmark (B for doctors) | Peru (C) |
| Netherlands (B for doctors and hospitals) | Switzerland (B for doctors) |

(4) Countries covering all residents, including pensioners, under a comprehensive medical care or sickness insurance program:

| | |
|---|---|
| Australia (B for hospital and pharmacy) | Norway (B for doctors) |
| Bulgaria (C) | Sweden (A for doctors and wards in public hospitals) |

---

[39] The letters were inserted by the author on the basis of the description by Gerig and Farman.

Iceland (B for doctors)       U.S.S.R. (C)
New Zealand (A for general    United Kingdom (B for doc-
 practitioner and private    tors; C for hospital)
 hospital)

(5) Countries covering pensioners under other arrangements:

Ireland (benefits chiefly to lower income groups through facilities belonging to local health authorities)
Canada (hospital benefits through Provincial systems of hospitalization insurance)[40]
Japan (compulsory National Health Insurance for householders not covered by compulsory system for the employed. C; A in some areas)

(6) Countries maintaining both old-age and sickness insurance programs, but not covering old-age beneficiaries under the latter:

Bolivia                 Ecuador
Brazil                  Iran
China (Nationalist)     Nicaragua
China (Communist)       Paraguay
Costa Rica              Portugal
Dominican Republic      Turkey

(7) Countries with an old-age benefit or pension program, but without a sickness insurance program:

Argentina               Malaya
Ceylon                  Philippines
Cuba                    Union of South Africa
Finland                 United Arab Republic
Iraq                    Uruguay
Israel

Extensive voluntary insurance operations are active in Israel and Cuba.

The varied approaches taken by other countries to provide or insure medical care for their aged are patterned to suit

---

[40] A. W. Brewster, "Canada's Federal-Provincial Program of Hospitalization Insurance," *Social Security Bulletin,* July, 1959; S. M. Gelber, "Hospital Insurance in Canada," *International Labour Review,* Vol. 79, p. 244 (March, 1959).

their particular cultures. The descriptions of these approaches have nothing to say concerning the quality of the services, nor their actual availability. With regard to medical care for the general population, irrespective of age, in no other country has voluntary health insurance developed as extensively as in the United States, not only by way of proportion of population covered but also as to scope of benefits and experimentation to adapt to medical progress.

# Toward A Goal                                                    8

THE MECHANISMS for providing medical care in the United States are being studied not only by their administrators, but also by the providers of medical care through their professional associations, by universities, by employers, by labor unions, by consumer organizations, by governmental agencies, and by legislative bodies at all levels of government. This general interest has led to a wide variety of proposals and activity to forward the process of development. Some of the legislative proposals regarding health insurance for the aged will be referred to later. This is preceded by a brief discussion of some general and economic factors relating to the medical care of the aged.

## SOME GENERAL FACTORS RELATED TO MEDICAL CARE OF THE AGED

*The Right to Medical Care.* Medical care is today regarded as a right of the individual comparable with the right to food, shelter, and clothing.[1] In the United States, the individual bears the responsibility of meeting these needs from his own resources; only when his resources are inadequate may he claim his right to whatever resources his community has available.[2] For those in need of medical care, but without

---

[1] Some distinctions and analogies between medical care and food as necessities are made by M. M. Davis, *Medical Care for Tomorrow* (New York: Harper & Bros., 1955), pp. 16–18. For an interesting discussion of health as a birthright, see R. Dubos, *Mirage of Health* (New York: Harper & Bros., 1959), chap. i.

[2] H. M. Somers and A. R. Somers, "Private Health Insurance: Part I, Changing Patterns of Medical Care Demand and Supply in Relation to Health Insurance," *California Law Review,* Vol. 46, p. 376 (August, 1958); this source discusses medical care as a civic right.

resources of their own, federal, state, and local governments and voluntary agencies have developed the programs described in the preceding chapter.

Government also provides medical care to some population groups under special circumstances, the prime example being veterans of the armed forces with service-connected disabilities. Other examples are the health services for Indians on reservations, the hospitals and clinics of the Public Health Service which provide services to the Merchant Marine, and the hospital and out-patient facilities of the Defense Department which serve dependents of the armed forces and certain other classes of civilians; another agency of the Defense Department operated for dependents of the armed forces is the Medicare Program.[3] Government may also be asked to provide medical care services on a fee basis to those living in isolated sections, as is the case for many Alaskans, other than Eskimos and Indians who receive free care.[4] There have been, furthermore, several instances where the federal government sponsored special programs of personal health services to specified categories of population for a few years, the best known example being the Emergency Maternal and Infant Care Program of World War II.[5]

*The Changing Characteristics of the Aged.* To fulfill its purposes, an insurance program must be sufficiently flexible

---

[3] P. I. Robinson, "Medicare: Uniformed Services Program for Dependents," *Social Security Bulletin,* July, 1957, and "Dependents' Medical Care Act," *U.S. Armed Forces Medical Journal,* Vol. 8, p. 82 (January, 1957); F. L. Wergeland, "The Medicare Program—Problems in Perspective," *Journal of the American Medical Association,* Vol. 171, p. 1485 (November 14, 1959); and "Restoration of Certain Care Authorized Under the Dependents' Medical Care Program," ODMC Letter No. 12–59, Office of the Surgeon General, U.S. Army, Washington, D.C., 25 November 1959. These sources describe the original Medicare Program, its restriction because of budget limitations and the wish of Congress that optimum use be made of service hospitals, and the subsequent restoration of benefits.

[4] Social Legislation Information Service, Washington, D.C., April 6, 1959.

[5] A. W. Brewster, *Health Insurance and Related Proposals for Financing Personal Health Services . . . A Digest of Major Legislation and Proposals for Federal Action, 1935–1957,* Division of Program Research, Social Security Administration, Washington, D.C., 1958, pp. 34–39.

to adapt itself to the changing characteristics of the population served and of the risk covered. Voluntary insurance promises ready adjustments as a consequence of community[6] and competitive pressures. A compulsory insurance program, geared to conditions current at its start, depends upon legislation and political expediency for its adjustments. The requirement of flexibility is particularly important for health insurance because of the rapidity of developments in medical science, practice, and facilities. Equally significant are the rapid changes in the characteristics of the aged; these are summarized here from earlier chapters.

In many aspects bearing upon their medical care problems, the aged of the near future will be far different from the current aged. Along with their growth in number and in proportion to the total population, there will be an increasing concentration at the extreme ages of life, where the complexities of illness are greatest. Females will become increasingly predominant over males among the aged. Most of these aged women will be widows, some living apart from relatives with a consequent complication of their medical care needs by their social problems.

However, each succession of new members to the ranks of the aged and retired in coming years will undoubtedly be increasingly prepared for the social and health problems of later life. This will be a consequence of trends already evident among those currently in midlife. Chief among these are rising educational attainments of the population; an improving economic status flowing from greater savings by home ownership, life insurance, pensions, and other means; an increasing awareness of what medical care offers; and a growing appreciation of the advantages of health insurance to meet the cost of medical care. With a population more health-conscious and benefiting more than ever before from a high standard of living, an improving health status may be expected among those entering old age and retirement in the

---

[6] This refers to a community of interests as well as to a geographic community.

years ahead. On the other hand, at the higher ages a growing proportion of persons with chronic illness is likely as medical progress increasingly prolongs the lifetime of those who become physicially impaired.

## SOME ECONOMIC FACTORS RELATED TO MEDICAL CARE OF THE AGED

The concern here is chiefly with factors related to the demand and supply of medical care for the aged, aside from those described previously.

*The Demand for Medical Care.* Viewed generally:

The demand for medical care is influenced by many factors, some of which increase and others of which decrease the number of people who can be cared for by a physician. Among these are demographic changes, changes in therapy, urbanization and suburbanization, use of ancillary personnel, the nature of facilities for medical care, shifts in the causes of morbidity and death, extension of prepaid medical care programs, and the effectiveness of preventive medicine.[7]

A few of these and other factors may be considered in relation to the aged.[8]

Individuals vary greatly in their reactions to physical discomfort and evidence of illness. As noted in Chapter 3, some elderly persons may disregard a mild symptom if its general recognition would involve loss of status, particularly a job or position in the community, or if access to medical care is not readily convenient; the same effect is produced by a stubborn reaction to pain and by negligence. Contrariwise, other aged may magnify a minor indisposition in order to attract a

---

[7] *The Advancement of Medical Research and Education Through the Department of Health, Education, and Welfare,* Final Report of the Secretary's Consultants on Medical Research and Education, Office of the Secretary, Washington, D.C., June 27, 1958, p. 33.

[8] For a general discussion without regard to age, see M. Roberts, *Trends in the Supply and Demand of Medical Care* (Study Paper No. 5, Joint Economic Committee, 86th Cong., 1st sess., November 10, 1959), p. 47.

family or neighborly attention otherwise lacking; for those living alone, it may provide an opportunity for social contact.

Whatever the case, highly subjective elements, in addition to needs created by actual morbid conditions, may affect the demand for medical care by the aged. The subjective elements tending toward greater utilization will very likely grow in importance in time as the aged become more health-conscious and as the proportion among them living alone or apart from relatives mounts. In other words, the aged, who are generally more introspective with regard to their health than younger persons, may become even more so. There is, of course, a beneficial effect if this trend encourages the habits of periodic check-up, preventive care, and early remedial care. Although subjective elements are also present at the younger ages, their influence may be smaller because of the need of the earner to work, the housewife to tend to her chores, and the child to attend school.

Because medicine is an art as well as a science, a large subjective element is also necessarily present in its practice. Much depends upon the training of the physician, his skill, and his temperament in relation to that of his patient. Although standards have been established for many diagnoses and treatments, there may be variations in the understanding that physicians have of them. For some diagnoses and treatments objective criteria may be lacking.[9] With patients at the older ages, a greater degree of subjectivity may be present on the part of the physician in view of the complexity of diseases that arise. The convenience of the physician may be a further influencing factor in the medical care of the patient. For example, to conserve his time and energy a busy

---

[9] Although the issues of the organization and quality of medical care are pertinent, they are not discussed here; recent references are G. Rosen, "Provision of Medical Care. History, Sociology, Innovation," *Public Health Reports,* Vol. 74, p. 199 (March, 1959); and P. M. Densen, "Approaches to the Problem of Measuring the Quality of Medical Care," *Proceedings, Group Health Institute of 1959,* Group Health Association of America, Chicago, p. 61.

physician may consider hospitalization for a patient living in a remote area who would otherwise be treated at home.

Each advance in medicine and the allied sciences elicits additional demands for medical care.[10] New diagnostic techniques and improvements upon the old make possible an earlier and more penetrating recognition of morbid conditions. Likewise, new therapies, surgical procedures, and techniques of rehabilitation have greatly enlarged the opportunities for medical care and therefore the demand for it. Even in the light of current knowledge, many are unaware of latent conditions they are harboring, as observed in the Hunterdon County Survey by Trussell and his associates. The Baltimore Study of the Commission on Chronic Illness found that where morbid conditions are known to the individuals affected, the medical needs often exceed the care sought. Thus, with scientific advance and an increasingly favorable attitude toward preventive care and meeting health needs, a constantly expanding demand for medical care is possible, particularly in old age. Its control within the bounds of necessity, as always, is the responsibility of the individual and his physician.[11] For the aged especially, this joint responsibility will grow as their improving economic status and expanding health insurance coverage gives them more ready access to medical care.

A problem of great moral significance is being created by the increased chances of survival to extreme old age and the rapid growth in numbers at that stage of life. An individual may arrive in these terminal years in a state of such mental and physical deterioration that he is helpless, and with no hope for improvement. Nevertheless, with modern medical knowledge life may be continued for a long time in that state. The physician, dedicated to the conservation of human life,

---

[10] F. Roberts states that ". . . the further medicine advances, the greater is the amount of work which it makes for itself," in *The Cost of Health* (London: Turnstile Press [succeeded by Phoenix House, Limited], 1952), p. 93.

[11] D. P. Barr, "Principles Relating to the Success of a Medical Care Plan," *Proceedings, Group Health Institute of 1959, op. cit.*, p. 4.

has no choice. However, he must depend upon resources available to him. Dean Clark referred to this matter:[12]

> The second and even more difficult aspect of this problem of the aged is the care of those of them who are chronically ill. . . . Part of this issue . . . is keeping people alive who, not to put too fine a point upon it, would be happier if allowed to die. . . . Not long ago I heard a minister talk on the various freedoms he would like to see available to all mankind. After reviewing the more familiar ones, he added a new one: Freedom to die.

*The Supply of Medical Care.* The consensus is that there is a shortage of personnel and facilities in relation to the potential demands for medical care. A succinct statement is found in a report of the Secretary of Health, Education, and Welfare:[13]

> There has been and continues to be a serious shortage not only of physicians but also of all other types of health personnel— nurses, occupational and physical therapists, medical and psychiatric social workers, medical technologists, dieticians, and also practical nurses, aids, technicians, and homemakers.

Almost two thirds of a total of nearly 2,000,000 employed in occupations related to health in 1955 were classed as professional, technical, and kindred workers.[14] Among them were 225,000 physicians and surgeons and 98,000 dentists (both including those retired and not in practice), 430,000 professional nurses and 113,000 student nurses, 111,000 pharmacists, 126,000 medical and dental technicians, and 22,000 dieticians. The one third not classified as professional or technical included 175,000 practical nurses, 337,000 attendants in hospitals and institutions, and 130,000 attendants in physicians' and dentists' offices.

[12] D. A. Clark, "Where Does the Nation's Health Stand Today?" *Proceedings of the 1957 Annual Conference,* Milbank Memorial Fund, New York, pp. 240–41.

[13] *Hospitalization Insurance for OASDI Beneficiaries,* Report submitted to the Committee on Ways and Means by the Secretary of Health, Education, and Welfare, Washington, D.C., April 3, 1959, p. 34.

[14] G. St. J. Perrott and M. Y. Pennell, *Health Manpower Chart Book,* Division of Public Health Methods, Public Health Service, Washington, D.C., 1957, p. 1.

In order to maintain the 1959 ratio of 141 physicians per 100,000 population, it has been estimated that the number of graduates would have to be increased to 9,600 in 1970, compared with 7,400 in 1959.[15] An increase to about 6,200 graduates in dentistry annually would be needed over the same period, or about 2,700 more than in recent years. The resources of the country with regard to these and other health personnel have been studied on several occasions.[16] Commenting on the outlook, The President's Commission on the Health Needs of the Nation made the point:[17]

We see no prospect for a great increase in the number of health workers in the near future. The lengthening of the training period for our health professionals, an indispensable element in raising the quality of medical care, makes this expansion process a slow one. We cannot appropriate today and have more health personnel tomorrow.

Notwithstanding intensive efforts to build needed medical care facilities throughout the country, appreciable gaps are still evident. The current (1959) situation was described in these terms:[18]

Eleven years ago we had about 60 percent of the general hospital beds we needed. Today, with the help of almost $1 billion in Federal funds and more than $2 billion in State, local, and private matching funds, 75 percent of the need for general hospital beds has been met. In addition, we now have 73 percent of the tuberculosis beds needed, as compared with 46 percent in 1948. In men-

---

[15] *Physicians for a Growing America,* Report of the Surgeon General's Consultant Group on Medical Education, Public Health Service, Washington, D.C., October, 1959, pp. 2, 3 and 67. The data for physicians include both doctors of medicine and of osteopathy.

[16] The President's Commission on the Health Needs of the Nation, *Building America's Health,* Washington, D.C., 1951, Vol. 2, pp. 114-91; D. Wolfle, *America's Resources of Specialized Talent* (New York: Harper and Bros., 1954); G. St. J. Perrott and M. Y. Pennell, *Health Manpower Chart Book, op. cit.; The Advancement of Medical Research and Education Through the Department of Health, Education, and Welfare, op. cit.*

[17] *Building America's Health, op. cit.,* Vol. 1, p. 11; G. St. J. Perrott and M. Y. Pennell, "Physicians in the United States: Projections 1955-75," *Journal of Medical Education,* Vol. 33, p. 638 (September, 1958).

[18] E. L. Richardson, "The Federal Role in the Nation's Health," *Public Health Reports,* Vol. 74, p. 661 (August, 1959).

tal hospital beds we have slipped from 55 percent of the need in 1948 to 53 percent today. All in all, State plans show a remaining deficit of 888,000 hospital beds of all types and 323,000 nursing home beds.

The role of personnel in this situation is exemplified by the statements that,[19] "There is at present a serious shortage of high quality nursing home beds of all types . . ." and, "The shortage of nurses imposes a major limitation on rapid expansion of skilled nursing homes and of high quality homes of all types."

The extent of these deficiencies in health personnel and facilities varies widely within the country, being generally greatest in the South. Thus, in 1957, the ratio of physicians per 100,000 population ranged from 100 in the South to 112 in the North Central area, 141 in the West, and 161 in the Northeast.[20] The variation for medical specialists may be even greater. At the beginning of 1959, the additional hospital beds needed in the United States and its Territories averaged 5.07 per 1,000 population.[21] This average ranged from about 4 per 1,000 in the Northeastern area of the country to more than 6 per 1,000 in the Southeast and Southwest.

Current shortages of health personnel, the limited potential for their increase, and the requisites for additional facilities have an important bearing on the development of programs to insure the costs of medical care. In the face of such gaps, an immediately introduced large-scale insurance program under government sponsorship, such as one for the aged, may produce appreciable dislocations in medical care

---

[19] *Hospitalization Insurance for OASDI Beneficiaries, op. cit.,* pp. 71 and 84. See also *The Aged and Aging in the United States: A National Problem* (Hearings before the Subcommittee on Problems of the Aged and Aging, U.S. Senate, 86th Cong., 2d sess., 1960), p. 131.

[20] *Health Manpower Source Book, Section 9, Physicians, Dentists, Nurses,* Division of Public Health Methods, Public Health Service, Washington, D.C., 1959, p. 10.

[21] "Hospital and Medical Facilities in the United States According to Approved State Plans Under Title VI of the Public Health Service Act as of January 1, 1959," Division of Hospital and Medical Facilities, Public Health Service, Washington, D.C.

services because of the higher utilization rates of insured persons.[22] This does not mean, of course, that much of this higher utilization may not represent actual need. In any event, such dislocations of medical care may be most severe where the shortages of personnel and facilities are greatest.

## THE POSSIBLE PATHS IN PROVIDING MEDICAL CARE FOR THE AGED

The possible paths in providing medical care for the aged form a broad spectrum. On the one hand, there is the present program for developing voluntary health insurance, with public and general assistance for the needy. At the diametric opposite is a complete national health service, fully tax-supported, with medical care available to persons of all ages and without any fee for specific services. Between the two, a great variety of melds of voluntary and government programs is possible, as may be noted in the preceding chapter.

*Voluntary Health Insurance.* For the purpose of encouraging private health insurers to experiment with new coverages for substandard risks, including the aged, several bills were introduced in the Congresses of 1956 and 1957 which would have permitted them to form reinsurance pools.[23] Such legislation was considered necessary by the current federal administration in view of existing antitrust laws. However, these legislative proposals were not enthusiastically received by the private insurance companies who felt that there was no need for such reinsurance facilities. There was also the feeling that the essential problems in covering sub-

---

[22] It has been noted that for several countries introducing health insurance into their social security programs, "Typically, benefits are first provided in the capital city and perhaps certain other centers, and are then gradually extended to other urban or rural areas. The pace of the extension is usually controlled by the rapidity with which new clinics and hospitals can be financed and erected in different regions, for the furnishing of medical benefits," *Social Security Programs Throughout the World, 1958,* Division of Program Research, Social Security Administration, Washington, D.C., 1958, p. xiv.

[23] A. W. Brewster, *op. cit.,* p. 1.

standard risks were to find a statistical basis for adequate premiums and to market the policies. The developments with these problems as far as the aged are concerned have already been described.

All categories of voluntary insurers—private companies; Blue Cross, Blue Shield, and other medical society approved plans; and most of the wide variety of independent plans— are actively promoting and experimenting with broadened coverages to protect the aged against their heavy costs of medical care. The position of the insurance companies in meeting the growing medical care needs of the nation, and particularly the aged, is contained in the following resolution introduced at a special meeting of the Health Insurance Association of America on December 8, 1958:

THEREFORE BE IT RESOLVED that the member companies of the Health Insurance Association of America examine the following principles designed to enable voluntary health insurance to meet the problems of financing the cost of medical care, and that each company independently carefully consider the implementation of these recommendations:

1. Insurers offering individual and family coverage of the cost of health care under contracts which are renewable at the option of the insurer should continue and accelerate their progress in minimizing the refusal of renewal solely because of deterioration of health after issuance.
2. Every insurer offering health care coverages should, among the types of insurance contracts it offers, promptly make available to insurable adults policies which are guaranteed renewable for life.
3. Every insurer should develop sales programs designed to encourage the sale of permanent health care insurance where the need for this type of coverage exists.
4. Every insurer offering individual and family hospital, surgical, and medical care coverages should promptly take steps if it is not presently doing so to offer insurance coverage to persons now over age 65.
5. It is essential that adequate voluntary health insurance be available to broad classes of physically impaired people. Initial insurance underwriting standards essential to fulfilling the first two of these recommendations increase the

need for insurance for the physically impaired. Otherwise, in the future, these people may be deprived of insurance coverage. It is recommended that each company carefully consider how it can contribute to the achievement of this objective.

6. Every insurer writing coverage on a group basis should develop and aggressively promote soundly financed coverages that will continue after retirement.

7. Every insurer offering coverage on a group basis should encourage the inclusion in the group contract of the right to convert to an individual contract on termination of employment.

For the workers and their dependents, voluntary health insurance has established a record for rapid growth in numbers covered and the broadened scope of benefits. This pattern is expected to be followed in extending protection against the costs of medical care at the older ages. On the basis of the trend in health insurance coverage of OASDI beneficiaries between 1951 and 1957, a report of the Secretary of Health, Education, and Welfare estimated that "about 70 per cent of the aged beneficiary group will have some form of health insurance by 1965."[24] However, the report has an estimate that only 56 per cent of *all* aged persons 65 and over will have hospital insurance by 1965. A somewhat more optimistic outlook is taken by the Health Insurance Association of America which bases its projection not only on an annual growth of about 3 per cent in coverage of all aged between 1952 and 1957, but also upon a rapidly growing public appreciation of health insurance and the most recent activities by the insurers. Their projection, when related only to those who "need and want" health insurance, thereby excluding those who can meet their medical care costs by other means or who have religious scruples against it, comes to 80 per cent.[25]

The future of voluntary health insurance for the aged will

---

[24] *Hospitalization Insurance for OASDI Beneficiaries, op. cit.,* p. 2.

[25] J. F. Follmann, Jr., "Present and Future Prospects of Health Insurance Protection for the Retired," presented before the National Health Forum, Chicago, March 18, 1959.

depend not only upon growth in the proportion covered, but also upon an expansion in the scope and quality of the benefits provided. Insurers are already giving consideration to plans which would broaden their more usual programs by including such coverages as nursing home care, nursing and home care, homemaker services, and other services that enter into a comprehensive medical care program. Out of the greatly varied plans being developed during the experimental period, a few basic patterns should emerge that may be adapted to suit most individual circumstances. As with life insurance, planning for health insurance for the later years is a continuing process, beginning in the early productive years.

Although an expansion of voluntary health insurance among the aged would mitigate some of the burden of the indigent and medically indigent in the community, a certain measure of the problem will remain. For such cases, there is an obvious need for strengthened medical care services on the part of both public and voluntary agencies in many areas of the country.

*National Health Service.* Of the several countries that maintain a complete national health service available to all residents, none has been studied and commented on as intensively as that of the United Kingdom.[26] Their system is complete in that it offers, under government administration, a full complement of medical, hospital, dental, and nursing home services. A small charge is made for drugs and some appliances and also for dental treatment to adults, except for pregnant women. The British National Health Service has won wide public acceptance and any material restriction in its present program appears unlikely, although it was necessary to introduce charges for some services and goods to control costs. However, an indication that this Service has not

---

[26] See, for example, H. Eckstein, *The English Health Service* (Cambridge, Mass.: Harvard University Press, 1958), and the special supplement on the National Health Service in the *British Medical Journal,* July 5, 1958.

been wholly satisfactory to all segments of the British population is found in the steady growth of voluntary health insurance in that country since 1949, the first full year since the Service was started.[27] The appeal of this insurance is the freedom it gives in the choice of medical specialist and the ready arrangement generally made possible for private hospital accommodation. Under the National Health Service, a lengthy waiting period is usual before admission to hospital. For general surgical cases, the average waiting time ranged from 53 days in nonteaching hospitals to 70 days in provincial teaching hospitals; urgent cases, of course, receive ready admission to a hospital, as would happen under any medical care program.

As far as the aged are concerned, the British National Health Service is still confronted with significant problems in fulfilling its purposes. One of the goals for the social security program contained in the Beveridge Report is to have "Comprehensive health and rehabilitation services for the prevention and cure of disease and restoration of capacity for work, available to all members of the community."[28] Against this goal for all persons may be set some observations regarding the status of health services for the aged in two reports made in 1956.

Thus, the *Report of the Committee of Enquiry into the Cost of the National Health Service* states that:[29]

We have heard a good deal of evidence about the difficulties which have arisen since the Appointed Day in the provision of adequate services for the treatment and care of the aged under

---

[27] J. F. Follmann, Jr., "Surprising Growth of Voluntary Health Insurance in Great Britain," *Journal of the American Medical Association,* Vol. 168, p. 1641 (November 22, 1958), and *A Study of the Growth of Voluntary Health Insurance in Great Britain,* Health Insurance Association of America, September, 1958; G. Bugbee, "Comments on Government Medicine in England and France," *Journal of the American Medical Association,* Vol. 166, p. 1474 (March 22, 1958).

[28] Sir William Beveridge, *Social Insurance and Allied Services* (London: H. M. Stationery Office, 1942), p. 120.

[29] *Report of the Committee of Enquiry into the Costs of the National Health Service* (London: H. M. Stationery Office, 1956), pp. 214–19.

the National Health Service Acts and the National Assistance Act.

## In further comment:

Other witnesses have maintained that the problems now arising in the services for the treatment and care of the aged arise not so much from the form of administrative organization as from the inadequacy of the services provided. The "gaps" in the Service have arisen not because of any loophole in the statutory duties imposed on the authorities, but because the demand for the services has greatly exceeded the supply. Moreover, the demands have been increasing—and will continue to increase—first because of the continued increase in the proportion of old persons in the community year by year . . . and secondly because the quality of the accommodation provided for old people both by hospital authorities and welfare authorities has been rising steadily since the Appointed Day and has in its turn stimulated the demand. There is less reluctance now to seek admission to many chronic sick hospitals or to small local authority old folks' homes of the modern pattern than there was before the war. These witnesses have added that the demand for institutional accommodation may have been increased still further in the postwar years by poor housing conditions, and by the fact that the housewife in many households is now going out to work and cannot devote her time to the care of an aged relative. We ourselves agree with the view that it is the "inadequacy" of the services . . . which is the root cause of the problems relating to the care of the aged. Clearly a great deal more of the country's resources would have to be devoted to the local authority and hospital services to make them fully "adequate" in this respect.

## The report goes on to say:

In conclusion we repeat the warning that it would be unrealistic to suppose that the deficiencies . . . for the treatment and care of the aged can be made good overnight. The responsible authorities can only aim to make good the deficiencies . . . as and when an increased proportion of the country's resources can be made available to the health and welfare services. We would add the proviso that the authorities concerned should make sure that the needs of the aged are given their due priority in the allocation of additional resources and are not overlooked amid the pressure of other competing needs.

The cost studies of the National Health Service by Abel-Smith and Titmuss led them to observe that:[30]

A second explanation of the relatively low costs of medical care for the elderly has to be sought in the field of quality and standard of service . . . But in so far as, by-and-large, the older age group are currently receiving a lower standard of service than the main body of consumers and that there are also substantial areas of unmet need among the elderly, then it would follow that the estimates we present are even less indicative of future trends in cost. The material we analyze . . . on the hospital population does suggest that, in terms of age groups, the scope for raising standards of service is greater among the elderly than among other groups in the population.

Apparently, after about a decade of operation, health services for the aged in Britain are still far from the goal set forth in the Beveridge Report.[31] And, significantly, many of the situations described in the foregoing quotations in the presence of a National Health Service are little different from those often cited for the United States.

**Health Insurance for OASDI Beneficiaries.**  Since 1952, a number of proposals have been made for federal legislation that would provide hospitalization, and sometimes additional medical care benefits, to beneficiaries of the Old-Age, Survivors, and Disability Insurance program, including their dependents.[32] More generally, the proposals would have extended the health insurance benefits to all persons currently eligible for OASDI benefits, whether or not they were then in receipt of the latter. The usual proposal provided for 60 days of semiprivate room hospitalization annually, including such other services and supplies as were customary for hospi-

---

[30] B. Abel-Smith and R. M. Titmuss, *The Cost of the National Health Service* (Cambridge, England: Cambridge University Press, 1956), p. 69.

[31] "These two obvious weak spots in the health service in its early years —affecting the aged and the chronic sick, and schoolchildren's teeth—were the direct result of trying to spread inadequate resources over the whole population," *The Economist* (London), July 5, 1958, p. 15.

[32] A. W. Brewster, *op. cit.*, pp. 23–24. See also *The Aged and Aging in the United States: A National Problem* (Hearings before the Subcommittee on Problems of the Aged and Aging, U.S. Senate, 86th Cong., 2d sess., 1960), p. 2.

tal-stay patients. However, one of the latest such proposals (1959) also provided benefits for nursing home care (with a prerequisite of one day of hospital stay) and for surgery; nursing home benefits would be payable for stays up to 120 days, less any days of hospital stay.[33] Proposals in this category contemplate that needed funds would be obtained by a rise in the Social Security payroll tax on both employers and employees and also on the self-employed (since they are included under OASDI). Such proposals raise two categories of issues: first, whether they are desirable as a matter of public policy; second, the problems of operation, including cost estimates. It will be convenient to start discussion with the latter.

The foremost question to be raised regarding operation is whether the promise of a hospital and nursing home benefit of good quality will be met whenever an entitlement arises, particularly with a nationwide program introduced on short order. On this score, there is considerable room for doubt in view of the present and potential inadequacies of medical care facilities and personnel indicated by various reports of the Department of Health, Education, and Welfare. Problems in providing such hospital and nursing home benefits may become especially acute in areas where the inadequacies are most acute. Also to be considered are possible dislocations in the utilization of medical services if the limited facilities of a community become more readily accessible, at one time, to one segment of the population than another. The Department of Health, Education, and Welfare recognizes the situation that could be created:[34]

Hospital insurance for OASDI beneficiaries would not directly affect existing variations in the number of hospital beds in relation to the total population of different communities or sections of the country, nor would it result in uniformly high standards of

---

[33] H. R. 4700, introduced February 18, 1959, during the 86th Cong., 1st sess. The proposed benefits would not be available to disability beneficiaries, although their dependents would be covered.

[34] *Hospitalization Insurance for OASDI Beneficiaries, op. cit.,* p. 68.

care in all hospitals. . . . It might also result in pressures for expansion of facilities in some areas. . . . The benefit could also be expected to have a greater impact on the future development of nursing home care and indeed of convalescent and chronic care facilities and arrangements generally.

Clearly, whatever deficiencies the United States has in this regard should be made up in substantial degree before benefits are promised en masse.

Operational problems also enter with regard to the hospital and nursing benefits to be offered under a social insurance program for OASDI beneficiaries. The report on these and other allied matters by the Secretary of Health, Education, and Welfare questions whether payments should be extended to such beneficiaries as are in receipt of care from federal general hospitals and those of the Veterans Administration and Public Health Service.[35] Although the report assumes, in making cost estimates, that care in tuberculosis and mental hospitals would not be covered by such a program, it also leaves open the decision in that regard. A discussion of nursing home care leads to the conclusion that: "Because of the increasing need for good nursing home care, and the difficulties of drawing a sharp line between skilled nursing home care and other types of care, it might prove difficult to limit a nursing home benefit under OASDI to short-term convalescent care." The question is then brought up whether such long-term care should be financed through a social insurance program or from general public revenues.

Although the HEW Report favors a service type of benefit over a cash indemnity for hospital room and board and certain special services, it goes on to point out administrative difficulties that would arise because of variations among hospitals in their special services and also in their charges. With a cash indemnity benefit most of these difficulties would disappear and, furthermore, there would be no need for negotiation with individual hospitals.

---

[35] *Hospitalization for OASDI Beneficiaries, op. cit.,* pp. 68–72; this will be referred to later as the HEW Report.

Several possibilities are considered in the HEW Report for arranging the payments to providers of hospital and nursing home services to OASDI beneficiaries.[36] With regard to the nursing home services, their lack of adequate accounting procedures and of general experience in arranging for payments for services are cited as difficulties that may be overcome in course of time. The purchase of insurance from private and nonprofit insurers on the basis of bids is questioned in the HEW Report. It is pointed out that state public welfare agencies generally were not successful with this approach for the purchase of hospital insurance for public assistance recipients. It is also believed that dealing with a group of insurers banded together would eventuate in an arrangement whereby the group would act simply as an administrative agent receiving only its cost of operation over claim costs. Such an arrangement would approximate that of the Medicare Plan with the use of a single administrative agent or perhaps several sharing responsibilities on some stipulated basis, geographic or otherwise. Although this is a possibility, the Medicare Plan has not produced experience with regard to those needs which are greatest among the aged; among the services it is not authorized to provide are those for chronic disease, nervous and mental disorders, and domiciliary care.[37]

The HEW Report also considers the possibility that state health or welfare agencies might act as administrators for an OASDI program on a cost-plus basis, in the same way as the approach indicated for private insurers. The Secretary of Health, Education, and Welfare would administer the program in those states not entering into such agreement. A last possibility considered in the HEW Report is direct administration by the Department of Health, Education, and Welfare. This would involve the Department in direct negotiations with individual hospitals and nursing homes. How-

---

[36] *Hospitalization Insurance for OASDI Beneficiaries, op. cit.*, pp. 72–76.

[37] Office for Dependents' Medical Care, *Medicare Manual and Schedule of Allowances*, Washington, D.C., p. 16.

ever, the Report suggests that the Secretary of Health, Education, and Welfare be given the option of dealing through voluntary insurers or representatives of providers of service. Consideration is given to including, under an OASDI health insurance program, the members of other public retirement systems and also Old-Age Assistance recipients.

The HEW Report recognizes that, whatever method might be adopted, "there should be no interference with the internal administration of hospitals or with the authority of the physician in medical matters." Yet it proposes a system of statistical checks as a guard against undue utilization of services and as a control on the handling of funds and the quality of care provided. Notwithstanding the disclaimer, such systems of guards and controls do introduce a possibility of increasing supervisory regulation that may extend beyond the original intention. Also, once inaugurated, it may prove difficult to confine the systems of guards and controls to the medical care of the aged alone. Since the aged take both a large and growing share of the nation's total medical care program, the systems may easily permeate the whole of it.

The history of social insurance has some notable instances in which projected estimates of cost fell below the experience actually developed.[38] Estimates of this kind are difficult

---

[38] Commenting on an estimate in the National Health Service bill presented to Parliament in 1946, Abel-Smith and Titmuss, *op. cit.*, p. 2, say, "It is now clear that this was a gross under-estimate of the prevailing costs of medical care; an under-estimate due in part to the extreme paucity of data before 1948 and to the use of unrealistic concepts of cost." The actuary serving a Parliamentary Committee of New Zealand to study a proposed National Health and Superannuation Scheme estimated its cost for the first full year as £17.85 million. Although the Scheme started operation in 1939, health benefits were not fully developed until later. The cost of the Scheme came to £17.1 million by 1944, of which £4.7 million were for health benefits; by 1957, the latter alone had increased to £16.8 million. (*The Growth and Development of Social Security in New Zealand*, Wellington, 1950, pp. 48 and 116; *Health Benefits in New Zealand*, New Zealand Department of Health, Wellington, 1 September 1957). In Canada, where a pension is provided every eligible person aged 70 and over without a means test and the fund is operated on a pay-as-you-go basis, the contribution formula has consistently produced total contributions that fall short of total pension payments (*House of Commons Debates*, Vol. 103, No. 54,

enough for the pension and survivorship benefits of a social security program, such as those under OASDI.[39] They become even more so when, to the ingredients essential for these estimates, are added those that enter into estimates for a health insurance program under social security. The HEW Report observes that "The long-range cost of hospital or other medical benefits will in addition be affected by changes in the organization of medical practice and new developments in scientific knowledge as well as by changes in labor costs and other charges." When data are practically nonexistent, as is the case for a nursing home benefit, the problem of estimation becomes practically insurmountable.

For the hospital benefit, the cost estimates for the aged in the HEW Report are based upon the sample survey made of beneficiaries of OASI during late 1957. An upward adjustment is made for the hospitalization of those beneficiaries who died during the survey period prior to interview. Unfortunately, the sampling variations of the survey findings are not given, so that it is not possible to gauge the corresponding sampling variation in the hospital cost estimates. A further difficulty with such survey data is that they depend upon the recollection of the respondent, with the error most likely on the side of understatement. A highly subjective factor is introduced in the HEW Report when it is assumed that the experience of the uninsured beneficiaries as observed in the survey will duplicate that of the insured after an OASDI health insurance program is introduced. At this point, many imponderables enter, some of which are considered in the HEW Report. However, account is not taken of allegations that present insurance benefits for the aged are inadequate, a situation which may be reflected in the survey

---

p. 2416 [April 9, 1959] and R. M. Clark, *Economic Security for the Aged in the United States and Canada,* Department of National Health and Welfare, Ottawa, 1959, sections 972–75).

[39] R. J. Myers, *Methodology Involved in Developing Long-Range Cost Estimates for the Old-Age, Survivors, and Disability Insurance Program,* Actuarial Study No. 49, Social Security Administration, May, 1959.

findings.[40] Also to be recognized are other social security experiences which showed a marked rise in hospitalization after introduction of an insurance benefit.[41] Caution would suggest that any cost estimate for health insurance in a social security program contain a liberal allowance for the imponderables.

**The Pressures for Extension of Health Insurance under OASDI.** As already noted, the HEW Report suggests the possibility that a nursing home benefit under OASDI may have to be extended beyond short-term convalescent care. Pressures for such and other extensions of initially limited benefits appear inevitable under a social health insurance program.[42] Thus, in due course, recognition may be given to the economies of home care[43] in connection with hospitalization and then to the advantage of full general medical care for reduction of hospital utilization.[44] A second suggestion in the HEW Report indicating a possible extension of the scope of health insurance under OASDI is the consideration that it might encompass members of other public retirement systems and OAA recipients.

The establishment of a governmental health insurance program for the aged on grounds of a high incidence of

---

[40] See, for example, a statement by N. H. Cruikshank: "In assessing statistics on the extent of voluntary health insurance, one must remember that every type of insurance is included, no matter how poor. It may cover only a few weeks of hospital care each year." U.S. House, Committee on Ways and Means, *Social Security Legislation* (Hearings . . . 85th Cong., 2d sess., on all titles of the Social Security Act, June, 1958), p. 761. Mr. Cruikshank is Director of the Social Security Department of the American Federation of Labor and Congress of Industrial Organizations.

[41] See, for example, p. 115 of Chapter 4.

[42] Thus, N. H. Cruikshank stated: "We believe your committee will want to explore additional types of benefits." U.S. House, Committee on Ways and Means, *Hospital, Nursing Home, and Surgical Benefits for OASI Beneficiaries* (Hearings . . . 86th Cong., 1st sess., July, 1959), p. 95.

[43] In this connection, see the resolution of the American Nurses' Association, p. 263.

[44] According to experience with general practitioner services in the British National Health Service, "It has not been found possible, however, to give any estimate of the cost of these services to old people," *Report of the Committee on the Economic and Financial Problems of the Provision for Old Age* (London: H. M. Stationery Office, 1954), p. 9.

costly illness and meager resources, with eligibility based only on age, may easily provide ground for further expansion of the system. Such a program obviously favors the older persons over those just below the critical age who are also afflicted with costly illness and have limited means. A basis is thereby created for pressure to lower the critical age and perhaps to its elimination. A precedent is evident in proposals to lower the age for eligibility to the disability benefit feature of the OASDI program.[45] Under pressures for extension of services, coverage, and eligibility on the ground of age, it may be claimed that the foundation is laid for a complete national health service.

In contrast to this outlook, Becker states, with regard to health insurance in general, that: "For more than a decade the issue of voluntary versus governmental insurance was debated extensively by all groups directly involved. . . . About ten years ago, for all practical purposes, this issue was resolved in favor of voluntary prepayment. The issue is not likely to be reopened unless voluntary prepayment fails to do the job it has undertaken."[46] In a similar vein, Pollack says that, if it fails, "then voluntary health insurance will be vulnerable to the pressures that will inevitably arise in a democratic society. On the other hand, it would be extremely difficult to convince people that a rational and well-functioning system should be replaced."[47] With such assurances it may be contended that further efforts of voluntary health insurance should be concentrated upon the productive ages, where it has been eminently successful, by leaving to a governmental program the problem of coverage at the older ages, where its efforts are just beginning. How such a course would weigh against the likely pressures for an expansion of

[45] See, for example, item 19c of *A Report of the Advisory Council on Public Assistance,* made to Congress and the Secretary of Health, Education, and Welfare, January 1, 1960, p. 41.

[46] H. Becker, "The Changing Scene in Health Care Economics," *New York State Journal of Medicine,* Vol. 59, p. 2044 (May 15, 1959).

[47] J. Pollack, "A Labor View of Health Insurance," *Monthly Labor Review,* Vol. 81, p. 626 (June, 1958).

a governmental program initiated for the aged alone is de-batable.[48] Accordingly, consideration of public policy toward governmental health insurance for OASDI beneficiaries can hardly be divorced in full from the issue of an eventual national health service of some form. What course public policy takes is a matter of community attitudes—that is, communities of interest as well as geographic communities.

Events in Canada may be indicative of trends and pressures. Following the development of Provincial hospital insurance plans, "Experience to date indicates that few employers have reduced their direct fringe benefit by the value of the government-underwritten hospital benefits. Through collective bargaining or otherwise, the slack has mostly been taken up by providing supplementary hospital benefits and/or extending medical, group life and sick pay benefits."[49] With regard to the outlook, Taylor said: "I am inclined to believe that the present hospital and diagnostic services programme may be the only part of the health care economy to be channelled through government. . . . I foresee a rapid expansion of voluntary prepayment and commercial insurance on a bolder scale. . . ."[50] However, an opinion was expressed that, "When the late government enacted the Hospital Insurance and Diagnostic Services Act, it began a

---

[48] During interrogation on H.R. 4700 by the House Committee on Ways and Means, Mr. Cruikshank stated that the AFL-CIO presently favors national compulsory health insurance. A similar attitude is contained in the statement, on the same occasion, by Walter P. Reuther, President of the United Automobile, Aircraft, and Agricultural Implement Workers of America (UAW). The National Association of Social Workers included a recommendation for a "comprehensive national health program, which will assure full health care to all individuals by applying the principles of group payment and tax support or the principles of compulsory national health insurance to a total range of health measures" in its goals of public social policy adopted May, 1958; this was made part of their statement in the hearings on H.R. 4700. *Op. cit.*, Hearings, 86th Cong., 1st sess., pp. 101, 403, 146.

[49] Health Insurance Association of America, *Medical Economics Briefs,* No. 2–59 (March 13, 1959), p. 3.

[50] M. G. Taylor, "Financing Health Insurance—What Lies Ahead?" *Report of Proceedings of the Eleventh Annual Tax Conference,* Canadian Tax Foundation, Toronto, March, 1958, p. 21.

process which is bound to end up in a comprehensive state-sponsored program of health care."[51]

## COMMUNITY ATTITUDES

The postwar era is witnessing a rapid growth of interest, in all segments of the nation, in the social, economic, and health problems of aging and the aged. This is expressed in a great variety of activity by private agencies of many kinds, by academic centers and by government at the local, state and federal levels.[52] Many of these activities outside of the area of medical care are related, directly or indirectly, to the health of the aged, such as those concerned with housing and living arrangements, nutrition, recreation, counseling and casework, social relations, and education.[53] By and large, these activities raise few issues; an important problem is that of resources. A similar situation prevails with regard to medical facilities for the aged. However, the problem of financing medical care for the aged has produced a wide divergence of opinion, the major issue being whether or not a health insurance mechanism should be introduced within the OASDI program.

A leading proponent of this approach is the American Federation of Labor-Congress of Industrial Organizations whose Executive Council, in February, 1957, made recom-

---

[51] A. Andras in "Symposium on the Future of Health Insurance in Canada," *Medical Services Journal,* Vol. 14, p. 173 (March, 1958). Mr. Andras is Director of Legislation, Canadian Labour Congress; the view expressed is stated to be his own.

[52] See, for example, footnote 13 to page 218. Also see *The Aged and the Aging in the United States (The Community Viewpoint)* (Hearings before the Subcommittee on Problems of the Aged and Aging of the Committee on Labor and Public Welfare, U.S. Senate, 86th Cong., 1st sess.), issued in several parts; *National Organizations in the Field of Aging,* August 4–6, 1959; and *A Survey of Major Problems and Solutions in the Field of the Aged and the Aging, 1959.* See also Committee on Labor and Public Welfare, *Studies of the Aged and Aging,* Vol. V, "Public and Private Services for Older People," and Vol. VI, "Care of the Aging by the Veterans Administration," 1956.

[53] O. A. Randall, "Health Related Services," *Public Health Reports,* Vol. 73, p. 982 (November, 1958).

mendations to the federal Congress for hospital, surgical, and nursing home benefits for all OASDI beneficiaries. In substance, these recommendations were included in H.R. 9467 introduced August 27, 1957 and again, with minor modifications, as H.R. 4700 on February 18, 1959; the nature of these proposals has already been indicated. Hearings on the first bill were held June, 1958 and on the second in July, 1959. The lists of proponents and opponents were practically the same on both occasions and, for the most part, the pattern of their statements was unchanged.

The statements presented by the AFL-CIO at these hearings referred to the low income and small resources of the aged and the high cost of illness, claimed that public assistance is not a satisfactory solution because of the means test and the low budgets provided by the states, and then indicated a lack of confidence in the potential of voluntary health insurance for the aged.[54] The AFL-CIO saw advantages in the use of the OASDI mechanism in that no premium charges would be required after retirement, since contributions would be made during the productive years,[55] benefits would be available during the remaining lifetime, and coverage would ultimately be practically universal, since a large proportion of the employed are now under OASI; stress was given to the need for immediate action on behalf of the aged. The leadership of the AFL-CIO is reflected in the statements of the UAW and other unions.

Support for the use of the OASDI mechanism was also given by a number of organizations, among whom were two —the American Public Welfare Association and the National Association of Social Workers—whose membership include many who are faced daily with the problems of providing medical care for aged persons.[56] The first of these organiza-

[54] Op. cit. (Hearings, 85th Cong., 2d sess.), p. 752, and (Hearings, 86th Cong., 1st sess.), p. 75.

[55] It should be noted that the retired eligible for benefits at the initiation of the plan would not have made any contributions at all.

[56] Op. cit. (Hearings, 85th Cong., 2d sess.), pp. 42 and 986, and (Hearings, 86th Cong., 1st sess.), pp. 139 and 310.

tions spoke from its experience with the administration of public assistance programs and the second from its experience in both private and public welfare and health agencies. The American Public Welfare Association (APWA) took the position in 1958:[57]

Health costs of old-age, survivors, and disability insurance beneficiaries should be financed through the OASDI program. Arrangements for achieving this objective should take into account the priority needs of the groups to be served; availability of facilities, personnel, and services; and protection and encouragement of high quality of care, including the organization of health and related services to effect appropriate utilization of services and facilities.

Suggested provisions for the OASDI program offered by the APWA at the 1959 hearings, in order that "there should not be unnecessary utilization of hospital care," include:

1. Diagnostic services which can be provided on an out-patient basis.
2. Skilled nursing service in the home, including visiting nurse service, under medical supervision.
3. Surgical services on an out-patient basis in the emergency room of the hospital, in a clinic, or in the physician's own office.

The next priority should be the provision of physicians' services in the home and office, and limited amounts of expensive drugs when prescribed by a physician and required by persons receiving care outside of hospitals.

At its 1958 convention, the American Nurses' Association passed a resolution in support of health insurance for beneficiaries of OASDI, and also recommended that "nursing services, including nursing care in the home, be included as a benefit of any prepaid health insurance program," apparently whether under voluntary or governmental auspices.[58]

The position of the current (1959) Federal Administration is contained in the statement by Arthur S. Flemming,

---

[57] *Federal Legislative Objectives, 1959,* Approved by the Board of Directors of the American Public Welfare Association, December 15, 1958.

[58] *American Journal of Nursing,* Vol. 58, p. 984 (July, 1958).

Secretary of Health, Education, and Welfare, at the 1959 hearings:[59]

> . . . The enactment of a compulsory hospital insurance law would represent an irreversible decision to abandon voluntary insurance for the aged in the hospital field and would probably mark the beginning of the end of voluntary insurance for the aged in the health field generally. [Furthermore], . . . as far as the administration of a program such as is envisioned by H.R. 4700 is concerned, I think that we do have to keep in mind the fact that this would be a new departure as far as social insurance is concerned.

The Secretary pointed to the rapid growth of hospital insurance among the aged and called for the further development of the voluntary approach.

In the forefront among the opponents to the provision of compulsory health insurance for OASDI beneficiaries is the American Medical Association.[60] The AMA regarded such a provision as a first step toward a national compulsory health insurance system with inevitable governmental control of standards and finances of medical care. Restrictions are foreseen on the relationship between the physician and his patient, an overcrowding of limited hospital facilities was anticipated, and a deterioration in the quality of medical care seemed inevitable. On the other hand, the AMA proposal of December, 1958 gave emphasis to the potentials in the rapid growth of voluntary health insurance for the aged, and pointed to the rapid growth of Blue Shield programs.[61] The AMA stated further that the needs of the aged are complex, that practically no diseases are exclusively characteristic of the aging process, and that many important physiological functions change little, if at all, with advance in age. The allied professional groups in opposition to the proposal for compulsory health insurance for OASDI beneficiaries included the Blue Shield Medical Care Plans, the American

---

[59] *Op. cit.* (Hearings, 86th Cong., 1st sess.), p. 9.

[60] *Op. cit.* (Hearings, 85th Cong., 2d sess.), p. 887, and (Hearings, 86th Cong., 1st sess.), p. 273.

[61] See p. 193 of Chapter 6.

Dental Association, the American Pharmaceutical Association, and the American Nursing Home Association.

Rising costs and increased utilization, without commensurate growth in resources, have placed a severe financial strain on voluntary hospitals.[62] This critical situation, their concern with the issue of government control when tax funds are used and, possibly, their close relations with the medical profession, are reflected in the policy of the American Hospital Association toward the use of the OASDI mechanism in providing health insurance for the aged:[63]

After extensive study, . . . we concluded that there are at least three dangers in the use of the social security mechanism which cannot be avoided. . . . First, that the Government as a purchaser of so much hospital care would exert the power of the purse in ways detrimental to the interests of hospital patients. . . . The use of the social security mechanism implies a commitment by the Federal Government of such a magnitude that there is little possibility of later retraction. It is an irrevocable step. . . . Second, that there is a real danger that the provision by Government of prepaid hospital benefits would lead to overutilization that could not be controlled and thus to runaway costs, with consequences that could be disastrous to hospitals and the public. . . . Third, that the acceptance of compulsory health insurance for one group of the population would foster its extension to other groups, and perhaps ultimately to the whole population.

Also, a joint resolution of the Boards of Trustees of the American Hospital Association and the American Medical Association concerned with the development of health care programs for needy persons claims that, "Such proposals as H.R. 4700 (Forand Bill) are not designed especially to assist the needy, since they apply to all Social Security beneficiaries and exclude the majority of needy persons who are not eligible for Social Security benefits, . . ."[64]

The Chamber of Commerce of the United States opposed

---

[62] "Financing the Hospital Needs of the Retired Aged," *Hospitals,* Vol. 32, p. 34 (May 16, 1958).

[63] *Op. cit.* (Hearings, 86th Cong., 1st sess.), p. 350, and (Hearings, 85th Cong., 2d sess.), p. 851.

[64] Resolution dated December 3, 1959.

the extension of the OASDI mechanism to include a program of compulsory health insurance for the aged because, "For good reason, Congress decided that the benefits should not be sufficient to cover the most extreme needs of a relatively small portion of the older population, but should be adequate to provide a floor of protection against want and destitution for the vast majority."[65] OAA was expected to provide for "the relatively few whose needs are unusually large because of chronic illness or other reasons, . . ." A point was also made that the approach of H.R. 4700 "ignores those aged most in need, the 2 millions who are now receiving old-age assistance alone." Also, "We find no justification for setting up a vast national program paying specified kinds of health care to fill a possible need for only a part of our low-income people, only some of whom are aged beneficiaries." The National Association of Manufacturers raised considerations of administrative complexities, cost, a likely expansion of the program, and proposed leaving as a federal government responsibility that which study showed cannot be done by the individual for himself, by private agencies, by state and local authorities and by federal grants to states.[66]

The American Bar Association, which recorded itself in opposition to the Forand Bill of 1958, took a similar stand in 1959.[67] The Standing Committee on Unemployment and Social Security of the Association took the position:

(1) That the payment of social security funds for personal services rather than providing cash payments conflicts with the basic concept of the social security system; (2) that since the payments are to be made directly to the hospital, nursing home, surgeon or dentist rendering the service, there is danger of the federal government, through regulations determining eligibility for payments, exercising an element of control over the operations of hospitals and the practice of medicine and dentistry; (3) that

---

[65] *Op. cit.* (Hearings, 86th Cong., 1st sess.), p. 120, and (Hearings, 85th Cong., 2d sess.), p. 553.

[66] *Op. cit.* (Hearings, 85th Cong., 2d sess.), p. 737, and (Hearings, 86th Cong., 1st sess.), p. 691.

[67] *Op. cit.* (Hearings, 86th Cong., 1st sess.), p. 695.

there is serious doubt that the proposals for funding (financing) the payments for these benefits are actuarially sound because there is really no method of determining the cost of the protection contemplated by these provisions of the bill; and (4) that private plans have not yet been given adequate time to solve the problem to which the bill is directed and that if such plans can be expanded to cover more of the aged, this solution, supplemented where necessary by local assistance, is preferable to a federal system within the framework of the OASI program.[68]

Insurance companies opposed extension of the Social Security Act to include obligatory health insurance for OASDI beneficiaries[69] because:

1. Such measures are premised on the false assumption that most of the aged are unable to finance their health costs or to secure adequate voluntary health insurance.

2. The proposal would impair, if not destroy, the present social security system, and voluntary health insurance.

3. It would fail to alleviate the only real problems—that of the presently aged who require assistance to meet their health care costs.

4. Such proposals would impose a new, uncertain, growing and crushing burden on an already heavily taxed citizenry.

5. Such proposals would develop enormous pressures for a complete compulsory health insurance plan.

6. Such proposals would aggravate and intensify the present and future economic and fiscal problems of the country.

7. Such measures are unnecessary since voluntary health insurance has the capacity and will to provide the aged, as well as the other segments of the population, with a sound and economic means of paying health care expenses.

8. Such proposals might very well promise and impose a tax for benefits, which, based on presently available facilities, could not be delivered.

Altogether, many groups with specialized interests in the problems of the aged have expressed their opinions regarding the introduction of a health insurance mechanism within the OASDI program to provide medical care for the aged. How-

---

[68] Report dated August, 1959, No. 45.

[69] *Op. cit.* (Hearings, 86th Cong., 1st sess.), p. 449, and (Hearings, 85th Cong., 2d sess.), p. 598.

ever, little has been heard from a representative sample of the aged themselves. One piece of evidence, derived from a 1957 sample survey of the aged in the general population by the National Opinion Research Center, was cited earlier; the inquiry was related to government health insurance in general, and not specifically to a program for the aged.[70] Well under one third of the aged respondents favored government health insurance for all persons, almost one fifth favored it only for those with an economic need, and well over two fifths expressed themselves against it.

## CONCLUSION

During the postwar period, the rapid progress of medicine and a growth in health-consciousness has made all segments of the population aware of the advantages of good medical care. For the population at the productive ages and its dependents, the problem thus created is being resolved in large measure by the record growth of voluntary health insurance. Although health insurance plans for the aged were later in their development, the number covered is growing at a greater rate than the coverage of the general population. The problem of insuring the aged differs from that of younger persons because older people have a relatively high prevalence of costly chronic illness, a greater degree of introspection with regard to their health status, and are subject to marked changes in their social and economic milieu.

The individual, the employer, the labor union, and the community must maintain a broad perspective with regard to medical care in old age. The individual, planning for his later years, weighs the possibilities for current consumption against the likely needs of the future. In our economy, the means of providing for the later years can take many forms, such as home ownership, pensions, savings bank deposits, and the purchase of life insurance and health insurance. The

---

[70] See p. 161 of Chapter 5.

employer, acting alone or with the labor union through collective bargaining, will consider how much of the resources
available for fringe benefits can be devoted to financing a
medical care program for retired workers. Likewise, in the
community, "consideration of the older person's needs must
be balanced with the needs of all members of the community,
regardless of age or status."[71] Thus, the individual, the employer, the labor union, and the community must give careful consideration to the medical care needs of old age in allocating available resources.

Medical care has shared fully in the postwar development of science and technology. The goods, services, and
facilities required currently for a high quality of medical care
are much different from those of the immediate prewar period. The training of personnel in the medical and allied professions has been greatly improved. Concentration on the
medical care of the aged has brought a better understanding of their problems and, in turn, changes in the patterns of
their care. The aged are also changing rapidly in their characteristics as they become more health-conscious, better educated, and improve their economic status. To keep abreast
of both these changing characteristics and the dynamism in
medical care for the aged, the mechanisms for providing this
care must be sufficiently flexible to adapt to new situations
as they arise.

The proposal for a program of compulsory health insurance for beneficiaries of the OASDI system represents a de-
parture from the pattern of voluntary health insurance
which has been so widely accepted in the United States. Of
the many issues raised by the proponents and opponents
of the proposal, two stand out. First is the question whether
the existing system of voluntary health insurance can do the
job. Second, the leading proponents of the proposal have also
expressed themselves in favor of a national compulsory
health insurance for the entire population, while the op-

---

[71] A. L. Chapman, "Considering the Aged," *Public Health Reports,* Vol.
74, p. 333 (April, 1959).

ponents have declared themselves fearful of such an eventuality. So far as the first issue is concerned, voluntary health insurance for the aged is now in its developmental stage. Given the same opportunity to develop programs for the aged as it has for the working population, the voluntary insurers express confidence in their capacity to meet the problem; this confidence is shared by the leading professions in the actual provision of medical care, but not by the proponents for an insurance program within OASDI. The second issue—namely, the implication of an eventual national program of compulsory health insurance—can hardly be avoided. On this matter, public policy will be formulated not only by taking into account current problems and their outlook, but also the cultural patterns and traditions of our society.

# Name Index

## A

Abbe, L. M., 83, 88, 99, 132, 141
Abdellah, F. G., 83
Abel-Smith, B., 111, 252, 256
Acker, M. S., 107
Altman, I., 88, 150
Anderson, O. W., 65, 120, 124, 129, 138, 149, 150, 188, 212
Andras, A., 261
Andrus, E. P., 179
Apple, D., 64, 80

## B

Balamuth, E., 202
Baney, A. M., 83, 86, 87, 88
Barr, D. P., 242
Barron, M. L., 80
Bartels, K. G., 121
Becker, H., 165, 259
Bellin, S. S., 111
Belloc, N. B., 94
Bennett, B. M., 126
Berke, M., 84
Beveridge, Sir W., 250
Bierman, P., 224, 227
Blaetus, G. J., 219
Bloodgood, R., 189
Borsky, P. N., 73
Braddock, J. H., 179
Brady, D. S., 21
Brauntuch, J., 85
Brewster, A. W., 45, 88, 94, 95, 99, 100, 109, 112, 139, 150, 189, 190, 192, 195, 199, 200, 205, 206, 207, 208, 212, 214, 218, 231, 235, 238, 246, 252
Brown, F. R., 86, 148
Brown, R. G., 9
Bugbee, G., 74, 250
Burgess, E. W., 4

## C

Campbell, J. R., 232
Campbell, Z., 39, 149
Cannon, J. E., 82

Cannon, K. J., 232
Caruso, U. F., 165
Caudill, W., 66
Cavan, R. S., 4
Chapman, A. L., 269
Chen, E., 55
Chiang, C. L., 48
Civic, M., 37
Clark, D. A., 243
Clark, R. M., 257
Cobb, S., 55
Cohen, B. R., 83
Cohen, E., 64
Cohen, W. J., 2
Collins, S. D., 45, 120
Covalt, N. K., 80
Crocetti, G. M., 85
Crowther, B., 135
Cruikshank, N. H., 258, 260

## D

Dacso, M. M., 83, 92
Davis, M. M., 237
Deardorff, N. R., 202
Densen, P. M., 202, 241
DiCicco, L., 64, 80
Dickerson, O. D., 186
Dickinson, F. G., 93
Donabedian, A., 59
Donahue, W., 14
Dorfman, R., 16, 18, 29, 30, 139, 140
Dubos, R., 237

## E

Eckstein, H., 249
Einhorn, M., 120, 124, 202, 203
Elinson, J., 45
Epstein, L. A., 13, 20

## F

Falk, I. S., 94, 99, 207, 212, 214
Fanshel, D., 68, 72
Farman, C. H., 233, 234
Faulkner, E. J., 165, 215
Feigenbaum, A., 86

271

# Subject Index

## A

Accident and Health Underwriters, Bureau of, 175; *see also* Health Insurance Association of America

Acute conditions, 48–53

Advisory Council on Public Assistance, 219, 220, 259

Aetna Life Insurance Company, 120

Age limitations, health insurance, 175, 180, 184–85, 189–90, 193–94

Aged, characteristics of
age and sex distribution, 4–7
assets, 25–35
debts, 27–28
education, 8, 10–11
employment status, 14–19
income, 12–14, 18, 19–25
labor force status, 14–19
living arrangements, 6–9, 29
marital status, 6–8
residence and migration, 7, 9–10
retirement and health, 14–19
veterans, 11

Aged, health attitudes, 64–80

Aging, influence of heredity, 44

American Association of Retired Persons, 179, 195 n

American Bar Association, 266

American Dental Association, 130–32, 264–65

American Federation of Labor–Congress of Industrial Organizations, 261–62

American Hospital Association, 82, 186, 190, 265

American Labor Health Association, 198 n

American Medical Association, 84 n, 87 n, 91 n, 92, 93, 134 n, 150 n, 164 n, 192 n, 193 n, 198 n, 222 n, 264, 265

American Nurses Association, 258 n, 263

American Nursing Home Association, 87 n, 265

American Pharmaceutical Association, 265

American Public Welfare Association, 220 n, 224 n, 262–63

Associated Hospital Service of New York, 85 n, 191

Associated Hospital Service of Philadelphia, 102, 103–4

## B

Basic Surgical Expense Table, 120

Basic Table for Hospital Expense, 101–3

Blue Cross
Associated Hospital Service of New York, 85 n, 191
Associated Hospital Service of Philadelphia, 102, 103–4
Health Service, Incorporated, 188
Inter-Plan Service Benefit Bank, 188
Inter-Plan Transfer Program, 188

Blue Cross Association, 188

Blue Cross Commission of the American Hospital Association, 188, 189 n, 190

Blue Cross Plans; *see also* Blue Shield and other Medical Society Plans; Health insurance benefits, 187, 188, 189–91
conversion privilege, 189
enrollment
age limitations, 189, 190
number of aged, 188–89, 205
trend, 187
type of coverage, 186, 187
experience, 102, 103–4, 120, 121, 191
nursing service, 189–91
retirement, 189

Blue Shield Medical Care Plans, Inc., 192, 193, 264

Blue Shield and other Medical Society Plans; *see also* Blue Cross Plans; Health insurance benefits, 192–93

275

**F**

Federal Council on Aging, 218 n
Federal Reserve Board, Survey of
    Consumer Finances, 21 n, 26–28
Forand Bills, 253, 260 n, 262, 265,
    266
Foreign countries; see Health insur-
    ance, government programs;
    Medical care, government pro-
    grams

**G**

Government programs; see Health
    insurance, government pro-
    grams; Medical care, govern-
    ment programs
Group conversion; see Conversion
    privilege, health insurance
Group insurance plans; see Health
    insurance, plans, group

**H**

Health Information Foundation, 31,
    46, 47, 65, 66, 70, 74 n, 77, 78 n,
    115 n, 124, 126 n, 132 n, 136, 137,
    141–42, 147, 154, 158 196, 211,
    212
Health insurance; see also Blue
    Cross Plans; Blue Shield Plans
    and other Medical Society
    Plans
  age limitations, 175, 180, 184–85,
    189, 190, 193, 194
  attitude toward, 150–61
  benefits, 175–86, 187, 188, 189–93,
    196–97, 198 n, 199–204, 249
  comprehensive medical expense
    insurance, 170
  coverage
    age, 205–18, 248
    family status, 207–9
    income status, 208–9, 217–18
    labor force status, 206, 207–8,
      213–14
    marital status, 206, 207, 216–18
    race and sex, 205–7, 213–15, 215–
      18
    region, 207
    trend, 171, 173, 174, 182, 187,
      198, 210–15
    type of coverage, 166–70, 170–72,
      172–74, 187, 198
    urban and rural, 207

Health insurance—*Cont.*
  government programs
    administrative problems, 254–56
    attitude toward, 158, 161, 261–
      68
    Canada; see Canada, health in-
      surance
    estimating cost, 256–58
    expansion of benefits, 258–61
    foreign countries, 105–9, 113–16,
      233–36, 249–52, 260–61
    Old-Age and Survivors Disa-
      bility Insurance, proposals,
      252–60
  growth and development, 164–66,
    170–72, 173, 187, 198
  hospital insurance, 166–67, 171,
    172–73, 177, 186–91, 196–97,
    198
  indigents, 226–28
  individual; see Health insurance
    plans, nongroup
  institutional population, 215
  legislative proposals, 252–60
  major medical expense insurance,
    168–70, 171, 172, 173, 177
  medical expense insurance, 168,
    170, 171, 172, 173, 177, 187,
    197, 198
  Old-Age and Survivors Insurance
    beneficiaries, 35, 117–19, 158–
      59, 209, 215–18, 248, 252–60
  plans, group
    age limitations, 175, 180
    benefits, 175–82
    cancellation, 180–81
    conversion privilege, 180–82,
      201–4, 210
    cost, 175, 178–79
    retired employees, 176–80, 248
    trend, 173
  plans, independent
    benefits, 196–97, 198 n, 199–204
    conversion privilege, 201–4
    enrollment, 195–200, 205
    industrial, 197–201
    nonindustrial, 196, 201–4
    retired employees, 197–204
    trend, 198
  plans, nongroup
    age limitations, 184–85
    benefits, 182–86
    cancellation, 180–81, 183–84

*This book has been set on the Linotype in 11 point Modern No. 21, leaded 2 points and 10 point Modern No. 21, leaded 1 point. Chapter numbers are in 24 point Caslon Open nad chapter titles in 18 point Bernhard Cursive Bold. The size of the type page is 24 by 42 picas.*

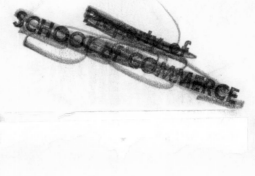